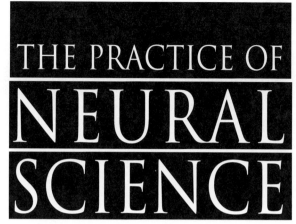

THE PRACTICE OF NEURAL SCIENCE

From Synapses to Symptoms

John C. M. Brust, MD
Professor of Clinical Neurology
College of Physicians and Surgeons of Columbia University
Director, Department of Neurology
Harlem Hospital Center
New York, New York

McGraw-Hill
Health Professions Division

New York   St. Louis   San Francisco   Auckland   Bogotá   Caracas   Lisbon   London
Madrid   Mexico City   Milan   Montreal   New Delhi   San Juan
Singapore   Sydney   Tokyo   Toronto

McGraw-Hill

A Division of The McGraw·Hill Companies

Notice

Medicine is an ever-changing science. As new research and clinical experience broaden our knowledge, changes in treatment and drug therapy are required. The author and the publisher of this work have checked with sources believed to be reliable in their efforts to provide information that is complete and generally in accord with the standards accepted at the time of publication. However, in view of the possibility of human error or changes in medical sciences, neither the author nor the publisher nor any other party who has been involved in the preparation or publication of this work warrants that the information contained herein is in every respect accurate or complete, and they are not responsible for any errors or omissions or for the results obtained from use of such information. Readers are encouraged to confirm the information contained herein with other sources. For example and in particular, readers are advised to check the product information sheet included in the package of each drug they plan to administer to be certain that the information contained in this book is accurate and that changes have not been made in the recommended dose or in the contraindications for administration. This recommendation is of particular importance in connection with new or infrequently used drugs.

This book was set in Palatino Roman by Rainbow Graphics, LLC.
The editors were John Butler, Janet Foltin, and Harriet Lebowitz.
The production supervisor was Shirley Dahlgren.
The production service was Rainbow Graphics, LLC.
The art coordinator was Eve Siegel.
The illustrators were Network Graphics.
The cover designer was Janice Barsevich Bielawa.
The interior designer was Aimee Nordin.
The index was prepared by Oneida Indexing Services.

Hamilton Printing was printer and binder.

This book is printed on acid-free paper.

Once more, for Meridee, Mary, Frederick, and James.

Contents

Preface

Students of neurobiology, especially medical students, often experience a wheat–chaff problem: amidst an onrushing deluge of facts and concepts, how does one tell which information has clinical relevance? Do physicians actually encounter symptoms and signs that reflect the difference between ligand-gated and voltage-gated ion channels? Does the proper choice of diagnostic studies ever require awareness that the spinothalamic tract is a crossed ascending system whereas the dorsal column is not? Does it matter that a protein called tau binds to microtubules? It was with such questions in mind that Dr. Eric Kandel invited me to write a companion volume to Kandel, Schwartz, and Jessell's *Principles of Neural Science,* with the broad aim of demonstrating the applicability of neurobiology to clinical decision making. In addition, it was thought readers might discover that understanding clinical phenomena in neurobiological terms can be good fun.

Although this book is designed especially for students and residents, seasoned clinicians and investigators are welcome. Part I includes a mostly neuroanatomical description of the neurological examination. Part II consists of 79 clinical vignettes, which are discussed neuroanatomically and neurophysiologically. Each case makes a cameo appearance somewhere within the Neurological Examination section, so that the reader can relate that part of the examination to a real world situation. Conversely, the cases are arranged systematically (eg, somatosensory, visual, auditory, olfactory, motor, or autonomic impairment; disorders of consciousness, language, cognition, or be-havior), allowing a reader who wishes to start with the vignettes to refer back to the appropriate section of the Neurological Examination.

Students in neurobiology courses can use this book for previews of coming attractions; they will, I hope, be reassured that so much of what they are slogging through really matters. Students in neurobiology clerkships or residents can use the book to refresh their memories—-or perhaps, in some instances, to update their fund of information.

This is not a comprehensive textbook. Cases have been selected to cover a broad array of neurological and neurobiological phenomena, but they are, after all, only 79 in number. Some involve patients I have known over the years. Others are from case reports in the literature.

Many thank yous are in order. Manuscript reviews by Eric Kandel, Steven Siegelbaum, Lewis P. Rowland, Timothy A. Pedley, and Robert E. Lovelace nipped a number of gaffes in the bud. John Butler, Harriet Lebowitz, and Eve Siegel of Appleton & Lange were professional, sympathetic, and flexible. Sarah Mack was more than accommodating with some of the artwork. Shirley Myers-Jones created a manuscript, and Arline Keithe polished my prose. As always, Dr. Edward B. Healton and Ellen Giesow of the Columbia University Affiliation at Harlem Hospital provided essential support.

Finally, to return to the original questions posed above, the answers can be found in Part II, Cases 19, 45, and 77.

John C.M. Brust

I

The Neurological Examination

1

Overview

▶ Strategic Principles

The human brain is the most complicated biological system; Ramón y Cajal referred to it as the "masterpiece of life." Not surprisingly, neurological disease produces very diverse symptoms and signs. (*Symptoms* are what a patient experiences; *signs* are what an examiner observes.) To assess a patient's "chief complaint," a clinician elicits a neurological history and performs a neurological examination addressing three basic questions: (1) Do the symptoms and signs signify neurological disease or injury? (2) What part of the nervous system is affected? (3) What is the disease process?

Neurological illness can be direct—from primary disease of the nervous system such as glial tumors or multiple sclerosis—or indirect—secondary to disease outside the nervous system, such as renal failure, which can cause altered mentation, or cardiac disease, which can result in embolic stroke. The terms *organic* and *functional*, used to distinguish neurological from psychiatric symptoms, are well entrenched but misleading; psychiatric illness is as organic as neurological illness. Indeed, psychiatry has been described as "neurology without signs." Certain symptoms—particularly headache and dizziness—often have a psychiatric origin, usually anxiety or depression. Psychiatric illness also directly produces neurobehavioral symptoms, for example, schizophrenic hallucinations. Sometimes symptoms turn out to be fabricated by patients for secondary gain (malingering).

Whether direct or indirect, symptomatic nervous system lesions can be diffuse or focal, can be single or multiple, and can involve the peripheral nervous system (muscle, neuromuscular junction, peripheral or cranial nerve, nerve plexus, and nerve root) or the central nervous system (spinal cord, brain stem, cerebellum, diencephalon, and cerebrum). A competent neurological history and examination thus require a basic understanding of the anatomy and physiology of the nervous system.

Fortunately, such an undertaking is less daunting than might be supposed. For all its complexity, the nervous system is highly organized; different combinations of regions subserve different functions, allowing a clinician to localize lesions with considerable accuracy. Moreover, in the great majority of cases the history and examination not only will define the problem as neurological and localize it accurately within the nervous system but also will generate a reasonable hypothesis as to the underlying disease process (Table 1–1). Laboratory or imaging studies

Table 1–1. Major categories of disease.

Congenital (genetic and nongenetic)
Infectious
Toxic-metabolic
Traumatic
Neoplastic
Vascular
Degenerative
Immunologic
Idiopathic (cryptogenic)
Psychiatric
Malingering

are then selected to confirm or exclude the tentative working diagnosis.

▶ Neurological History-taking: The Answers Are in the Details

History-taking should allow patients to describe symptoms in their own words. The clinician's questions should not lead the patient, yet should be sufficiently directed to determine precisely what the patient means. Many terms are used differently by different people. For example, dizziness might refer to near-syncope, vertigo, imbalance, or simply a hard-to-describe subjective feeling. Numbness might mean just that or it might refer to paresthesias (spontaneous somatic sensation in the absence of an external stimulus). *Weakness* might mean loss of power, slowness of movement, or fatigue. Some patients say numb when they mean weak and weak when they mean numb. Similar elaboration is required for terms such as *blackout* (which might mean syncope, a seizure, an amnestic episode, or loss of vision) and *disorientation* (which might describe impairment of recent memory, perceptual disturbance, or a psychiatric dissociative state).

Details as to location, duration, quality, and pattern are crucial to neurological diagnosis. Low back pain, described without further detail, could indicate change to any of a number of structures, whereas low back pain that first appears in a young adult during heavy lifting and is subsequently triggered by bending, twisting, or coughing, with radiation down the posterior leg into the heel, suggests compression of the first sacral (S1) nerve root, probably by a herniated intervertebral disk. Similarly, pain in the left side of the face could be of nonneurological origin, such as maxillary sinusitis or a tooth abscess, whereas spontaneous jabs of severe pain lasting only a few seconds, sharply restricted to the region supplied by the second or third division of the trigeminal nerve and triggered by lightly touching the upper lip or gum, describes trigeminal neuralgia.

Even more complex symptoms are often localizable. An episode of confusion or talking out of one's head could signify drug intoxication or a seizure originating in the limbic system of the brain; more detailed descriptions such as "I knew what I wanted to say but I couldn't think of the right words," or "When I tried to say something the wrong words came out," suggests aphasia, in turn implying (at least in a right-handed person) a structural lesion in the left cerebral hemisphere.

A neurological history is of course not obtained in isolation, but is interpreted in the context of a general medical history (including previous illnesses, injuries, hospitalizations, medications, and use of alcohol, tobacco, or recreational drugs), family history, occupational and social background, and review of nonneurological systems (head, eyes, ears, nose, throat, respiratory, cardiovascular, gastrointestinal, renal or urinary, genital, musculoskeletal, skin, endocrine, and hematologic). Sudden hemiplegia is probably of cerebrovascular origin, whether in a 70-year-old person with hypertension and diabetes or in an otherwise healthy 22-year-old person who smokes "crack" cocaine; the underlying causes of their strokes, however, are likely very different.

▶ The Neurological Examination: Content and Focus

The neurological examination usually follows the medical and neurological history and the general physical examination, by which time a working diagnosis, or at least a differential diagnosis of several possibili-

Table 1–2. The five components of the neurological examination.

Mental status
Cranial nerves
Motor function (including coordination and gait)
Sensory function
Reflexes

ties, has been formulated. The examination consists of five parts (Table 1–2). The thoroughness with which the clinician addresses each part will be influenced by the history as well as by other systemic or neurological signs. For example, olfactory testing would usually be superfluous in someone with a peroneal nerve injury but should be performed in anyone with significant head trauma. Reading and writing do not usually need to be assessed in someone suspected of having myasthenia gravis but should—if possible—be tested in anyone with cognitive or behavioral disturbance. Proprioception obviously cannot be tested in the presence of delirium, and gait may be difficult to assess in someone with postural syncope. Vigorous strength testing should be deferred in a patient whose myocardial infarction occurred the day before. Chapters 2–6 review the five parts of the neurological examination.

2

Mental Status:
The Components of Thinking Are Not Easily Isolated

The parts of the mental status examination are listed in Table 2–1; the order in which they are most appropriately performed varies from patient to patient. Language function cannot be properly assessed in someone who is stuporous, and memory cannot be assessed in someone who is severely aphasic. How a mental status examination is conducted thus depends on what is abnormal.

▶ Alertness and Attentiveness

The mental status examination usually begins with an assessment of alertness and attentiveness, for if either of these faculties is more than mildly compromised, a complete neurological examination becomes impossible (see Chapter 7). A number of terms describe degrees of nonalertness, for example, lethargy (the patient responds to verbal stimuli but tends to nod off when the stimulus is removed), obtundation (at least shouting or shaking is required to produce a response, which is then incomplete), stupor (the patient responds only to pain), and

Table 2–1. The mental status examination.

Alertness and attentiveness
Behavior, mood, and thought content
Orientation and memory
Cognitive abilities
Language
Praxis
Gnosia and spatial manipulation

coma (there is no response, even to pain). Because these terms are not used identically by all clinicians, the examiner should note both the minimal stimulus required to elicit a response and the response elicited.

An impaired attention span is usually apparent during history-taking. It may emerge or worsen as the examination proceeds. Attention span can be more formally tested by having the patient repeat a series of numbers. Most normal adults can repeat seven digits forward and five backward after a single hearing. Sequential digit testing is sensitive but not specific; difficulty may connote impairment of immediate ("working") memory rather than inattentiveness per se. Certain parts of the neurological examination, for example, visual field and proprioceptive testing are more likely to be compromised by inattentiveness than by impaired working memory.

The term *delirium* denotes inattentiveness sometimes so severe that meaningful interaction with the environment is impossible. Mental content, if assessable, is usually abnormal. Such patients are often agitated or less than alert (sometimes rapidly alternating between agitation and obtundation), and in some delirious states, such as delirium tremens of alcohol withdrawal, tremor and hallucinations are prominent.

SEE CASE 59 | p. 231

"Hospitalized for bronchopneumonia, a 55-year-old unemployed accountant becomes anxious and tremulous."

► Behavior, Mood, and Thought Content

Neuropsychiatric abnormalities can be identified in this part of the mental status examination. Affect, the outward expression of mood, may be manifested in clothing, facial expression, amount and type of activity, and stream of conversation.

Mood may be more disturbed than affect suggests, however; patients should be specifically questioned about depression and, if appropriate, suicidal ideation. Patients with cyclothymic mood swings may demonstrate irritation, pressured speech, euphoria, or psychotic mania.

SEE CASE 79 | p. 283

"For several months a 53-year-old lawyer has experienced increasing insomnia and fatigue."

Schizophrenic patients may demonstrate indifference, flattening of affect, or mood inappropriate for a given topic. They may appear hostile and paranoid, with ideas of reference, obsessions, or delusions. Behavior sometimes suggests hallucinations even when they are denied. Schizophrenic speech may reveal distractibility, blocking, stereotypy, loosening of associations, or incoherence superficially resembling jargon aphasia.

SEE CASE 78 | p. 278

"A 17-year-old high school student, always considered by his classmates to be a loner, becomes increasingly withdrawn."

Slowing of speech and activity is also a manifestation of medial frontal lobe damage (abulia). Lesions of the frontal lobe also produce social disinhibition, inappropriate jocularity, and difficulty sustaining goal-directed behavior.

SEE CASE 77 | p. 276

"A 57-year-old high school teacher undergoes a change in personality."

Intermittent or paroxysmal changes in behavior or mood should always raise the possibility of a seizure disorder.

SEE CASE 71 | p. 259

"For 11 years, a 21-year-old woman has had attacks of incapacitating fearfulness."

SEE CASE 72 | p. 263

"A 14-year-old boy has had episodes of altered behavior since sustaining a head injury with loss of consciousness at the age of 3."

► Orientation and Memory

People aware of their own identity as well as basic facts of their present surroundings (hospital, home address, city, state; time of day, day of week, month, year) are said to be "oriented to person, place, and time." Memory impairment secondary to brain injury or a dementing illness is usually greater for recent than remote events; such patients are disoriented to place and time but not to person. Disorientation is neither a sensitive nor a specific marker of amnesia, however. Patients with mild-to-moderate memory loss may be fully oriented yet perform poorly on more sensitive testing. Disorientation, moreover, can have causes other than deficient memory or simply impaired recall. Patients who insist that their hospital room is actually their apartment or home have paramnesia, a more complex disturbance; patients oriented to place and time who cannot remember who they are have hysterical amnesia, a psychiatric dissociative state; and patients who identify themselves as Joan of Arc are either psychotic or excessively whimsical.

Memory is conventionally categorized as immediate (working), recent, and remote. As noted, impaired working memory can be inferred in a seemingly attentive patient unable to repeat six or seven digits forward (the same skill that allows a person to look up a phone number and then dial it). A sensitive test for recent memory is to have the patient repeat three unrelated words (eg, Chicago, orange, thirty-three) and then repeat them again after 5 minutes. If unable to recall the words, the patient is asked to select each word from a list. Amnestic disorders tend to affect spontaneous recall more than recognition.

Long-term memory can be tested by having the patient recall people or events from the past (eg, Where were you born? Where did you attend school? When did you get married?), but the answers must then be verified. Also problematic is using current or historical events such as presidents, sports figures, or television performers to test memory; the examiner should have a good idea of a patient's expected fund of information.

Amnestic patients sometimes fill their gaps in memory with fabricated yet plausible events, so-called confabulation. Although most often encountered in alcoholic patients with nutritional deficiency (Korsakoff syndrome), confabulation occurs in other amnestic disorders as well. Conversely, some alcoholics have profound memory loss without confabulation.

SEE CASE 74 | p. 269

"A homeless middle-aged man is brought to an emergency room having been found sitting on the sidewalk in a daze."

Conventional testing identifies disturbances of *episodic* memory, the recall of particular autobiographical events in time. Other memory systems include *semantic memory* (remembering what things are, such as a knife, a fork, or an automobile) and *procedural* memory (remembering how to perform a skilled motor act). Procedural memory tends to be relatively preserved in most patients with amnestic or dementing disorders. A patient with moderately severe Alzheimer disease is unlikely to have forgotten how to use table utensils or drive a car.

SEE CASE 73 | p. 265

"A 75-year-old right-handed college graduate becomes forgetful."

▶ Cognitive Abilities: Manipulation of Old Knowledge

The intellectual skills assessed in this part of the mental status examination, formally assessable in standardized IQ tests, are subject to educational and cultural bias. Questions directed at a patient's general fund of knowledge will produce useful clinical information only if the examiner has a reasonable idea of what to expect. Somewhat more useful are tests of simple calculation (in which performance sometimes improves when the questions are posed in terms of dollars and cents), similarities (eg, How is a dog like a lion? How is a bicycle like an automobile? How is yesterday like tomorrow?), opposites (eg, What word is the opposite of up, summer, north, quick, full?), or proverb interpretation (eg, A rolling stone gathers no moss). Concrete responses such as "A bicycle and an automobile both have wheels" may or may not signify cognitive impairment in a particular patient, but absurd answers or the reply "I don't know" likely indicate that something is wrong.

With mental retardation (failure to achieve normal cognitive development from birth or early childhood), verbal and performance skills tend to be equally affected, and even casual conversation usually reveals that intellectual function is subnormal. With dementia (loss of previously existing cognitive ability), vocabulary tends to be relatively preserved unless there is an obvious aphasic component, and the degree of disability in such patients is often unrecognized until specific tests of memory and other cognitive function are performed. Such dissociation would be reflected in IQ testing; demented patients tend to achieve better verbal than performance scores.

▶ Language

Aphasia is a disturbance of language that, in contrast to dysarthria, is explained neither by weakness or incoordination of the muscles of articulation nor by impaired hearing or vision. Impairment in nonlanguage cognitive spheres often coexists, and aphasic features are frequently encountered in dementing illnesses such as Alzheimer disease. The pathology responsible for aphasia is in the left cerebral hemisphere in over 98% of right-handed and around 60% of left-handed people. Cortical opercular structures (bordering the sylvian fissure) are usually involved, but aphasia has also followed damage to the thalamus, caudate, or cerebral white matter. The location and extent of the lesion differentiate the clinical subtypes of aphasia, which can be identified by assessing six basic components of language: spontaneous speech, speech comprehension, naming, repetition, writing, and reading.

Spontaneous Speech

Spontaneous speech is assessed by posing questions or remarks designed to elicit full-sentence replies. (Asking "Is your right arm weak?" does not accomplish this goal. Asking "What happened that caused you to come to the hospital?" does.) Fluency refers to the amount of speech produced over time (normally more than 50 words per minute). Word-finding difficulty can produce nonfluent hesitations, but except with very severe anomia the patient is usually able to produce several consecutive words or syllables at a normal rate. By contrast, the speech of Broca aphasia is severely and consistently nonfluent independent of word-finding and is often marked by long delays in initiation and hesitations between words and syllables.

Prosody refers to the musical qualities of speech, including rhythm, accent, and pitch. It gives languages and dialects their special oral character and serves different functions. Prosody can convey the emotional quality of speech (*sad, glad, mad;* this probably depends on right hemispheric processing), can provide propositional information (eg, the pitch inflections that characterize a sentence as interrogative or imperative), and, in languages such as Chinese or Thai, can convey semantic meaning.

The term *paraphasia* describes the unintentional substitution of incorrect for correct words. There are two types of paraphasic errors, literal and verbal. *Literal* (or phonemic) paraphasias involve words that phonetically resemble the intended word but contain one or more substituted syllables (eg, *bistbatch* for *wristwatch*). When such alterations have the character of real words, they are called *neologisms*. *Verbal* (or semantic) paraphasias involve real but unintended words (eg, *clock* for *wristwatch*); the substituted word is often semantically close to the intended word. In some patients, paraphasic errors are occasional contaminants of speech. In others, they almost entirely replace it; such incomprehensible speech is called *jargon*.

Even in the absence of paraphasias, the content of aphasic speech may be difficult to grasp. Severely restricted vocabulary may cause logorrheic but empty speech rather than word-finding hesitations. *Paragrammatism* refers to seemingly preserved syntax amid such profoundly restricted semantic content. By contrast, syntactic or relational words (such as prepositions, conjunctions, possessives, or verb tenses) are sometimes conspicuously absent in aphasic speech, particularly with Broca aphasia; such speech, practically reduced to nouns and verbs, is called *agrammatic* or *telegrammatic*.

SEE CASE 63 | p. 245

"A 55-year-old right-handed man suddenly develops difficulty speaking and weakness of his right side."

Speech Comprehension

If a patient's speech comprehension is impaired, the rest of the examination must be restructured. Strikingly abnormal speech comprehension may become apparent only on shifting from open-ended conversation to specific testing. Moreover, abnormalities of speech comprehension (like any neurological sign) may be mild or severe, or may become more severe as the examination progresses.

Assessment of speech comprehension should not depend on the patient's own verbal output; a wrong answer to a question could signify a paraphasic error rather than failure to understand the question. Asking the patient to follow spoken commands is also potentially problematic. If a command, simple or complex, is followed, and if the examiner has avoided nonverbal cues, it can be presumed that the command was understood. Failure to follow a command, however, could have different possible explanations, for example, paralysis, apraxia, pain, or negativism.

A more reliable method of testing speech comprehension is to ask yes–no questions. Even patients with severely restricted speech output can usually indicate affirmative or negative. The correct answers must of course be known to both the patient and the examiner. Still another way of testing speech comprehension is to ask the patient to point to objects or body parts.

These strategies detect disorders of semantic comprehension. As with abnormal speech output, semantic and syntactic (relational) comprehension can be dissociated. Syntactic comprehension can be assessed (in patients with adequate motor ability) by object manipulation. First identifying a comb, a pen, and a key, the patient is asked to put the key on top of the comb or the comb between the key and the pen. Alternatively, the patient can be given a statement such as "Tom's uncle's wife has blue eyes," and then asked, "Is the person with blue eyes a man or a woman?"

SEE CASE 64 | p. 247

"A 53-year-old woman abruptly begins 'talking out of her head.' "

Naming

Naming ability is tested in patients with adequate vision by showing them objects, body parts, colors, or pictures of actions (confrontation naming). Patients with impaired speech comprehension may not grasp the nature of the task. A variety of abnormal responses indicate anomia. Some patients produce literal or verbal paraphasias, which may or may not then be self-corrected. Some hesitate and effortfully grope for the correct word (tip-of-the-tongue phenomenon); such patients, though unable to come up with the word on their own, may correctly select it from a spoken list or say it correctly after being given its first letter. Other patients describe rather than name the object. For example, instead of saying "necktie," the patient says, "It's what you wear around your neck."

Repetition

Repetition is tested by having the patient repeat several sentences such as "Today is a sunny day" or "In the winter the President lives in Washington." Syntactically loaded sentences may be particularly difficult (eg, "If he were to come, I would go out"). Repetition errors most often consist of paraphasic substitutions.

Writing

Testing of writing begins by having patients sign their names. If that cannot be accomplished, more elaborate tests will almost surely fail. (Writing one's name does not necessarily rely on language processing per se; in many people it is an "overlearned motor act" more akin to a golf swing than true graphia.) More specific tests of writing include dictated sentences, words, or letters, as well as spontaneous writing, for example, describing what is seen in a room. Right hemiparesis need not deter such testing; most people can write, however awkwardly, with their left hand, and it is language, not penmanship, that is being tested.

Reading

Reading is tested both orally and for comprehension. Using large print, the patient reads aloud simple sentences, words, or letters. Reading comprehension can be tested by having the patient follow written commands that were successfully executed as oral commands or by having the patient answer written yes–no questions.

Dissociations between oral reading and reading comprehension can be striking. Some patients understand what they read quite well, yet oral reading quickly disintegrates into incomprehensible *paralexia*. Others can read aloud with unexpected accuracy even though they comprehend little of what they read.

SEE CASE 65 | *p. 249*

"Awakening in the morning, a college-educated 62-year-old right-handed man discovers that he cannot see in the right half of his visual field and that written words make no sense to him."

▶ **Praxis**

Praxis refers to the performance of a learned motor act. The term *apraxia* describes a number of different phenomena. In its broadest sense, apraxia refers to impaired motor activity not explained by weakness, incoordination, abnormal tone, bradykinesia, movement disorder, dementia, aphasia, or poor cooperation. Failure to perform an act is not apractic; to be apractic the act needs to be performed incorrectly or components of the act need to be performed imprecisely. Parts of the act might be omitted, sequenced abnormally, or incorrectly oriented in space. There are three types of testing: (1) gesture ("Show me how you

would . . ."), imitation ("Watch how I . . . , then you do it"), and (3) use of an actual object ("Here is a . . . . Show me how you would use it"). Tests for buccofacial apraxia include sticking out the tongue or blowing out a match. Tests for limb apraxia include hitchhiking, opening a door with a key, or flipping a coin. Serial acts can be tested, for example, folding a letter, putting it in an envelope, sealing the envelope, and placing a stamp.

Patients with *ideomotor* apraxia are unable to perform a learned motor act, although they understand what the act should be and are able to perform the individual movements that comprise the act. An example would be someone unable to pretend to strike a match, although able to explain the act, to perform its separate components, and even, when given a match and matchbook, to perform the act in its entirety. The disturbance can be viewed as a functional disconnection between the idea of the act (its physiological memory trace or *engram*) and the act's final execution. Other less clearly defined forms of apraxia are considered to involve the engram itself (*ideational* apraxia) or its executive apparatus (*limbkinetic* apraxia).

SEE CASE 66 | *p. 250*

"A 59-year-old right-handed man suddenly develops right leg weakness."

▶ **Gnosia and Spatial Manipulation**

Gnosia refers to recognition. *Agnosia* is a failure of recognition not explained by impaired primary sensation (tactile, visual, auditory) or cognitive impairment. It has been described as "perception stripped of its meaning." Agnosia differs from anomia in that the patient not only fails to name the confronted object but cannot select it from a group or match it to a likeness. In tactile agnosia (*astereognosis*), touch threshold is normal, yet patients cannot identify what they are touching. (See the Sensory Examination, Chapter 5.)

Comparable agnosias exist in the visual and auditory spheres. Responsible lesions are likely to be bilateral, and so visual and auditory agnosias are rare. *Simultanagnosia* is inability to recognize the meaning of a whole scene or object, even though its individual components are correctly perceived and recognized. Auditory agnosia can involve spoken words, music, or nonverbal, nonmusical sounds.

SEE CASE 67 | p. 252

"A 58-year-old right-handed man suddenly develops left hemiparesis and complains that both words and music sound like noise to him."

Prosopagnosia is selective inability to recognize familiar faces. The problem seems to be one of fine tuning; affected patients can recognize a face as a face (or a dog as a dog) but are unable to identify which one. Nearly all patients examined at autopsy have had bilateral temporooccipital lesions.

SEE CASE 69 | p. 256

"A 55-year-old woman suddenly develops impaired vision, and computerized tomographic (CT) scan reveals bilateral temporooccipital infarcts."

Whereas the left hemisphere usually processes language (and related analytic skills), the right hemisphere processes spatial information. Right hemispheric lesions (particularly parietal) cause impairment of spatial perception and manipulation. There may be difficulty reading maps or finding one's way about (topographagnosia), copying simple pictures or shapes, or drawing simple objects such as a flower or a clock face (constructional apraxia or *apractagnosia*).

Even more striking is *hemineglect*. Patients with damage to the right hemisphere may ignore any object to the left of midline,

even the left side of their own body. They may fail to recognize severe hemiplegia (*anosognosia*) or even to acknowledge left body parts as their own (*asomatognosia*), insisting, for example, that a paralyzed limb belongs to someone else. Objects or voices in contralateral space are ignored, and grooming or dressing may be restricted to the right half of the body. Asked to bisect a line, such patients indicate a point to the right of midline. A copied picture might be missing the left half, and a drawn clock face might have all the numbers neatly arranged on the right. As with aphasia, when this syndrome is severe there is usually additional cognitive impairment, but not enough to explain the spatial disturbance. Neither is hemineglect the result of homonymous hemianopia (see later).

SEE CASE 68 | p. 254

"A 57-year-old woman is brought to the hospital after being found at home unable to move her left arm."

A subtle manifestation of hemineglect is *extinction*, the ability to recognize a stimulus (visual, auditory, or tactile) on either side when it is presented alone, with inability to feel the stimulus on one side when it is accompanied by stimulation of the opposite side. As with other forms of hemineglect, extinction suggests a lesion of the contralateral parietal lobe.

Some patients demonstrate anosognosia for neurological impairment other than hemiparesis. Anosognosia is a common accompaniment of severe Wernicke aphasia and Korsakoff amnesia. Less often it is encountered in patients who are blind or deaf.

SEE CASE 70 | p. 258

"A 58-year-old woman is brought to the hospital by her husband, who reports that several hours earlier she began acting strangely."

3

Cranial Nerves:
Twelve Is a Misleading Number

Variably afferent and efferent, somatic and visceral, the 12 cranial nerves are functionally more complex than their ordered number would suggest (Table 3–1). Cranial nerves 4, 6, and 12 are solely somatic efferent. Cranial nerves 1 and 8 are solely afferent, but 8 conveys two very different kinds of sensory information. Cranial nerve 2, while solely afferent, is actually a central nervous system tract (accounting, among other things, for its frequent involvement in multiple sclerosis). Cranial nerve 11, while solely efferent, is anatomically an aberrant spinal nerve; its motor neurons reside in the upper cervical spinal cord, accounting for its involvement by lesions at or just below the foramen magnum. The other cranial nerves—3, 5, 7, 9, and 10—are multifunc-

tional. Nonetheless, for clinical purposes the examination of the cranial nerves is usually straightforward. How many components of each nerve are assessed will depend on the clinician's diagnostic index of suspicion.

▶ The Olfactory Nerve

The first cranial nerve is concerned with the sense of smell. Chemoreceptors of the olfactory epithelium are located high in the nasopharynx (Figure 3–1), and the first step in assessing olfaction is to look into the nose for possible obstruction of airflow. Each nostril is then tested separately, using nonnoxious odorants such as coffee, peppermint, or soap. (Pungent substances such as ammonia

Table 3–1. The cranial nerves.

Cranial Nerve	Cranial Foramen	Function
1. Olfactory	Cribriform plate	Sensory
2. Optic	Optic foramen	Sensory
3. Oculomotor	Superior orbital fissure	Motor, autonomic
4. Trochlear	Superior orbital fissure	Motor
5. Trigeminal	Superior orbital fissure; foramen rotundum; foramen ovale	Motor, sensory
6. Abducens	Superior orbital fissure	Motor
7. Facial	Internal auditory meatus	Motor, sensory, autonomic
8. Vestibulocochlear	Internal auditory meatus	Sensory
9. Glossopharyngeal	Jugular foramen	Motor, sensory, autonomic
10. Vagus	Jugular foramen	Motor, sensory, autonomic
11. Accessory	Jugular foramen	Motor
12. Hypoglossal	Hypoglossal foramen	Motor

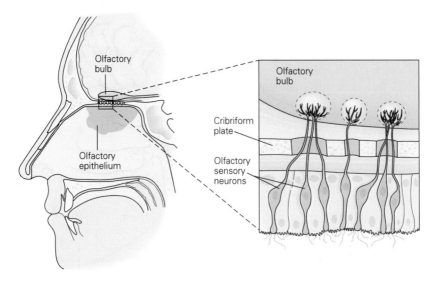

Figure 3–1. Olfactory sensory neurons are within the epithelium of the dorsal posterior nasal cavity. Axons of these neurons project onto neurons of the olfactory bulb, which rests on the cribriform plate of the ethmoid bone. (Reproduced with permission from Kandel ER, Schwartz JH, Jessell TM. 1999. *Principles of Neural Science,* 4th ed. New York: McGraw-Hill.)

will stimulate trigeminal nociceptors.) Failure to smell anything is termed *anosmia.* Unpleasant distortion of the stimulus is termed *parosmia.* Inability to identify the stimulus more likely reflects inexperience than true olfactory agnosia.

The cerebral representations for olfaction are multiple, and anosmia is most often secondary to local nasal disease, infectious or neoplastic. Anosmia following head trauma is attributed to severance of centrally projecting axons of primary olfactory neurons as they pass through the cribriform plate of the ethmoid bone. Intracranial causes of anosmia include neoplasm (eg, a meningioma overlying the cribriform plate) and infection (eg, neurosyphilis or an aftermath of bacterial or tuberculous meningitis).

It is not unusual for anosmic patients—particularly those accustomed to more subtle fare than fast food—to report their disability as loss of taste.

SEE CASE 15 | p. 119

"For several months a 57-year-old woman has noticed that food seems to have less taste."

Structural lesions of either the orbitofrontal or inferomedial temporal cortex can cause seizures consisting of olfactory hallucinations. In such patients the sense of smell is otherwise usually normal.

SEE CASE 16 | p. 120

"A 12-year-old boy suffers concussion and a skull fracture."

▶ The Optic Nerve

The second cranial nerve is concerned with vision, assessment of which requires familiarity with the anatomy of the visual pathways. The examination includes testing of visual acuity, testing of the visual field, and examination of the fundus.

Anatomy

Crucial to lesion localization is knowledge of the anatomy of the optic nerve, the optic chiasm, and the visual pathways posterior to the chiasm. Projections from the nasal retina (subserving the temporal visual fields) cross at the chiasm whereas projections from the temporal retina (subserving the nasal visual fields) do not. Therefore, a unilateral lesion anterior to the chiasm will produce monocular visual impairment, a unilateral lesion posterior to the chiasm will produce contralateral homonymous hemianopia, and a lesion transecting the chiasm will produce bitemporal hemianopia.

The optic radiations, projecting from the lateral geniculate nucleus of the thalamus to the occipital visual cortex, have an inferior component within the temporal lobe and a superior component within the parietal lobe. A unilateral lesion of the inferior component (or of the inferior lip of the occipital visual cortex) will produce contralateral superior homonymous quadrantanopia. A unilateral lesion of the superior component (or of the superior lip of the occipital visual cortex) will produce contralateral inferior homonymous quadrantanopia.

Visual Acuity

Visual acuity is tested with a Snellin chart (at 20 ft) or a hand-held card (at 14 in). The eyes are tested separately, and if acuity is reduced below the upper line of the chart, the examiner assesses finger counting, detection of hand movement, or light perception. Refractive errors are identified by having patients wear their glasses or look through a pinhole. Inspection of the eyes and funduscopic examination will often identify ocular lesions accounting for reduced acuity, such as corneal scarring, cataracts, glaucoma, diabetic retinopathy, or macular degeneration.

Visual Fields

Bedside or office visual field examination is usually by confrontation. The patient and examiner face each other, and the eyes are tested separately. With one eye covered, the patient and the examiner fixate on each other's open eye and, with the examiner's visual field being used as a comparison, the stimulus to be detected is held equidistant between them. It can be a small object moving slowly inward from the periphery, with the patient being asked to indicate when it is first seen. Alternatively, the patient can be told to count fingers held successively in different visual quadrants. If testing indicates that the visual fields are grossly normal and a cerebral lesion is suspected, stimuli are presented simultaneously to the right and left fields to identify visual hemineglect (*extinction*—see section on Agnosia). Subtle defects are sometimes identified using a red rather than a white stimulus. If confrontation testing is normal in a patient with unexplained visual impairment, formal ophthalmologic testing is performed, including perimetry.

Visual field testing provides very accurate localization of structural lesions (Figure 3–2). Monocular visual impairment, including either field defect or *scotoma* (an area of visual loss surrounded by preserved vision), localizes a lesion to the optic nerve, the retina, or other ocular structures. Bitemporal hemianopia, if caused by a single lesion, places that lesion at the optic chiasm. Homonymous hemianopia, quadrantanopia, or bilateral congruent scotomas place the lesion behind the chiasm in the contralateral optic tract, lateral geniculate nucleus of the thalamus, optic radiation, or primary visual cortex.

SEE CASE 8 | p. 103

"For several months a 37-year-old woman has had progressively severe bifrontal headaches."

SEE CASE 9 | p. 105

"A 66-year-old man with a history of childhood rheumatic fever abruptly develops difficulty seeing to the left."

Funduscopy

An effective funduscopic examination requires a good ophthalmoscope and clinical experience. Focusing successively on the

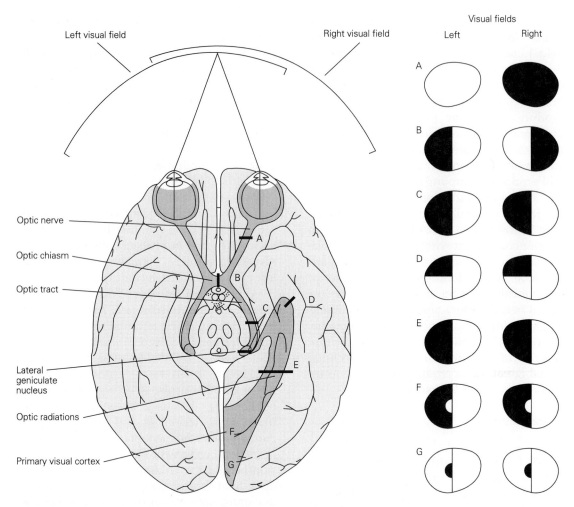

Figure 3–2. Visual field defects from lesions along the visual pathway. **A.** Lesion of the right optic nerve, with right eye blindness. **B.** Lesion of the optic chiasm, with bitemporal hemianopia. **C.** Lesions of the right optic tract or lateral geniculate nucleus, with left homonymous hemianopia. **D.** Lesion of the right inferior temporal optic radiation, with left homonymous superior quantrantanopia. **E.** Lesion of the right inferior and superior optic radiation, with left homonymous hemianopia. **F.** Lesion of the right primary visual cortex sparing the occipital pole, with left homonymous hemianopia and macular sparing. **G.** Lesion of the right occipital pole, with left homonymous paracentral scotomas. (Reproduced with permission from Martin JH. 1996. *Neuroanatomy Text and Atlas*, 2nd ed. Stamford, CT: Appleton & Lange. Adapted with permission from Patten H. 1977. *Neurological Differential Diagnosis*. New York: Springer-Verlag.)

cornea, the anterior chamber, the lens, and the vitreous, the examiner then surveys the optic disk, the retinal vessels, and the retina itself. *Optic atrophy* refers to disk pallor, and its myriad causes include glaucoma, neurotoxins, optic nerve compression by a neoplasm, infarction, trauma, heredodegenerative disease, multiple sclerosis, and longstanding papilledema. The temporal disk margin is paler than the nasal margin in most people with normal vision, and so subtle degrees of optic atrophy—for example, as seen in alcoholics with nutritional amblyopia—may be easily missed.

SEE CASE 7 | p. 102

"A 32-year-old woman awakens with impaired vision in her left eye and left retroorbital pain on eye movement."

Papilledema refers to optic disk swelling. It can be the result of local pathology, for example, the inflammatory demyelination of optic neuritis, in which case visual acuity is acutely impaired, often with a central scotoma. When papilledema is the result of increased intracranial pressure, the normal blind spot becomes enlarged, but visual acuity is not initially affected; over time, however, there is constriction of the visual fields and then impaired visual acuity, which can progress to blindness.

In papilledema the disk margins become blurred and elevated, the optic disk cup becomes less evident, and the disk color, normally paler and pinker than the retina, becomes closer to the color of the retina. When the cause is increased intracranial pressure, the ratio of the diameter of retinal veins to arteries (normally about 3:2) increases, and there may be retinal hemorrhages and whitish exudates.

A great variety of other abnormalities can be identified by funduscopy, including arterial narrowing (hypertension), different kinds of exudates (diabetes mellitus, blood dyscrasias), microaneurysms (diabetes mellitus), subhyaloid hemorrhages (located between the retina and the vitreous membrane and associated with subarachnoid hemorrhage), tubercles and other granulomas, phakomas (glial collections, associated with the hereditary diseases neurofibromatosis and tuberous sclerosis), pigmentary changes (retinitis pigmentosa), and emboli (seen within arteriolar branches of the central retinal artery and consisting of platelets, cholesterol, or calcific debris).

SEE CASE 6 | *p. 101*

"For the past 6 weeks a 52-year-old man has been having spells of transient monocular visual loss."

Normal variants that can be confused with papilledema are drusen (colloidal excrescences that deform the disk) and myelinated nerve fibers (which appear as white streaks or fans spreading a short distance beyond the disk).

In sum, funduscopy provides an extraordinary view of a unique structure. The optic nerve, arising from retinal ganglion cells and 1.5 mm in diameter, is the only part of the central nervous system that a clinician can directly observe.

Other Visual Abnormalities

Lesions of the occipital lobe or visual association areas can produce bizarre symptoms and signs, for example, loss of the ability to perceive motion or selective loss of depth or color vision.

SEE CASE 10 | *p. 107*

"A 64-year-old hypertensive man suddenly loses color vision."

Primary and association visual areas can also generate visual hallucinations in patients with either epilepsy or migraine.

SEE CASE 11 | *p. 109*

"For several years a 30-year-old woman has had headaches preceded by visual symptoms."

▶ The Oculomotor, Trochlear, and Abducens Nerves

The oculomotor nerve, in conjunction with the trochlear and the abducens nerves, controls eye movements. In addition, it provides parasympathetic supply to the pupils. The autonomic function of the oculomotor nerve will be considered first. Because the afferent end of the pupillary light reflex includes the optic nerve and because sympathetic innervation is responsible for pupillary dilatation, examination of the pupils involves assessment of these systems as well.

Pupils

Sympathetic input. If there is pupillary inequality (anisocoria), the abnormal pupil could be either the larger or the smaller. An abnormally small pupil can result from a lesion involving sympathetic projections anywhere along their extensive pathway—hypothalamus, brain stem, spinal cord as far down as the upper thoracic segments, spinal sympathetic chain and ganglia, pericarotid plexus, and sympathetic fibers entering the orbit with the first division of the trigeminal nerve. In fact, the most common cause of acquired unilateral miosis is probably lung cancer affecting the sympathetic cervical ganglia. Miosis resulting from sympathetic damage is often accompanied by mild ptosis (from denervation of smooth tarsal muscles within the eyelid) and absent sweating on the same side of the face; the triad is called *Horner syndrome.*

In a normal pupil, local instillation of either cocaine or hydroxyamphetamine onto the eye causes pupillary dilatation. However, a pupil in a patient with Horner syndrome will not dilate when cocaine is locally instilled. Cocaine acts as an adrenergic agonist by blocking presynaptic reuptake of norepinephrine; if the neuron has not fired, there is no synaptic neurotransmitter to block. By contrast, instillation of hydroxyamphetamine produces pupillary dilatation in a Horner pupil if the lesion is proximal to the superior cervical ganglion, but not if it involves the final neuron of the sympathetic pathway. Hydroxyamphetamine acts as an adrenergic agonist by releasing norepinephrine from nerve endings whether they are normally firing or not; if the nerve in contact with the iris is damaged, there is no longer a viable nerve ending from which to release neurotransmitter.

SEE CASE 39 | *p. 189*

"A 47-year-old woman, who has smoked a pack of cigarettes daily for 30 years, notices that her pupils are of unequal size."

Parasympathetic input. The sympathetic system does not directly participate in the pupillary light reflex, which becomes abnormal following damage to either the optic or the oculomotor nerve. When a pupillary abnormality is unilateral, the neurological examination readily reveals which system is at fault. In the presence of a lesion affecting the mesencephalic Edinger-Westphal nucleus or the parasympathetic component of the oculomotor nerve (including the intraorbital ciliary ganglion) the ipsilateral pupil will be larger and will have reduced constriction to light shone in either eye. With a lesion of the retina or optic nerve, there will be reduced constriction of both pupils to light shone in the affected eye but the pupils will remain equal in size at all times; an afferent lesion does not cause anisocoria.

The strict consensuality of the pupillary light reflex is easily understood when its anatomy is reviewed (Figure 3–3). After diverging from the visual pathway proximal to the thalamic lateral geniculate nucleus (a divergence that accounts for the preservation of the light reflex in patients with cortical blindness), fibers mediating the light reflex synapse in the midbrain pretectum. Each pretectal nucleus then sends fibers to both the ipsilateral and the contralateral Edinger-Westphal nuclei. As a result, under normal conditions light shone into one eye invariably produces an equal degree of miosis in both.

Pupillary constriction to near vision is tested by having the patient fixate on a distant object and then on an object held a few inches in front of the eyes. (A pencil usually suffices, but sometimes asking the patient to tell the time from a closely held watch more reliably produces a response.) Miosis is accompanied by convergence, which is observed, and accommodation of the lens (increased lens curvature), which is not observed but can be inferred if the closely held object remains in focus.

The afferent end of the near/accommodation reflex arc is in visual areas of the occipital lobe, which communicate with the Edinger-Westphal nucleus by a route sepa-

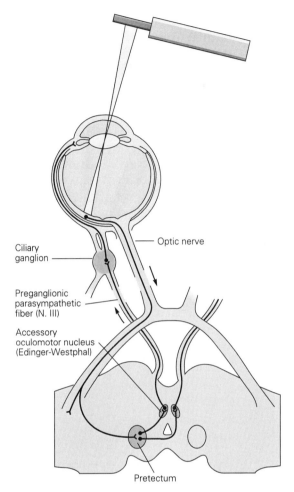

Optic nerve

Ciliary ganglion

Preganglionic parasympathetic fiber (N. III)

Accessory oculomotor nucleus (Edinger-Westphal)

Pretectum

Figure 3–3. The pathway mediating reflex constriction of the pupil to light includes retinal light receptors at the afferent end and pupilloconstrictor smooth muscle at the efferent end. The reflex is consensual because following synaptic relay in the midbrain pretectum there are bilateral projections to each Edinger-Westphal (parasympathetic) nucleus. (Reproduced with permission from Kandel ER, Schwartz JH, Jessell TM. 1999. *Principles of Neural Science*, 4th ed. New York: Mc-Graw-Hill.)

rate from the light reflex pathway. Pupillary light and near reflexes can therefore dissociate. *Argyll-Robertson pupils*, seen most often in patients with neurosyphilis, are bilaterally small and fail to react to light but become smaller with near vision. The lesion is presumed to be in the midbrain tegmentum, bilaterally interrupting the light reflex pathway but sparing the near/accommodation pathway and the Edinger-Westphal nucleus.

Light-near dissociation also occurs with an *Adie's pupil*, which is usually unilateral and larger than normal. On casual testing it appears unreactive to light and constricts to near vision, but if a bright light is shone long enough, a slow constriction often occurs. When the light is removed, miosis is maintained for up to a minute, followed by a slow return to mydriasis. The lesion is in the ciliary ganglion, and light-near dissociation (which would not be expected with damage to a final common pathway) occurs because the great majority of ciliary ganglion neurons mediate near/accommodation, providing greater reserve when degeneration affects the ganglion randomly. Consistent with this localization, an Adie's pupil constricts briskly to locally applied cholinomimetic agents (such as mecholyl or pilocarpine) in dilutions that do not constrict normal pupils, an example of denervation supersensitivity.

The parasympathetic innervation of the iris runs along the outer surface of the third nerve. Pupillary enlargement or unreactivity is therefore usual in compressive lesions of the oculomotor nerve (eg, a nearby ruptured saccular aneurysm or transtentorial herniation of the inferomedial temporal lobe secondary to a supratentorial mass). On the other hand, microinfarction of the third nerve—which is not unusual in patients with diabetes mellitus—tends to spare the nerve's outer rim, resulting in impaired eye movements with normal pupillary size and reactivity.

Extraocular Eye Movement

Nerves and muscles. The motor function of the oculomotor, trochlear, and abducens nerves is evaluated by examination of eye movements (Figure 3–4). The eyes are tested first for the presence of spontaneous, involuntary movements and then for the presence of disconjugate movement (identified either by obvious lagging in one or the other eye or by a report of diplopia) or gaze palsy

A

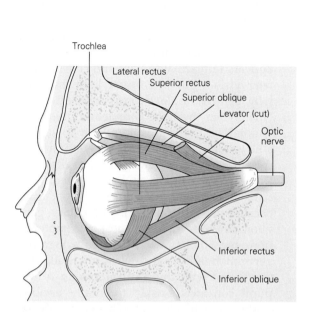

B

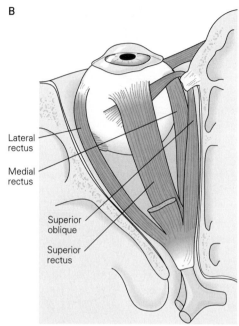

Figure 3–4. Lateral (**A**) and superior (**B**) views of the origins and insertions of the extraocular muscles. (Reproduced with permission from Kandel ER, Schwartz JH, Jessell TM. 1999. *Principles of Neural Science*, 4th ed. New York: Mc-Graw-Hill.)

(incomplete but conjugate limitation of movement of both eyes in a particular direction). To test for eye movement the patient follows a clearly defined object such as a pen tip or a fine point of light to the left and to the right and then upward and downward when the eyes are in the midline and when they are deviated to each side. Normal movement in each direction requires the following:

1. Lateral movement (abduction) is brought about by the lateral rectus muscle (sixth nerve).
2. Medial movement (adduction) is brought about by the medial rectus muscle (third nerve).
3. When the eye is abducted, it is elevated by the superior rectus muscle and depressed by the inferior rectus muscle (both third nerve).
4. When the eye is adducted, it is elevated by the inferior oblique muscle (third

nerve) and depressed by the superior oblique muscle (fourth nerve).

Therefore, if the eye cannot move outward, there is a lesion involving either the sixth nerve or the lateral rectus muscle; if the eye cannot move downward when deviated inward, there is a lesion of the fourth nerve or the superior oblique muscle; any other monocular limitations in movement are due to a lesion of the third nerve or one of its muscles of innervation. (An exception is internuclear ophthalmoplegia—see below.)

SEE CASE 52 | *p. 216*

"A 46-year-old man experiences horizontal diplopia when he reads."

The third nerve supplies the levator palpebrae muscle, and ptosis is a common feature of oculomotor nerve lesions. In addition to its usual association with an abnormally large rather than an abnormally small pupil, such ptosis differs from ptosis associated with Horner syndrome in its severity. Sympathetic denervation causes only mild ptosis; oculomotor denervation can result in total eye closure. Moreover, sympathetic lesions also affect the lower lid (upside down ptosis).

Because of their direction of insertion onto the globe, the oblique muscles mediate intorsion and extorsion when the eye is either in mid-position or abducted. A compensatory head tilt (away from the side of the lesion) is therefore a feature of fourth nerve palsy.

If a patient complains of diplopia but eye muscle weakness is not evident, a red glass test can help define the problem. A transparent red glass or plastic cover is placed over one eye while the patient looks at a point of light in each of the directions just described. If diplopia is reported, the examiner asks if it is horizontal or vertical and if the red image is to the left or right, and above or below, the white image. Diplopia will be produced or accentuated when looking in the direction of the weak muscle, and in any direction of gaze the most peripheral image will belong to the affected eye.

Normal are *exophoria* and *esophoria* (lazy eye), in which one eye is exo (outwardly) or eso (inwardly) deviated when not participating in fixation (as during fatigue or sleep or when the eye is covered); in such people the eyes are normally aligned during fixation. By contrast, *exotropia* and *esotropia* refer to an abnormal fixed divergence or convergence of the eyes in all directions of gaze. It is most often congenital, and an affected infant will preferentially fixate with one eye. The nonfixating eye is then at risk for permanently impaired vision (*amblyopia ex anopsia*) because occipital ocular dominance columns that receive input from that eye will fail to develop. Such an outcome can be prevented by covering each eye on alternate days until surgical correction of the malalignment can be accomplished.

Acquired hypertropia (*skew*), with one eye above the other in all directions of gaze, signifies a lesion of the brain stem, most often the pontine tegmenum. Skew is probably the result of an imbalance of vestibular input to the two oculomotor nerve nuclei.

Horizontal gaze palsy. Eye movements are normally conjugate, and most lesions causing diplopia involve either cranial nerves (peripherally or within the brain stem) or extrinsic eye muscles. Certain central nervous system lesions produce *gaze palsy*—the eyes remain conjugate and there is no diplopia, but neither eye moves fully in a particular direction.

Rapid (saccadic) eye movements are triggered by the frontal eye fields, anterior to the motor cortex on the cerebral convexity (Figure 3–5). Stimulation of this area (as during a seizure) produces conjugate horizontal eye movements in a direction contralateral to the side of the stimulus. Destruction of the area produces conjugate deviation of the eyes toward the side of the lesion and inability to move them voluntarily to the opposite side. Descending through the anterior limb and genu of the internal capsule, projections from the frontal eye fields cross in the lower midbrain and communicate with the paramedian pontine reticular formation (PPRF), stimulation of which causes conjugate horizontal eye movements ipsilaterally. Destruction of the PPRF causes contralateral deviation and inability to move the eyes conjugately in the direction of the lesion.

Subtle features sometimes help to determine whether a horizontal gaze palsy is due to a cerebral or a brain stem lesion (Figure 3–6). For example, frontal lesions are more likely to spare reflexive pursuit movements, as when patients fixate on a target and then do not lose fixation when their head is moved passively and unpredictably in various directions. Pursuit (slow, nonsaccadic) eye movements appear to be controlled by areas of the posterior temporal lobe, which send projections through the posterior limb of the internal capsule that ultimately communicate with cerebellar structures and vestibular nuclei but not with the PPRF. In most cases, however, the

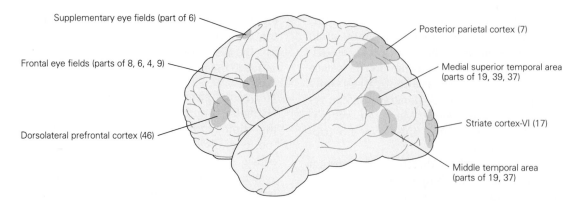

Figure 3–5. Cortical areas involved in eye movements. The frontal eye fields, the supplementary eye fields, and the dorsolateral prefrontal cortex participate in generating saccadic (rapid) eye movements. Pursuit (slow) eye movements require visual motion processing and are dependent on the occipital visual (striate) cortex and regions of the posterior temporal lobe. The posterior parietal cortex is necessary for visual attentional processing in the generation of saccades. Numbers in parentheses correspond to Brodmann areas. (Reproduced with permission from Kandel ER, Schwartz JH, Jessell TM. 1991. *Principles of Neural Science*, 3rd ed. Norwalk, CT: Appleton & Lange.)

anatomical basis of a horizontal gaze palsy is surmised by accompanying signs. For example, a patient unable to gaze leftward who also has a left hemiparesis probably has a right frontal lobe lesion; a patient unable to gaze leftward who has a right hemiparesis probably has a left brain stem lesion (Figure 3–7).

Internuclear ophthalmoplegia. From the PPRF the circuitry controlling horizontal gaze projects to the abducens nucleus (lesions of which produce horizontal gaze palsy, not simply abduction palsy) and then, via the contralateral median longitudinal fasciculus (MLF), to the oculomotor nucleus supplying the medial rectus muscle of the opposite eye. Lesions of the MLF disrupt horizontal conjugate gaze. In such internuclear ophthalmoplegia there is restricted voluntary adduction ipsilateral to the lesion; however, if the oculomotor nucleus is undamaged, the medial rectus muscle continues to perform normally during convergence (see Figure 3–6). When bilateral, internuclear ophthalmoplegia is most often due to multiple sclerosis and when unilateral, is most often due to infarction.

SEE CASE 51 | p. 213

"Two weeks after being treated for a myocardial infarction a 48-year-old man suddenly develops left hemiparesis, left lateral deviation of gaze, double vision, and right facial weakness."

Vertical gaze palsy. In experimental animals bilateral simultaneous stimulation of the frontal eye fields produces vertical conjugate eye movements, and involuntary upward eye deviation is sometimes a feature of major motor (grand mal) seizures. It also occurs as a dystonic side effect of antipsychotic medications. Vertical gaze palsies are not associated with cerebral cortical lesions, however. (Inability to look upward is common in patients with Parkinson disease, the major pathology of which is in the substantia nigra.) Impaired vertical gaze, particularly upward, follows lesions of the midbrain's rostral interstitial nucleus of the MLF, a control area for vertical gaze comparable to the PPRF's control of horizontal gaze. Projections from the rostral interstitial nucleus to the oculomotor nuclei for the superior rectus and inferior oblique muscles pass through the posterior commissure; hence, lesions in that area (such as compression by a pineal

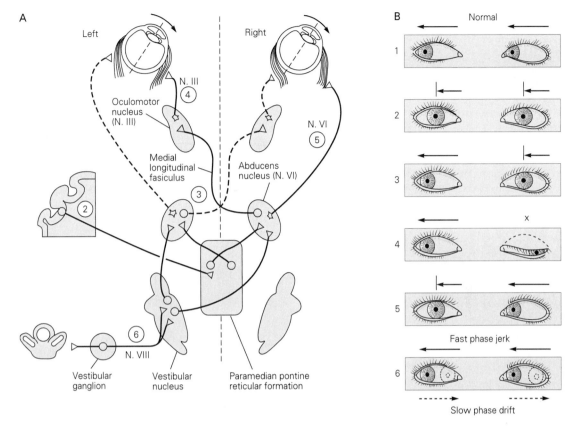

Figure 3–6. A. Pathways for horizontal gaze. **B.** Abnormalities of eye movements on attempted gaze to the right correspond to the numbered lesions in the horizontal gaze system shown in A. A normal right gaze (**1**). A lesion of the left frontal cortex (**2**) causes impaired gaze to the right. A lesion of the left medial longitudinal fasciculus (**3**) causes impaired voluntary or pursuit adduction of the left eye with preserved adduction on convergence. A lesion of the left oculomotor nerve (**4**) causes weakness of the left medial rectus muscle (plus weakness of the left superior rectus, inferior rectus, inferior oblique, and levator palpebrae muscles). A lesion of the right abducens nerve (**5**) causes weakness of the right lateral rectus muscle. A lesion of the left vestibulocochlear nerve (**6**) causes horizontal rightward-jerking nystagmus (often with a rotatory component). [Reproduced with permission from Kandel ER, Schwartz JH, Jessell TM. 1991. *Principles of Neural Science*, 3rd ed. Norwalk, CT: Appleton & Lange. Adapted with permission from Sears ES, Franklin GM. 1980. Diseases of the cranial nerves. In: Rosenberg RN (ed): *The Science and Practice of Clinical Medicine*, Vol. 5: *Neurology.* New York: Grune & Stratton, pp. 471–494.]

tumor) can impair upward gaze without affecting downward gaze.

Nystagmus. Nystagmus—rhythmic oscillatory eye movements—can be either unilateral or bilateral. *Pendular* nystagmus, with roughly equal velocity in either direction, is most often the result of severe visual impairment during early childhood. *Jerk* nystagmus, with a slow drift in one direction and a rapid corrective movement in the other, can be present with the eyes at rest, but tends to be accentuated by ocular deviation, with the fast component in the direction of gaze. Horizontal or rotatory nystagmus is most often associated with vestibular lesions, peripheral or central (see Figure 3–6). Vertical nystagmus (the fast component directed upward or downward) suggests a brain stem lesion, either intrinsic (eg, multiple sclerosis or syringobulbia) or extrinsic (eg, compression by a cerebellar tumor or an Arnold-Chiari malformation). Patients with lesions of the MLF often have horizontal

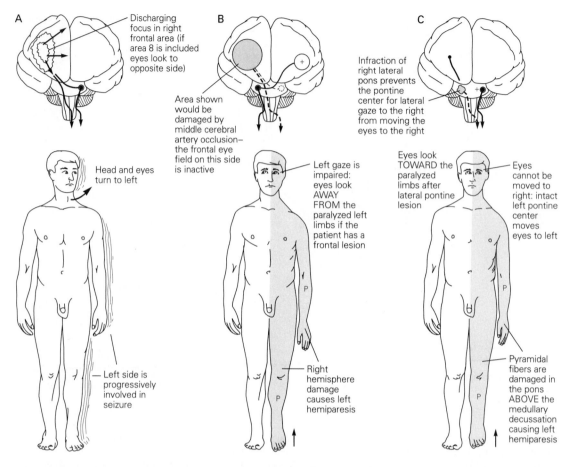

Figure 3–7. Disorders of gaze combined with other impairments can localize the lesion. **A.** Right frontal irritative (epileptic) lesion. **B.** Right frontal destructive lesion. C. Right pontine destructive lesion. +, Functioning gaze center; P, paretic limbs; arrow, Babinski sign. (Reproduced with permission from Kandel ER, Schwartz JH, Jessell TM. 1991. *Principles of Neural Science,* 3rd ed. Norwalk, CT: Appleton & Lange. Adapted with permission from Patten H. 1977. *Neurological Differential Diagnosis.* New York: Springer-Verlag.)

nystagmus in the contralateral abducting eye. Nystagmus on lateral gaze is a benign side effect of certain drugs, particularly barbiturates and the anticonvulsant phenytoin.

Nystagmus is reflexly produced by opticokinetic testing. When a vertically striped tape is passed horizontally in front of the eyes, a normal response consists of nystagmus with the fast component directed opposite to the direction in which the tape is moving. Nystagmus occurs because the visual stimulus of the tape elicits reflexic pursuit eye movements in the same direction, which in turn produce corrective saccades in

the opposite direction. Opticokinetic testing may fail to produce nystagmus with either anterior or posterior cerebral lesions: With anterior lesions it is because there are no corrective saccades; with posterior lesions it is because there is no initial pursuit (see Figure 3–5).

Other abnormal eye movements. There are many other abnormal involuntary eye movements, some with localizing value. For example, ocular bobbing, with rapid conjugate downward movements of the eyes several times per minute, indicates a lesion of the pontine tegmenum. Ping pong gaze, with the eyes moving conjugately, rapidly, and continuously from side to side, indicates bilateral severe damage rostral to the pons. Both abnormalities carry a poor prognosis.

▶ The Trigeminal Nerve

The fifth cranial nerve carries sensation from the face, anterior scalp, eye, and much of the nasal and oral cavities. Fibers in its mandibular division also provide motor innervation to the muscles of mastication, including the temporalis and masseter (jaw closure), the lateral pterygoid (protraction and contralateral deviation of the jaw), and the mylohyoid (jaw opening).

Anatomy

Familiarity with trigeminal neuroanatomy is necessary for interpreting abnormalities of facial sensation (Figures 3–8 and 3–9).

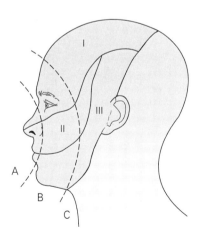

Figure 3–8. Distribution of the three sensory branches of the trigeminal nerve. Dashed concentric lines indicate rostrocaudal distribution within the spinal trigeminal nucleus. The area within A is most rostral; the area within C is most caudal. (Reproduced with permission from Kandel ER, Schwartz JH, Jessell TM. 1991. *Principles of Neural Science*, 3rd ed. Norwalk, CT: Appleton & Lange. Adapted with permission from Brodal A. 1981. *Neurological Anatomy in Relation to Clinical Medicine*, 3rd ed. New York: Oxford University Press, pp. 508–532.)

1. The trigeminal (semilunar, gasserian) ganglion, containing neurons that convey touch, temperature, and pain sensation, resides in Meckel's cave, an indentation in the petrous bone. It gives off three peripheral divisions. The ophthalmic division (V_1) exits the middle cranial fossa through the superior orbital fissure, the maxillary division (V_2) through the foramen rotundum, and the mandibular division (V_3) through the foramen ovale.
2. V_1 supplies the forehead as far back as the vertex, the upper lateral nose, the cornea, and most of the nasal mucosa. V_2 supplies the malar region; the lower lateral nose; the upper lip, teeth, and gums; the palate; and the inner cheek. V_3 supplies the chin, the area anterior to and above the ear, the anterior two thirds of the tongue, and the lower teeth and gums. The skin of the ear and the angle of the jaw are not supplied by the trigeminal nerve.
3. In the pons light touch and tactile discrimination are relayed by way of the primary (principal) sensory nucleus to the ventral posterior medial nucleus of the thalamus (mostly contralaterally) and from there to the postrolandic sensory cortex of the parietal lobe. Projections for pain and temperature sensation, however, descend into the medulla and upper cervical cord, synapsing along the way onto the spinal trigeminal nucleus, axons of which ascend (mostly contralaterally) to a different subdivision of the ventral posterior medial nucleus of the thalamus.
4. Fibers carrying afferent information from muscle spindles in the jaw bypass the extraparenchymal ganglion; their cell bodies are intraparenchymal in the mesencephalic trigeminal nucleus.
5. The efferent trigeminal motor nucleus supplies jaw and masticatory muscles.

Examination

For a general discussion of sensory testing, see later. The examiner initially checks the forehead, the malar region, and the chin, defining the outer borders of any deficit found. Decreased sensation confined to the

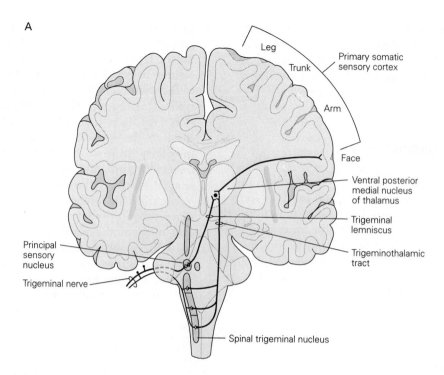

A

Leg

Trunk

Arm

Primary somatic
sensory cortex

Face

Ventral posterior
medial nucleus
of thalamus

Trigeminal
lemniscus

Trigeminothalamic
tract

Principal
sensory
nucleus

Trigeminal nerve

Spinal trigeminal nucleus

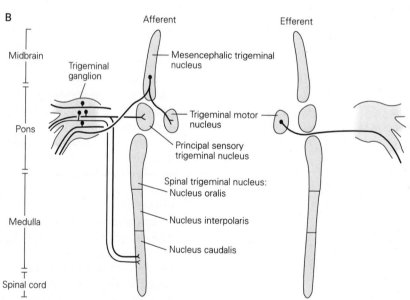

B

Afferent

Efferent

Midbrain

Trigeminal
ganglion

Mesencephalic trigeminal
nucleus

Trigeminal motor
nucleus

Pons

Principal sensory
trigeminal nucleus

Spinal trigeminal nucleus:
Nucleus oralis

Medulla

Nucleus interpolaris

Nucleus caudalis

Spinal cord

Figure 3–9. A. Central projections of the afferent component of the trigeminal system. **B.** Afferent and efferent components of the trigeminal system within the brain stem and cervical spinal cord. (Reproduced with permission from Kandel ER, Schwartz JH, Jessell TM. 1991. *Principles of Neural Science,* 3rd ed. Norwalk, CT: Appleton & Lange. Adapted with permission from Brodal A. 1981. *Neurological Anatomy in Relation to Clinical Medicine,* 3rd ed. New York: Oxford University Press, pp. 508–532.)

entire trigeminal area indicates a peripheral lesion involving the nerve root or the trigeminal ganglion. Decreased sensation confined to one division suggests a more distal lesion. If pain and temperature are decreased but touch is preserved, the lesion is in the lower brain stem or upper cervical cord involving the spinal trigeminal tract and nucleus. If only touch is lost, the lesion is in the pons involving the principal trigeminal nucleus. If impaired sensation extends beyond the borders of the trigeminal, the lesion is suprasegmental in the upper brain stem, thalamus, or parietal lobe.

The corneal reflex, the efferent end of which is mediated by the facial (seventh) nerve, is censensual. A purely trigeminal lesion will therefore result in a decreased response in both eyes when the affected side is stimulated and a normal response in both eyes when the unaffected side is stimulated. Unilateral weakness of eye closure, whether upper or lower motor neuron in type (see below), will produce a decreased response in the affected eye when either cornea is stimulated. Unexpectedly, the corneal reflex can be decreased on an afferent basis with suprasegmental lesions, as high as the parietal lobe.

Examination of trigeminally innervated muscles begins with inspection. Atrophy, with hollowing of the temples, is seen in motor neuron diseases such as amyotrophic lateral sclerosis or neuromuscular diseases such as myotonic dystrophy. The masseter and temporalis muscles are palpated and compared when the jaw is tightly clenched. In unilateral lesions, lateral pterygoid muscle weakness causes the opened and protracted jaw to deviate toward the weak side. A jaw that falls open but recovers with rest suggests myasthenia gravis. Like other components of the special visceral motor cell column, each trigeminal motor nucleus receives bilateral innervation from the primary motor cortex, and so unilateral suprasegmental lesions—such as an infarct involving the internal capsule or the perirolandic cortex—usually produce little or no jaw weakness.

The jaw jerk is a stretch reflex produced by tapping downward on the chin when the jaw is slightly open. Its afferent end is mediated through the mesencephalic trigeminal nucleus, and it can be abolished by lesions involving the trigeminal nerve or the brain stem. (In many normal people, however, a response is not produced.) Upper-motor-neuron lesions produce a hyperactive jaw jerk, a useful clue in patients with brisk limb reflexes that the lesion is rostral to the spinal cord.

Another trigeminally innervated muscle—the tensor tympani of the middle ear—is not specifically tested on the neurological examination, but when it is affected by trigeminal nerve damage, the patient may report impaired hearing for low-pitched sounds.

SEE CASE 54 | p. 220

"A 56-year-old woman has had 6 weeks of left facial numbness and intermittent left-sided headaches."

In patients with trigeminal neuralgia, facial sensation is usually normal except for the presence of trigger zones—sharply localized areas on the skin, gum, or inner cheek that, when touched, precipitate lancinating pain.

SEE CASE 5 | p. 98

"A 60-year-old woman develops paroxysms of sharp stabbing pain in her right malar area and upper lip, gums, and teeth."

▶ The Facial Nerve

The facial (seventh) nerve subserves motor, sensory, and autonomic functions, and familiarity with its anatomy allows a clinician not only to identify facial weakness as central or peripheral in origin but also, if peripheral, to localize the lesion along the nerve's pathway (Figure 3–10).

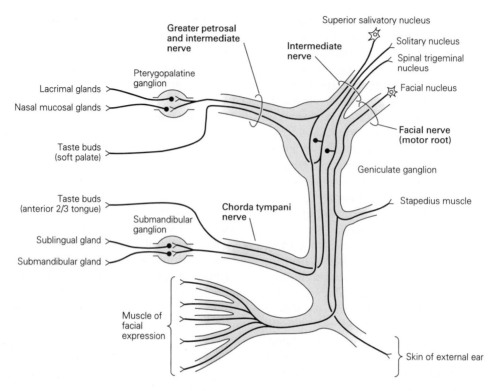

Figure 3–10. The facial nerve is comprised of the motor root, innervating the stapedius muscle and muscles of the face, and the intermediate root, which has autonomic and sensory functions. (Reproduced with permission from Kandel ER, Schwartz JH, Jessell TM. 1991. *Principles of Neural Science*, 3rd ed. Norwalk, CT: Appleton & Lange.)

Motor Innervation

Passing through the internal acoustic meatus into the petrous bone, the somatic efferent facial nerve supplies the stapedius muscle of the middle ear and then emerges through the stylomastoid foramen to supply facial muscles, including the frontalis ("wrinkle your forehead"), orbicularis oculi ("close your eyes tightly"), orbicularis oris ("press your lips together"), levator anguli oris ("smile or show your teeth"), and platysma ("show your teeth with your jaw partly open"). Inspection may be more revealing than specific testing; subtle facial weakness can result in reduced forehead wrinkles, incomplete involuntary blinking, widening of the palpebral fissure or a drooping lower lid, flattening of the naso-labial fold, or a tendency to talk out of one side of the mouth. With mild bilateral facial weakness such findings will be inapparent, making diagnosis difficult.

In most people motor neurons innervating the upper facial muscles, particularly the frontalis, receive projections from the motor cortex of both hemispheres, whereas those innervating the lower facial muscles receive only contralateral projections. Suprasegmental lesions—such as a stroke or a brain tumor—thus tend to spare the frontalis and sometimes eye closure (upper-motor-neuron facial weakness), whereas lower brain stem or nerve damage—such as a cerebellopontine angle neoplasm or idiopathic spontaneous facial paralysis (Bell palsy)—tends to involve all the facial muscles (lower-motor-neuron facial weakness).

With facial weakness secondary to a lesion of the motor cortex there may be preservation of facial movements that show emotions—that is, attempts to show the teeth reveal obvious unilateral weakness yet a spontaneously generated smile is quite symmetric. Less often lesions involving the limbic system produce the converse—strength is normal, but an emotionally produced smile is crooked. In Parkinson disease there may be a complete loss of facial movements that show emotions as well as reduced blinking,

Following peripheral nerve injury such as Bell palsy or trauma, aberrant reinnervation may produce *synkinesis*—eye closure results in involuntary elevation of the angle of the mouth on the affected side, and baring the teeth results in involuntary ipsilateral eye closure. Proposed mechanisms for synkinesis include aberrant regeneration (damaged axons regrow distally but make wrong turns as they do so) and ephaptic transmission (damaged axons make nonsynaptic electrical contact with one another—so-called cross-talk).

Denervation of the stapedius muscle of the middle ear causes impaired reflex dampening of ossicle movement during loud noise. The result is louder-than-normal sound perception (*hyperacusis*).

Sensory and Autonomic Innervation

Sensory and autonomic functions of the seventh nerve are carried in its intermedius portion. On entering the petrous bone, it gives off the greater superficial petrosal nerve, which, via the pterygopalatine ganglion, innervates the lacrimal gland and glands in the nasal mucosa. The intermedius next gives off its chorda tympani branch, which, via the submandibular ganglion, innervates the submaxillary and submandibular salivary glands. The chorda tympani also conveys taste from the anterior two thirds of the tongue. Additional small branches of the intermedius convey general sensation from skin in the external auditory canal. (Although this region is not specifically tested on the sensory examination, the presence of vesicles there in a patient with unexplained acute facial palsy strongly suggests a viral cause, most likely herpes zoster.) Primary neurons of the seventh nerve subserving taste and general sensation reside in the geniculate ganglion within the petrous bone.

Unilaterally decreased lacrimation or salivation is not usually recognized by patients with facial nerve lesions, for the parotid gland still functions, and weakness of eye closure can cause tears (epiphora) if some lacrimation is preserved, creating the impression of increased tear production. Applying filter paper to the conjunctivum of each eye allows comparison of lacrimation on the two sides, and following recovery from Bell palsy there may be lacrimal-salivatory synkinesis with ipsilateral lacrimation stimulated by eating (crocodile tears).

Gustatory receptors in the tongue and tonsillar area recognize four primary tastes: salt, sweet, sour (vinegar), and bitter (quinine). Testing is usually performed with salt or sugar, applied to the anterior lateral tongue, with comparison of the two sides.

Localization

Knowledge of facial nerve anatomy allows the clinician to understand the following localizations:

1. If unilateral facial weakness spares the forehead, and particularly if there is accompanying ipsilateral limb weakness, the lesion is in the contralateral motor cortex or its descending corticobulbar projection.
2. If unilateral facial weakness involves the forehead and is accompanied by ipsilateral abducens weakness, the lesion is in the pons. (Hemiparesis, if present, will in this case be contralateral.)
3. If unilateral facial weakness involves the forehead and if taste, salivation, and lacrimation are affected, the lesion involves the seventh nerve before the takeoff of the greater superficial petrosal and chorda tympani branches. If in such a patient the fifth and eighth nerves are also affected, the lesion is at the cerebellopontine angle (and is likely a neoplasm).
4. If unilateral facial weakness involves the forehead and is unaccompanied by other abnormalities, the lesion probably involves either the facial nucleus in the pons or the nerve distal to the takeoff of the chorda tympani.

5. If only a few facial muscles are involved—particularly the frontalis—the lesion probably is in the facial nerve distal to its emergence from the stylomastoid foramen, or else it directly involves the facial muscles.

One other point: Persons able to raise one eyebrow voluntarily probably have mostly contralateral facial representation in the motor cortex. In such subjects upper-motor-neuron facial weakness might well include the frontalis.

See Case 53 | p. 218

"A 34-year-old woman awakens with continuous dull pain behind her left ear and the following day notices that her left face is droopy."

▶ The Vestibulocochlear (Auditory) Nerve

The eighth cranial nerve is really two nerves running together, the auditory and the vestibular. Both carry information from the labyrinths of the inner ear. The auditory (cochlear) nerve conveys sound information from the cochlea. The vestibular nerve conveys equilibratory information from the utricle, saccule, and semiciccular canals (Figure 3–11).

Auditory

The cochlear nerve carries sound impulses from the tonotopically organized cochlea through the spiral ganglion to the cochlear nuclei in the medulla. A mostly crossed pathway then ascends, via the lateral lemniscus, the inferior colliculus, and the medial geniculate nucleus of the thalamus, to Heschl's gyrus in the temporal lobe. Interpretation of auditory stimuli involves association areas adjacent to Heschl's gyrus. (In the language-dominant hemisphere one of these areas is referred to as Wernicke area.) An additional auditory system, projecting bilaterally via the superior olivary complex in the pons, is concerned with sound localization (Figure 3–12).

Although damage to Heschl's gyrus results in decreased auditory acuity, particularly contralaterally, the impairment is likely

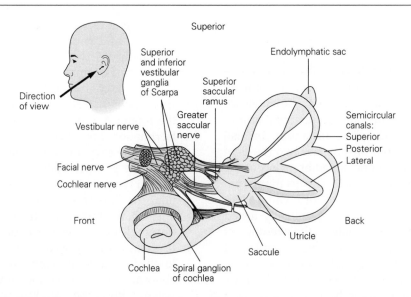

Figure 3–11. The labyrinths of the inner ear include the cochlea, the utricle, the saccule, and the semicircular canals. (Reproduced with permission from Kandel ER, Schwartz JH, Jessell TM. 1999. *Principles of Neural Science*, 4th ed. New York: McGraw-Hill.)

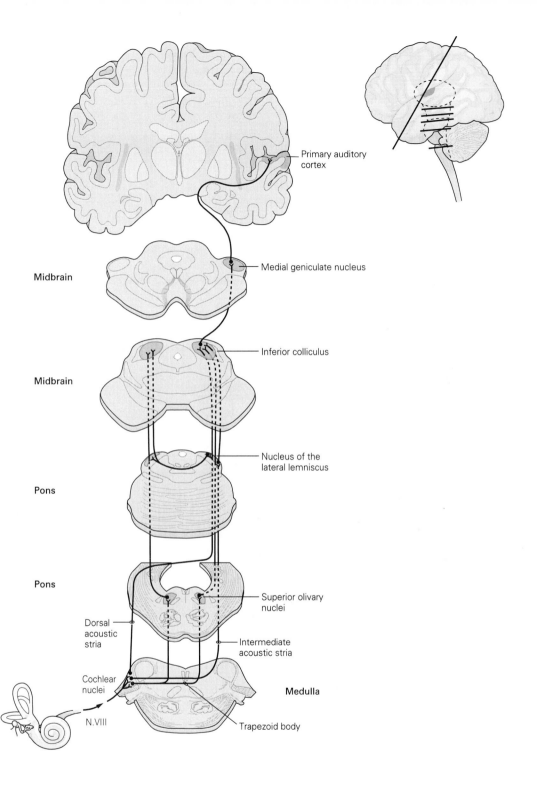

Figure 3–12. Central auditory projections from the cochlear nuclei in the medulla to the primary auditory cortex in the temporal lobe. Each cochlear nucleus projects, mostly contralaterally, to the inferior colliculus in the midbrain, as well as bilaterally to the superior olivary nuclei in the pons. The bilateral interactions of this system mean that unilateral lesions rostral to the cochlear nuclei will not produce unilateral deafness, although there may be loss of sound localization, tinnitus, or partial hearing loss. (Reproduced with permission from Kandel ER, Schwartz JH, Jessell TM. 1999. *Principles of Neural Science,* 4th ed. New York: McGraw-Hill. Adapted with permission from Brodal A. 1981. The auditory system. In: *Neurological Anatomy in Relation to Clinical Medicine,* 3rd ed. New York: Oxford University Press.)

to go unnoticed by the patient. In fact, even unilaterally impaired hearing from eighth nerve or cochlea lesions may be unrecognized unless it affects the ear customarily used for telephoning.

Deafness from peripheral lesions is of two types. *Conduction* deafness is the result of obstruction or disease of the external auditory canal, the tympanic membrane, or the middle ear. *Sensorineural* deafness is the result of damage to the cochlea, the cochlea nerve, or the cochlear nuclei. Conduction deafness preferentially affects low tones; sensorineural deafness preferentially affects high tones. Patients with bilateral conduction deafness tend to speak softly; those with bilateral sensorineural deafness tend to speak loudly. Patients with cochlea lesions often have loudness recruitment—sounds of low volume are not heard well, but the same sound at a higher volume is heard normally. Patients with eighth nerve or cochlea nucleus lesions may have only mildly impaired hearing for pure tones yet severe difficulty in discriminating speech. Both peripheral and central lesions cause *tinnitus*, a hissing, buzzing, or whistling sound in the ear. Tinnitus can be present without evident hearing loss.

The auditory examination begins with the simple screening maneuver in which the ability of each ear to detect a watch ticking or two fingers rubbed together is compared. The Weber and Rinné tests help to distinguish conduction from nerve deafness. In the Weber test a 512-Hz tuning fork is placed midline on the forehead. (If a 128-Hz tuning fork is used, the patient may be confused by the perception of vibration.) With conduction deafness the sound will be heard best on the hearing-impaired side and with nerve deafness the sound will be heard best on the normal side. In the Rinné test the tuning fork is placed over the mastoid; when the patient reports that it is no longer heard, it is held close to the external auditory meatus. In normal subjects and in those with nerve deafness, air conduction will outlast bone conduction. With conduction deafness, bone conduction will outlast air conduction. The Weber test is most useful when deafness

is unilateral and the Rinné test when deafness is bilateral. The clinical picture may warrant more sophisticated procedures such as audiometry, stapedius reflex testing, or brain stem auditory evoked response testing. The latter can localize lesions to specific points along the auditory pathway from cochlea to temporal lobe.

Conduction deafness is most often the result of obstruction (cerumen, Eustachian tube blockage, or neoplasm) or middle ear infection. Cochlea lesions include Ménière disease, advanced otosclerosis, drug toxicity (eg, aminoglycoside antibiotics), infarction secondary to internal auditory artery occlusion, and trauma (including prolonged loud noise). Eighth nerve lesions can be secondary to neoplasms (particularly acoustic neuroma), meningitis, and trauma. The most common brain stem lesions responsible for impaired hearing are infarction, neoplasm, and multiple sclerosis. Deafness of old age (presbyacusis) is of both cochlea and nerve origin.

Vestibular

The vestibular nerve carries impulses to the brain stem vestibular nuclei from hair cells in the semicircular canals, the saccule, and the utricle when those receptors are stimulated by displacement of endolymph. Widespread projections from the vestibular nuclei communicate with the spinal cord, the cerebellum, eye movement control centers, and the forebrain (Figure 3–13). Via the ventral posterior nucleus of the thalamus a pathway reaches the contralateral parietal lobe (the vestibular cortex, probably contributing to conscious awareness of head position, motion, and balance).

Tests of vestibular function involve labyrinthine stimulation, either by head movement, head positioning, or temperature. In some patients, vertigo, nystagmus, and sometimes nausea and vomiting are precipitated by any rapid movement of the head. In others—particularly those with benign positional vertigo—vertigo is triggered, after a latency of up to half a minute, by ly-

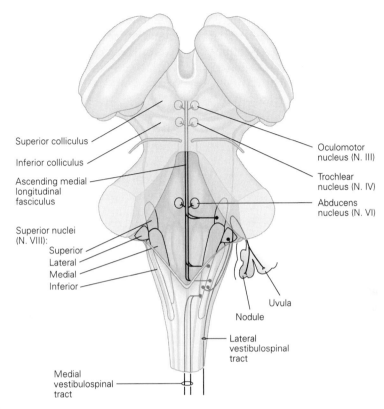

Figure 3–13. Central connections of the vestibular nuclei. (Reproduced with permission from Kandel ER, Schwartz JH, Jessell TM. 1991. *Principles of Neural Science*, 3rd ed. Norwalk, CT: Appleton & Lange.)

ing on the affected ear (the Nylen-Barany maneuver). Compared to vertigo of central origin (brain stem or higher), vertigo associated with peripheral lesions is more likely to be positional after a latent period, to display rapid adaptation, and to be severe.

When vestibular disease is suspected, the examination includes assessment of normal vestibular responses to rotation and temperature. With caloric testing, water several degrees centigrade above and below body temperature is run into the external ear canal; with the head elevated 30°, a normal response consists of nystagmus (and vertigo) with the fast component directed away from the cold stimulus and toward the warm stimulus. (The mnemonic COWS stands for "cold-opposite/warm-same," referring to the fast component of the nystagmus.) There are two main patterns of abnor-

mal response. An absence or decreased duration of nystagmus when either a cold or a warm stimulus is applied to one ear is called canal paresis. A reduced response when either cold water is instilled into one ear or warm water is instilled into the other is called directional preponderance. Canal paresis is associated with peripheral vestibular lesions and directional preponderance is associated with lesions of central vestibular pathways.

Vertiginous patients whose eyes are closed tend, when pointing to objects, to deviate toward the side of the lesion (past-pointing). Similarly, when walking in place with closed eyes, they tend to rotate toward the affected side.

Some patients with nystagmus have *oscillopsia*, the subjective sensation that the visual world seems to be rhythmically jerking back and forth. More common, however, is rotatory vertigo, a sense of continuous uninterrupted movement of objects in one direction. The reason is that subjective vision is usually obliterated during rapid eye movements, whether normal saccades or the rapid phase of nystagmus.

SEE CASE 12 | p. 113

"For over a year a 47-year-old woman has been having attacks of dizziness and tinnitus."

SEE CASE 13 | p. 114

"For several months a 50-year-old woman has had increasing difficulty understanding what people are saying over the phone, which she customarily holds over her left ear."

SEE CASE 14 | p. 116

"A 63-year-old man suddenly develops vertigo, nausea, and vomiting and is unable to stand."

▶ The Glossopharyngeal and Vagus Nerves

The ninth and the tenth cranial nerves have functional overlap, and so they are customarily considered together.

Anatomy

The complex functional anatomy of these nerves includes the following:

1. Neurons in the nucleus ambiguus innervate muscles in the palate (10), pharynx (mostly 10), and larynx (10) (Figure 3–14). Each nucleus ambiguus receives bilateral projections from the motor cortex.
2. Neurons in the salivatory nucleus (9) supply, via the otic ganglion, the parotid gland.
3. Visceral efferent fibers from the dorsal motor nucleus of the vagus form plexuses within the thorax and abdomen that ulti-

mately innervate the heart, lungs, gut, and other organs, producing bradycardia, bronchial constriction, alimentary secretion, and peristalsis.

4. In contrast to sympathetic afferents, which convey pain and other consciously recognized sensations, visceral afferents of the glossopharyngeal and vagus nerves are mostly concerned with visceromotor, vasomotor, and secretory reflexes, which, if they reach consciousness, do so only vaguely.
5. The main afferent pathways for control of the circulation originate in mechanoreceptors (baroreceptors) in the carotid sinus and aortic arch (conveyed by the glossopharyngeal nerve) and the heart and lungs (conveyed by the vagus nerve). A fall in blood pressure produces decreased firing in these nerves, resulting in reflex vasoconstriction (sympathetically mediated) and increased heart rate (from combined sympathetic stimulation and vagal inhibition).
6. Peripherally located neurons convey taste sensation from the posterior tongue (9) and general sensation from the posterior tongue (9), pharynx (9 and 10), larynx (10), and thoracic and visceral structures including lungs, aorta, heart, and gut as far as the splenic flexure of the colon (10). Centrally directed fibers conveying visceral afferent information synapse in the nucleus solitarius of the lower brain stem.
7. Peripherally located neurons of both the ninth and the tenth nerves supply general sensation to part of the external ear; fibers conveying this somatic afferent information synapse in the spinal trigeminal nucleus.

Examination and Localization

Despite this complexity, assessment of the ninth and tenth cranial nerves is usually limited to examination of the palate and pharynx. Nasal speech (or a history of nasal regurgitation of fluids) suggests palatal weakness. Hoarseness or a reduced cough suggests laryngeal weakness. In myasthenia gravis, dysphonia may increase toward the end of each sentence.

Choking on saliva while talking suggests pharyngeal weakness. Difficulty swallowing (dysphagia) limited to solid food suggests mechanical obstruction such as esophageal carcinoma; dysphagia for liquids as well as solids or for only liquids suggests neurological dysfunction. Dysphagia can be checked by asking the patient to swallow a small amount of water.

When the patient says, "Ah," with the mouth open and the tongue relaxed, the palate should rise symmetrically, the uvula should remain in the midline, and the pharyngeal walls should contract symmetrically. With unilateral palatal or pharyngeal weakness, phonaton causes the uvula to deviate toward the normal side. (An asymmetric palate at rest may be the result of tonsillar swelling or old tonsillar surgery.) The gag reflex is tested by gently touching each side of the pharynx with a cotton-tipped applicator. As with the pupillary and corneal reflexes the response is bilateral. The response of the palatal and pharyngeal muscles to phonation and to tactile stimulation therefore reveals whether a lesion is unilateral or bilateral and whether it is efferent, afferent, or both. Abnormalities include the following:

1. Bilateral weakness with preserved sensation suggests motor neuron disease (such as amyotrophic lateral sclerosis or poliomyelitis), a neuromuscular junction disorder (such as myasthenia gravis), or a myopathy (such as polymyositis).
2. Unilateral motor and sensory loss suggests an ipsilateral lesion of the lower brain stem (such as lateral medullary infarction) or combined lesions of the glossopharyngeal and vagus nerves either in the posterior fossa or as they exit together through the jugular foramen.
3. Bilateral motor and sensory loss suggests an intraparenchymal medullary lesion (such as syringobulbia), in which case other cranial nerves and long tract signs are probably present.

4. Bilateral sensory loss with normal movement on phonation is so rare as to suggest psychiatric disease (hysterical insensitivity of the pharynx), but it is important to remember that some normal people have little or no gag reflex.

Laryngeal weakness can also be unilateral or bilateral. With unilateral lesions the abnormal vocal cord may be positioned in adduction, in which case there may be no symptoms, or it may be positioned in abduction, in which case there will be hoarseness but normal breathing. With bilateral lesions the vocal cords may be positioned in abduction, in which case there will be hoarseness or aphonia but normal breathing, or they may be positioned in adduction, in which case there will be inspiratory phonation (*stridor*) and life-threatening respiratory obstruction. Dysphonia in the absence of other symptoms usually indicates a lesion involving the larynx or one or both recurrent laryngeal nerves (branches of the vagus). Possibilities include neoplasm, aortic aneurysm, and trauma.

In some patients, particularly those complaining of nonvertiginous dizziness or syncope, circulatory reflexes are assessed. Failure of heart rate to change with hypotension or hypertension or during the Valsalva maneuver indicates parasympathetic dysfunction. If heart rate does change appropriately with deep breathing (sinus arrhythmia) or following atropine, the problem is at the afferent end of the reflex arc. If it does not change in these settings, the problem is at the efferent end.

SEE CASE 38 | p. 185

"Following a year of impotence and nocturnal urinary frequency, a 57-year-old man experiences blurred vision during exercise."

▶ The Spinal Accessory Nerve

Anatomy

Supplying the sternocleidomastoid and upper trapezius muscles, the eleventh cranial

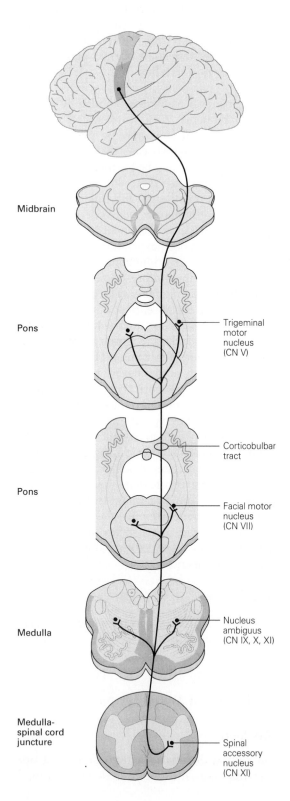

Midbrain

Pons

Trigeminal
motor
nucleus
(CN V)

Corticobulbar
tract

Pons

Facial motor
nucleus
(CN VII)

Medulla

Nucleus
ambiguus
(CN IX, X, XI)

Medulla-
spinal cord
juncture

Spinal
accessory
nucleus
(CN XI)

nerve arises from the upper cervical spinal cord, enters the posterior fossa through the foramen magnum, and then exits the cranium through the jugular foramen. It is therefore involved by intrinsic or extrinsic lesions of the upper cervical cord (such as syringomyelia or a foramen magnum meningioma) or by lesions within the posterior fossa or the jugular foramen (in which case the vagus and glossopharyngeal nerves are often affected as well). The so-called cranial root of the accessory nerve is actually an aberrant branch of the vagus, arising from the nucleus ambiguus and running for a short distance with the accessory nerve (see Figure 3–14).

The sternocleidomastoid is the only major striated muscle with ipsilateral cortical representation, accounting for contralateral head turning during seizures arising from the frontal lobe. Following destructive cerebral lesions sternocleidomastoid weakness is unusual, but ipsilateral sternocleidomastoid and contralateral trapezius weakness may be present.

Examination

The sternocleidomastoid is tested by having patients hold their chin against resistance in the direction of the contralateral shoulder. Bilateral involvement (as in motor neuron disease or muscular dystrophy) causes weakness of forward head flexion with the head lagging backward as the patient sits up from a supine position. Trapezius weakness is demonstrated by assessing shoulder elevation or shrugging or by observing winging of the upper scapula; at rest the involved shoulder may be set lower.

Figure 3–14. Rostrocaudal organization of the nucleus ambiguus (cranial nerves IX and X) and the spinal accessory nucleus (cranial nerve XI). Like the trigeminal motor nucleus and the facial motor nucleus, the nucleus ambiguus receives bilateral projections from the primary motor cortex. (Reproduced with permission from Martin JH. 1996. *Neuroanatomy Text and Atlas*, 2nd ed. Stamford, CT: Appleton & Lange.)

The significance of muscle bulk, tone, fasciculations, and abnormal involuntary movements will be considered in Chapter 4.

▶ The Hypoglossal Nerve

Anatomy

Supplying the muscles of the tongue, the twelfth cranial nerve arises near the midline of the medulla oblongata and exits the posterior fossa through the hypoglossal foramen. Each hypoglossal nucleus receives bilateral projections from the motor cortex (Figure 3–15).

Examination

Inspection of the tongue often reveals nonneurological abnormalities, such as enlargement (acromegaly), fungal infection (AIDS), or a smooth red surface (cobalamin deficiency). Inspection may also reveal atrophy, which if unilateral causes reduction in size with excessive ridging and wrinkling of the affected side. Atrophy indicates a lower-motor-neuron lesion, either centrally or peripherally. Fasciculations of the tongue can be difficult to tell from normal tongue movements or tremor; nonrhythmic and resembling a "bag of worms," they should be present when the tongue is completely at rest. In contrast to fasciculations of the trunk or limbs, which can be normal, tongue fasciculations strongly suggest motor neuron disease.

With unilateral weakness due to upper- or lower-motor-neuron lesions the tongue deviates toward the weak side. If there is no deviation, the patient is told to push the tongue into each cheek, and the examiner attempts to force it back. With unilateral upper-motor-neuron lesions there may be no deviation and little evident weakness, yet dysarthria may be prominent for lingual consonants (*tay* for the anterior tongue, *kay* for the posterior tongue). Bilateral tongue weakness causes dysarthria, dysphagia, and sometimes even difficulty breathing. Complete immobility produces *anarthria*. Unilateral lesions involving the frontal lobe of the language hemisphere—particularly those affecting the operculum or perisylvian cortex—also cause anarthria (called, in such a setting, *aphemia*) as well as *lingual apraxia*, in which the tongue cannot be protruded on command yet does protrude to less voluntary stimuli such as licking the lips during eating.

SEE CASE 24 | p. 149

"A 21-year-old man has noted hoarseness for 2 years, pain in the left side of his neck for several months, and slurred speech for several weeks."

▶ Bulbar and Pseudobulbar Palsy

Bilateral weakness of muscles innervated by cranial nerves of the lower brain stem is called *bulbar palsy*. Dysarthria and dysphagia are severe. The tongue is paralyzed, atrophic, and may display fasciculations. There is no movement of the palate or pharynx with phonation, and the gag reflex is absent. Because there is bilateral cerebral projection to lower brain stem motor neurons these muscles are often spared or only mildly involved with unilateral supranuclear lesions. Bilateral lesions of the cerebrum or upper brain stem, however, can result in severe dysarthria and dysphagia. The tongue is paralyzed but neither atrophic nor fasciculating. The palate and pharynx do not move with phonation, but the gag reflex is hyperactive. Such a patient is said to have *pseudobulbar palsy.* An interesting and unexplained feature of this syndrome is lability or hyperreflexia of emotional response. A remark that would normally produce a mild chuckle precipitates embarrassed peals of laughter, and asking a question such as "How are you feeling?" results in explosive weeping.

SEE CASE 29 | p. 159

"A 58-year-old business executive develops slurred speech and difficulty swallowing liquids."

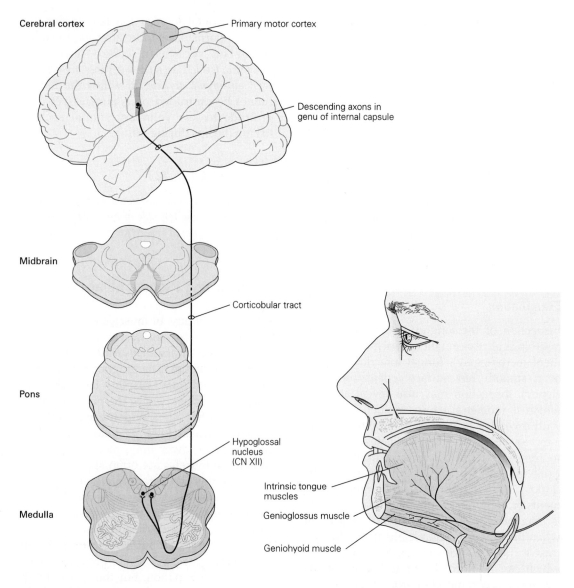

Figure 3–15. The region of the motor cortex controlling tongue movement projects bilaterally to both hypoglossal nuclei. (Reproduced with permission from Martin JH. 1996. *Neuroanatomy Text and Atlas*, 2nd ed. Stamford, CT: Appleton & Lange.)

4

The Motor Examination:
There Is Always More Than Weakness

The motor examination has many components, which should be performed systematically. A lesion causing weakness can affect any level of the corticospinal (pyramidal) system from the frontal lobe to the spinal cord (Figure 4–1). It can also affect anterior horn cells, motor nerve roots, peripheral nerves, the neuromuscular junction, or muscles themselves. By looking for abnormalities other than weakness, the examiner often identifies the level of the neuraxis that is involved. Weakness secondary to frontal lobe or corticospinal tract lesions (upper-motor-neuron–type weakness) may be accompanied acutely by reduced muscle tone (*flaccidity*), but over days or weeks muscle tone increases (*spasticity*) with hyperactive tendon reflexes. As a result of disuse, loss of muscle bulk (*atrophy*) can evolve over time, but marked atrophy would be unusual with upper-motor-neuron–type weakness, and chronic muscle fasciculations are not a feature. Weakness secondary to anterior horn cell, nerve root, nerve plexus, or peripheral nerve lesions (lower-motor-neuron–type weakness) is accompanied by reduced muscle tone and hypoactive tendon reflexes. After 2 or 3 weeks, atrophy develops, and if a muscle is completely denervated, atrophy rapidly becomes marked. Particularly with lesions directly involving anterior horn cells such as amyotrophic lateral sclerosis (ALS), muscle fasciculations may be prominent. (The fact that ALS involves both upper and lower motor neurons means that hyperreflexia, atrophy, and fasciculations can affect the same limb or even the same muscle, a nearly pathognomonic combination.)

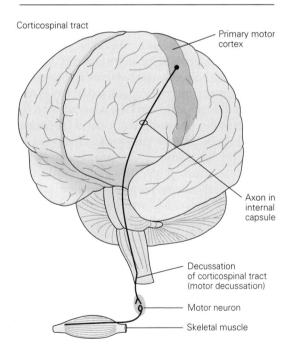

Figure 4–1. The lateral corticospinal tract arises from neurons in the motor cortex and descends through the internal capsule and the brain stem, crossing at the pyramidal decussation of the lower medulla. It projects somatotopically onto anterior horn cells of the spinal cord, which innervate voluntary muscles. (Reproduced with permission from Martin JH. 1996. *Neuroanatomy Text and Atlas*, 2nd ed. Stamford, CT: Appleton & Lange.)

SEE CASE 26 | p. 152

"A 55-year-old man notices difficulty buttoning and turning keys."

In myopathic disorders such as polymyositis or muscular dystrophy, atrophy can eventually develop, but usually over years, not weeks. In fact, in Duchenne muscular dystrophy (a hereditary sex-linked recessive disorder affecting boys) the muscles may appear larger than normal despite severe weakness.

SEE CASE 17 | p. 125

"A 15-year-old boy, weak since early childhood, has been wheelchair-bound for 3 years."

▶ Muscle Bulk

Cerebral injury during infancy can result in deficient growth of contralateral limbs, which may be weak and hypertonic but usually maintain normal muscle contours. Diffuse muscle atrophy can be a consequence of malnutrition or malignancy, and reduced muscle bulk follows prolonged disuse of a limb from any cause.

Muscle atrophy in association with neurological disease suggests denervation or myopathy. As noted, atrophy is usually an early sign with denervating diseases such as ALS, brachial plexitis, or peripheral neuropathy. Trophic changes in the hair or nails sometimes accompany denervation atrophy but are not a feature of disuse atrophy. With myopathic diseases such as muscular dystrophy or polymyositis, atrophy is usually of later development. Depending on the patient's body habitus, muscle atrophy might be suspected in the presence of a prominent tibial bone (anterior tibialis), concavity of the lower medial thigh (quadriceps), or a prominent scapular spine (infraspinatus and supraspinatus). Mild symmetric atrophy is difficult to recognize, and even mild asymmetric atrophy sometimes becomes evident only after measuring and comparing the circumference of each limb proximally and distally.

Pathological muscle hypertrophy is rare. It can be a consequence of chronic involuntary movements. In Duchenne muscular dystrophy the increased muscle bulk (often particularly prominent in the calves) is actually the result of fat and fibrous tissue deposits; the muscle fibers themselves are atrophic. Muscle enlargement follows supraphysiologic doses of androgen hormones.

▶ Passive Range of Motion and Muscle Tone

Neurological disease can adversely affect joints. Reduced pain sensation in patients with tabes dorsalis (a form of tertiary neurosyphilis) or syringomyelia can result in Charcot joints, which are swollen, painless, and crepitant on motion and radiographically display severely damaged articular surfaces. The cause is repeated trauma secondary to joint anesthesia; whether trophic abnormalities contribute is disputed. When a joint is kept immobile for a prolonged period, the muscles that move it become permanently shortened (contracture) and range of motion is limited. An example is the frozen shoulder or the tight heel cord that can follow a stroke with hemiplegia. Extensive physical therapy may be required to stretch the affected muscles back to their proper length. Contractures also result from lack of opposition to a muscle when its antagonist is paralyzed, for example, in poliomyelitis. Surgery may be necessary to restore full range of motion to the joint.

Clinicians define two kinds of increased muscle tone. *Spasticity,* from lesions of the frontal lobe or descending corticospinal projections, tends to affect primarily flexor muscles in the arms and extensor muscles in the legs. There is resistance to passive movement that increases with the speed of the movement, and toward the end of the movement the resistance often abruptly melts away—the so-called clasped knife response. *Rigidity,* particularly associated with Parkinson disease and other disorders of the basal ganglia, shows less preference for flexor or extensor muscles and consists of more plastic resistance (lead pipe rigidity) that is not velocity dependent and that continues throughout the range of movement. In Parkinson disease rigidity is often characterized by rapidly alternating contractions of agonist and antagonist muscles, producing a ratchet-like effect (cogwheel rigidity).

When a hypertonic muscle is abruptly stretched, reflex contraction is followed immediately by relaxation. Maintenance of the stretch sometimes elicits rapidly successive contractions and relaxations (*clonus*). In the legs, clonus is most easily elicited by dorsiflexing the foot at the ankle or by pushing the patella distally. Like brisk tendon reflexes (see later), clonus can be normally present in tense people. When clonus is asymmetric or when it is accompanied by spasticity or weakness, it is likely the consequence of a corticospinal tract lesion.

In addition to resisting passive stretch, hypertonic muscles are firm to palpation. Hypotonic muscles are easily stretched and lax. Muscles out of use become hypotonic, and the muscles of someone who is truly relaxed may appear so. Pathological hypotonia occurs with lesions interrupting the reflex arc either at the afferent end (the muscle spindle or its centrally projecting axons) or at the efferent end (the motor neuron, its peripherally projecting axons, or the muscle fibers they collectively innervate—the motor unit). Hypotonia is sometimes observed in patients with cerebellar lesions or with basal ganglia lesions causing chorea (see later). Following sudden severe injury to the spinal cord, a paraplegic patient may have hypotonic (and areflexic) legs for a week or two—so-called spinal shock. There follows a gradual return of tone and then progression to spasticity. The physiological basis of spinal shock is uncertain. A similar progression from hypotonia to spasticity sometimes accompanies hemiplegia in patients with cerebral infarction or hemorrhage.

SEE CASE 46 | p. 200

"A 17-year-old boy is shot through the midthoracic spine."

Myotonia refers to muscle contraction that persists longer than intended. For example, a patient giving a vigorous handshake and then being told to release it might not be able to do so for several seconds. Myotonic muscles demonstrate local contractions when percussed, for example, involuntary contraction of the opponens pollicis or dimpling of the tongue when they are gently tapped with a reflex hammer. Myotonia is a feature of certain myopathic disorders, notably myotonic dystrophy and myotonia congenita. In a condition called *paramyotonia,* myotonia is provoked by exposure to cold.

SEE CASE 18 | p. 128

"A man in his mid-20s insidiously develops mild ptosis, which slowly progresses over the next several years."

▶ Muscle Power

Anatomy

To assess muscle strength effectively, the examiner needs to know the actions of individual muscles, their segmental (nerve root) innervation, and their peripheral nerve innervation (Table 4–1). Illustrated monographs are available that demonstrate how to test each muscle. A routine examination includes the flexors and extensors of the neck; the abductors, adductors, and rotators of the shoulders; the flexors and extensors of the elbows, wrists, and fingers; thumb abduction and opposition; finger abduction; the abdominal muscles; and the flexors and extensors of the hips, knees, ankles, and toes. Precise localization of a nerve root or peripheral nerve lesion requires examination of *all* the muscles innervated by that root or nerve.

Table 4–1. Muscle innervation and principal function

Muscle	Root	Nerve	Function
Trapezius	C1, 2, 3, 4	Accessory	Elevation and adduction of scapula
Rhomboids	C4, 5	Dorsal scapular	Adduction of scapula
Serratus anterior	C5, 6, 7	Long thoracic	Lateral and forward movement of scapula
Supraspinatus	C5, 6	Suprascapular	Initiation of arm abduction
Infraspinatus	C5, 6	Suprascapular	External rotation of arm
Pectoralis major	C5, 6, 7, 8	Lateral pectoral	Adduction and medial rotation of arm
Latissimus dorsi	C6, 7, 8	Thoracodorsal	Adduction, extension, and medial rotation of arm
Deltoid	C5, 6	Axillary	Abduction of arm
Biceps	C5, 6	Musculocutaneous	Flexion and supination of forearm
Triceps	C7, 8	Radial	Extension of forearm
Brachioradialis	C5, 6	Radial	Flexion of forearm at elbow
Supinator	C5, 6, 7	Radial	Supination of forearm
Pronator teres	C6, 7	Median	Pronation of forearm
Extensor carpi radialis	C6, 7, 8	Radial	Wrist extension
Extensor carpi ulnaris	C7, 8	Radial	Wrist extension
Flexor carpi radialis	C6, 7	Median	Wrist flexion
Flexor carpi ulnaris	C7, 8	Ulnar	Wrist flexion
Extensor digitorum	C6, 7, 8	Radial	Finger extension at metacarpophalangeal joints
Abductor pollicis longus	C7, 8	Radial	Radial abduction of thumb
Extensor pollicis brevis	C7, 8	Radial	Extension of proximal phalanx of thumb
Extensor pollicis longus	C7, 8	Radial	Extension of distal phalanx of thumb
Flexor digitorum sublimis	C7, 8, T1	Median	Flexion of proximal and middle phalanges of fingers
Flexor digitorum profundus	C7, 8, T1	Median (digits 2 and 3) and ulnar (digits 4 and 5)	Flexion of distal phalanges of fingers
Flexor pollicis longus	C7, 8, T1	Median	Flexion of distal phalanx of thumb
Abductor pollicis brevis	C8, T1	Median	Palmar abduction of thumb
Opponens pollicis	C8, T1	Median	Movement of first metacarpal across palm
Flexor pollicis brevis	C8, T1	Median	Flexion of proximal phalanx of thumb
Interossei	C8, T1	Ulnar	Abduction and adduction of extended fingers
Lumbricals	C8, T1	Median (digits 2 and 3) and ulnar (digits 4 and 5)	Flexion of extended fingers at metacarpophalangeal joints
Iliopsoas	L2, 3, 4	Lumbar plexus	Flexion of hip
Thigh adductors	L2, 3, 4	Obturator	Adduction of hip
Gluteus maximus	L5, S1, 2	Inferior gluteal	Extension of hip
Gluteus medius	L4, 5, S1	Superior gluteal	Abduction of hip
Quadriceps femoris	L2, 3, 4	Femoral	Extension of leg at knee
Hamstrings	L4, 5, S1, 2	Sciatic	Flexion of leg at knee
Anterior tibial	L4, 5	Deep peroneal	Dorsiflexion of foot
Peronei	L4, 5	Deep peroneal	Eversion of foot
Gastrocnemius	S1, 2	Posterior tibial	Plantar flexion of foot
Posterior tibial	L5, S1	Posterior tibial	Inversion of foot
Extensor digitorum longus	L5, S1	Deep peroneal	Dorsiflexion of four lateral toes and of foot
Extensor digitorum brevis	L5, S1	Deep peroneal	Dorsiflexion of four medial toes
Extensor hallucis longus	L5, S1	Deep peroneal	Dorsiflexion of big toe and foot
Flexor digitorum longus	L5, S1	Posterior tibial	Plantar flexion of toes

Testing Strength

Strength is graded on a scale of one to five (Table 4–2). Some muscles, of course, normally have more power than others, but even the intrinsic muscles of the hand are difficult to overcome if the patient contracts them maximally. Large muscles may lose a considerable degree of power before weakness is appreciated. Reduced power can sometimes be best demonstrated by using the patient's own weight rather than the examiner's exertions as a counterforce, for example, climbing onto a chair or rising from a squatting position (gluteus maximus and quadriceps) or hopping (gastrocnemius). Having the patient walk on heels and toes may reveal subtle asymmetries in the anterior tibialis or gastrocnemius muscles. Gower's sign, the result of proximal leg and paraspinal weakness, is seen in children with muscular dystrophy; attempting to stand up from a lying flat position, the patients place their hands first on their lower legs and then more and more proximally—climbing up the legs—as they rise.

Upper Versus Lower Motor Neuron

With corticospinal tract (upper-motor-neuron) lesions, rate and amplitude of movement are often reduced out of proportion to the loss of strength. Weakness, like spasticity, is most marked in the abductors and extensors of the arm and the flexors of the leg. As with certain muscles innervated by cranial nerves, the paraspinal muscles are usually spared in upper-motor-neuron lesions,

Table 4–2. Grading strength.

Grade	Strength
0	No visible or palpable muscle contraction
1	Muscle seen or felt to contract but no movement across a joint
2	Full range of movement across a joint but not against gravity
3	Full range of movement against gravity, but any additional force overcomes resistance
4	More than minimal force required to overcome resistance
5	Normal

probably because, being supplied by the anterior uncrossed corticospinal tracts, they receive bilateral input through the ventral white commissure of the spinal cord. Mild corticospinal tract lesions may produce no demonstrable weakness, yet attempts to sustain a posture result in drift; the arm, outstretched with palm up, slowly pronates or falls downward, and when the patient lies prone with the knees flexed to 90°, the lower leg drifts slowly downward.

SEE CASE 28 | p. 157

"A 53-year-old hypertensive man awakens one morning with weakness of his right arm and leg and dysarthria."

With lower-motor-neuron lesions, rate and amplitude of movement tend to be reduced in proportion to weakness. The distribution of weakness and atrophy depends on whether there is a focal lesion affecting a particular spinal cord segment, nerve root, plexus, or peripheral nerve or whether the process is more widespread as with peripheral neuropathy or motor neuron disease. Probably related to disordered axonal transport, weakness (and sensory loss) in peripheral neuropathy tends to be maximal distally and to affect the feet before the hands. With the two most common peripheral neuropathies—secondary to alcoholism with nutritional deficiency or to diabetes mellitus—weakness is preceded by impaired sensation. Other peripheral neuropathies cause weakness early and predominantly; examples include immunologically mediated motor neuropathies, either acute (Guillain-Barré syndrome) or chronic (chronic inflammatory demyelinating polyneuropathy), and hereditary sensorimotor neuropathies (a group of genetic disorders collectively referred to as Charcot-Marie-Tooth disease).

SEE CASE 22 | p. 142

"Two weeks after a brief viral respiratory infection, a 62-year-old man develops mild paresthesias of his soles and achiness in his back and thighs."

SEE CASE 23 | p. 146

"A 5-year-old boy is noted by his parents to have high arches and curled-up toes (hammer toes)."

Some peripheral neuropathies affect strength and sensation to the same degree; patients with such neuropathies demonstrate distal limb weakness associated with "stocking-glove" sensory loss.

SEE CASE 40 | p. 191

"A 54-year-old man has had 6 years of slowly progressive numbness and weakness of his distal limbs."

Lesions of the brachial or lumbosacral plexus produce patterns of weakness that do not conform to single roots or peripheral nerves. By referring to the anatomy of these structures, the examiner can determine not only that the lesion is a *plexopathy* but where within the plexus (ie, upper versus lower, proximal versus distal) the damage has occurred.

SEE CASE 42 | p. 194

"Two weeks after a flu-like illness a 37-year-old man abruptly develops pain in his left shoulder, upper arm, and base of the neck."

With amyotrophic lateral sclerosis, weakness can be proximal or distal and symmetric or asymmetric. Early in the course it can be strikingly focal, but over time it becomes increasingly widespread.

Myopathy Versus Neuropathy

Myopathic weakness—for example, with polymyositis, dermatomyositis, alcoholic myopathy, or certain drug toxicities—is usually greatest proximally. Hereditary muscular dystrophies may also begin proximally, but some have more restricted distributions, such as facioscapulohumeral dystrophy (a dominantly inherited genetic disorder the name of which describes the weak muscles).

Proximal versus distal weakness helps to distinguish myopathic from neuropathic disorders, but exceptions exist. A rare myopathic disorder is appropriately known as *distal myopathy,* and of the several kinds of hereditary motor neuron disease, one group (called Kugelberg-Welander disease) causes mostly proximal weakness. In such conditions electrodiagnostic studies or nerve and muscle biopsies may be necessary for diagnosis.

SEE CASE 25 | p. 150

"A 22-year-old woman develops difficulty climbing stairs and running, and findings on examination include mild proximal weakness of her legs and arms, decreased tendon reflexes, and normal sensation."

Neuromuscular Junction

The weakness of myasthenia gravis is notable for its variability over time. It can be brought out by sustained or repetitive muscle contraction, for example, upward gaze to precipitate ptosis, squeezing a ball or an inflated blood pressure cuff to produce a weak grip, or counting to 50 or 100 to demonstrate weakness of respiratory muscles. Such characteristic fatigability is the result of damaged muscle acetylcholine receptors at the motor end-plate and rapid saturation of those that remain.

SEE CASE 19 | p. 131

"A 26-year-old woman notes the intermittent appearance of horizontal diplopia and bilateral ptosis."

In another neuromuscular junction disease, Lambert-Eaton syndrome (an immunologically mediated disorder of calcium channels at peripheral nerve terminals), there is more constant proximal weakness, and, in contrast to myasthenia gravis, muscles innervated by cranial nerves tend to be spared. Repetitive contractions of muscles in Lambert-Eaton syndrome may actually result in temporarily increased rather than decreased power, the result of a brief recruitment of acetylcholine stores in nerve endings.

A third neuromuscular junction disease, botulism, affects not only all striated muscles, including those that control eye movements and respiration, but also smooth muscle.

SEE CASE 21 | *p. 140*

"A 54-year-old woman develops abdominal cramps, nausea, and vomiting, followed a day later by diarrhea."

Botulism and neuromuscular blocking agents such as curare can produce complete paralysis of all voluntary muscles, making it impossible to determine the level of alertness. Bilateral destruction of the corticospinal/corticobulbar tracts in the upper brain stem produces comparably severe paralysis except that eye movements are spared (see Chapter 7).

Episodic Weakness

In some patients with episodic weakness the history is more informative than the examination, which may be normal. Fleeting loss of truncal power with abrupt falling but no loss of consciousness describes *drop attacks,* which can be either epileptic or ischemic (affecting the corticospinal tracts in the brain stem or spinal cord) in origin, but usually, except for the risk of fracture, represent a benign disorder of uncertain pathophysiology. Abrupt weakness associated with emotion, for example, sudden fright or laughter, suggests cataplexy, often encountered in patients with narcolepsy. More sustained but spontaneously resolving weakness is a feature of the periodic paralyses.

SEE CASE 20 | *p. 136*

"A 7-year-old boy has had attacks of limb weakness for several months."

Motor neglect refers to an apparent disinclination to use the limbs on one side of the body; when testing can be accomplished, strength and coordination are found to be normal or at least not very impaired. The lesion that is responsible often involves the contralateral mediofrontal cortex.

SEE CASE 32 | *p. 167*

"A 64-year-old hypertensive man suddenly develops difficulty speaking and using his left leg and arm."

Conversion/Malingering

Weakness is frequently feigned (conversion, hysteria, or malingering). An obvious clue is the observation (or report) that the patient is able to perform tasks that could not be performed if the weakness were real. More subtle clues are simultaneous contraction of agonists and antagonists when a muscle is tested and a tendency for the power exerted by the patient to be proportional to that exerted by the examiner; in other words, any degree of force elicits a comparable degree of weakness, or the muscle suddenly gives way. Feigned weakness will not be restricted to muscles innervated by a single nerve or root.

SEE CASE 56 | *p. 224*

"A 31-year-old woman slips and falls at home, landing on her sacrum."

▶ Coordination

Anatomy and Physiology

Although assessment of coordinated movement is considered part of the motor examination, abnormalities can have an afferent as well as an efferent origin. Properly executed movement requires exquisite coordination of different muscle groups, including appropriately timed relaxation of antagonists. The movement must be sufficient but not excessive in velocity and amplitude, and there must be awareness of precisely where the part is to be moved and where the part is positioned before, during, and at the end of the movement. These requirements are not met if normal phasic and static information from muscle spindles is unavailable to the spinal cord, the brain stem, the cerebellum, the extrapyramidal system, and the cerebral cortex. Incoordination or *ataxia* (literally, disorder) can thus be the consequence of damage at any level of the neuraxis, peripheral or central, including associative regions of the parietal lobe.

Examination

Standard tests of coordination include the following:

1. With the eyes closed, the arms are held outstretched, palms up. As noted, a downward or pronation drift suggests a lesion of the frontal cortex or corticospinal tract. With cerebellar lesions the ipsilateral arm may overshoot as it is raised (*dysmetria*) and when held out may waver about its axis. If the arm is deafferented and proprioception is deficient (see later), it may drift sideways or even upward, the patient unaware it is moving. The arm is then tapped repetitively or briefly forced downward. With weakness it may drift further or not normally bounce back. With cerebellar or proprioceptive disturbance it may bounce back with overshoot (rebound). In a comparable maneuver to detect this phenomenon patients hold both arms above the head and then bring them rapidly down to a horizontal position. The arm ipsilateral to a cerebellar lesion will overshoot and then rebound back to the intended position.

2. With the arm abducted to 90°, patients reach out and touch the examiner's finger and then place their fingertip on their own nose. Mild abnormalities can be revealed by having patients move their fingertip back and forth from the examiner's finger to their own nose, with the examiner's finger moved to a different position for each excursion. With a cerebellar lesion the ipsilateral arm may overshoot the target (again, dysmetria) or may demonstrate a coarse regular side-to-side tremor. With impaired proprioception the limb may move hesitatingly but reach the target so long as the eyes are open; when the eyes are closed, however, patients are no longer aware of where the limb is in space, and the target is missed, often widely. (With malingered ataxia, whether the eyes are open or closed, the fingertip may land confidently and consistently at a single spot on either side of the nose.)

3. Each arm is held above the head and, with eyes open and then closed, the patient's fingertip is brought down to touch the examiner's fingertip. A unilateral cerebellar lesion may cause past-pointing of the ipsilateral limb toward the side of the lesion (in contrast to a unilateral vestibular lesion, which will cause past-pointing of both limbs toward the side of the lesion). (See section on the Vestibulocochlear Nerve, Chapter 3.)

4. Lying supine, patients attempt to touch the examiner's finger with their big toe or to write a figure 8 in the air. They then place their heel on the opposite knee and run the heel down the shin to the top of the foot. These maneuvers may result in dysmetria or intention tremor, the latter demonstrated as a side-to-side oscillation. Again, with proprioceptive loss abnormalities are greatly accentuated when the eyes are closed. Rapid successive or alternating movements include rapidly rotating the hands at the wrists when the arms are held out, repetitively tapping the thumb and index finger or the palm of one hand on the back of the other, alternately touching the back of one hand with the palm and back of the other hand, and repetitively tapping the floor

with the toe or alternately with the toe and heel. As noted above, with weakness, particularly of upper-motor-neuron type, such movements are reduced in rate and amplitude but usually maintain a regular, if slowed, rhythm. Reduction in rate and amplitude is also encountered in Parkinson disease; such bradykinesia would usually be recognized on casual inspection as a reduction or slowing of the continuous conscious and unconscious movements that normal people make. With cerebellar lesions there is a breakdown in rate, amplitude, and rhythm of rapid successive and alternating movements, referred to as *dysdiadochokinesis,* as well as errors in timing of successive components of movement involving multiple joints (decomposition of movement).

SEE CASE 34 | *p. 172*

"A 16-year-old girl, who has had occasional ear infections since age 12, awakens with left postauricular pain."

▶ Stance and Gait

Stance

Posture is assessed as the patient stands in a natural position. Spinal abnormalities can be nonneurological in origin—for example, kyphosis of osteoarthritis, poker spine of Marie-Strumpel disease (ankylosing spondylitis), or kyphotic gibbus of Pott disease (tuberculous vertebral osteomyelitis). They can also be secondary to neurological disease—for example, scoliosis with syringomyelia or excessive lordosis with muscular dystrophy.

A stooped posture is common in elderly people. In Parkinson disease such a stoop can be marked, affecting primarily the upper spine; the head and neck are held forward and the arms hang with the backs of the hands facing forward (simian posture). Patients with Parkinson disease often have a striking impairment of postural reflexes.

When pushed while standing, they may fall without making appropriate arm or leg movements to maintain balance, or a mild push from behind elicits forward movement (propulsion).

With severe cerebellar lesions (such as hypertensive hemorrhage) or vestibular dysfunction (such as Ménière disease) standing and walking may be impossible (*astasia-abasia*). Patients able to stand are asked to do so with feet together and eyes open and then closed. Patients with cerebellar lesions prefer to stand with a wide base and may wobble or fall as they reluctantly move their feet closer together. With cerebellar hemispheric lesions (such as metastatic cancer) or unilateral vestibular lesions (such as labyrinthine infarction) there is a tendency to fall toward the side of the lesion. With cerebellar vermal lesions (such as alcoholic-nutritional cerebellar degeneration) or bilateral vestibular lesions (such as streptomycin toxicity) the patient is more likely to fall backward or to fall inconsistently in any direction.

Romberg's sign, referring to a patient's ability to stand unaided with eyes open but not with eyes closed, is often encountered in patients with impaired proprioception in the legs. Causative conditions include tabes dorsalis, the severe sensory polyneuropathy associated with lung cancer, the myelopathy associated with cobalamin deficiency, and certain genetic disorders such as Friedreich ataxia. In such a setting, as with tests of limb coordination, vision compensates for the inability of patients to determine the position of their legs. Romberg's sign is not specific for proprioceptive loss, however; a patient with disequilibrium from any cause may be helped by visual cues.

Gait

The most useful information on gait is often obtained by observing patients who are unaware they are being studied, for example, as they enter or leave the room. Normal people often walk unnaturally when asked to do so, and malingerers often forget to display their ataxia when they believe they are not being watched.

The patient is asked to walk a distance, turn around, and walk back, and then to walk tandem—heel-to-toe as on a tightrope. A number of abnormalities may be present.

1. As with stance, cerebellar disease produces a broad-based gait, with impaired tandem walking and a tendency to fall toward the side of a hemispheric lesion. Unsteadiness is often accentuated by turning, and there may be a coarse vertical tremor of the head and trunk (titubation). When the lesion is restricted to the cerebellar vermis, there may be marked gait ataxia with little or no dysmetria, tremor, or dysdiadochokinesis of the limbs.

2. A unilateral upper-motor-neuron lesion produces dragging of the contralateral foot; if weakness is marked, the leg will swing outward from the hip (circumduction). If the lesion is above the cervical spinal cord there may be a reduced arm swing on the same side as the circumduction, even in the absence of weakness.

3. Bilateral upper-motor-neuron lesions produce a stiff spastic gait, with dragging of both feet and, because there is often relatively preserved power in the hip adductors, a tendency of each foot to cross in front of the other (scissoring). Relatively preserved gastrocnemius power may result in toe-walking and eventual contracture in plantar flexion.

4. Damage to the fourth and fifth lumbar nerve roots (eg, from compression by a herniated intervertebral disc) or the peroneal nerve (eg, from trauma or with Charcot-Marie-Tooth–type hereditary polyneuropathy) causes paralysis of ankle dorsiflexion (foot drop) and a high-stepping gait. The foot is lifted high enough to clear the toe, which then hits the ground first.

5. With proprioceptive loss patients watch their feet as they walk (and may complain of special difficulty walking in the dark). The gait is uncontrolled, and the leg or legs tend to move randomly in different directions.

6. When asked to rise from a sitting position, patients with Parkinson disease may be unable to do so without using their arms. The gait is then stooped with flexed hips and knees and reduced arm swing, and the feet tend to shuffle, sometimes never leaving the ground. Often, steps become quicker as walking proceeds, and patients may be unable to stop before walking into a wall or a chair (festination).

7. Bilateral frontal lobe disease produces a magnetic gait. The legs tend to be broad based and the feet, never leaving the ground, take tiny steps or, despite visible efforts to walk, do not move at all (slipped clutch gait). In contrast to patients with Parkinson disease, those with frontal lobe lesions tend to stand upright, to lean backward, or to retropulse. This type of gait disorder is associated with chronic normal-pressure hydrocephalus, but its mechanism is unclear. One view is that the enlarged lateral ventricles stretch frontal lobe fibers projecting to nuclei in the basis pontis that give rise to the middle cerebellar peduncles.

8. Pelvic girdle weakness, as in myopathic diseases, causes a waddling gait, with the pelvis tilting from side to side with each step. The cause is bilateral weakness of gluteus medius muscles, which normally abduct the hip; when they are weak, the pelvis tends to tilt toward whichever leg is lifted off the ground.

9. Gait ataxia as a form of malingering is often bizarre without the stereotypic features of neurological illness. It may not be broad based despite much bobbing and weaving, and some patients even maintain tandem as they sway and flail their arms about. The gait is much improved when the patient is unaware of being observed, and stance may improve with distraction (eg, performing finger-to-nose testing while standing with feet together).

10. The gait is altered in many different ways by pain (antalgic gait). For example, a patient with hip arthritis will limp, attempting to keep weight on the pain-free leg. To relieve low back and leg pain, a patient with stenosis of the lumbar spinal canal and compression of lumbar nerve roots will walk with a forward stoop (lordosis further narrows the canal) and will stop to rest after walking a short distance (pseudoclaudication).

See Case 33 | p. 170

"A 50-year-old alcoholic man has had an unsteady gait for several years."

▶ Abnormal Involuntary Movements

In addition to identifying negative phenomena such as weakness, incoordination, and difficulty walking, the motor examination includes careful inspection for positive phenomena in the form of spontaneous involuntary movements not normally present.

Seizures

Epileptic seizures are either generalized or focal. A full-blown major motor (*grand mal, tonic-clonic*) convulsion consists of loss of consciousness, a minute or two of generalized rigidity, and then a minute or two of clonic jerking, plus tongue-biting and urinary incontinence; gradual awakening over minutes or hours follows. Such a display would not be missed, but other types of seizure are more subtle. *Petit mal absence* seizures, most often affecting small children, consist of staring and immobility for several seconds, with or without repetitive blinking; beginning and ending abruptly, such spells resemble normal daydreaming. Focal motor seizures can take such easily identifiable forms as clonic jerking that rapidly spreads proximally from one or more digits up a limb (a Jacksonian march) or continuous coarse clonic jerking of the face or a limb

(*epilepsia partialis continua*). Focal tonic or clonic movements can be very brief and restricted, however, perhaps involving one thumb or the corner of the mouth. Whether obvious or subtle, focal motor seizures usually signify an irritative structural lesion of the contralateral frontal cortex. Lesions of the frontal lobe sometimes cause generalized tonic-clonic seizures whose only focality is contralateral deviation of the head and eyes.

See Case 30 | p. 161

"A previously healthy 27-year-old woman suddenly experiences tonic contractions of her left fingers, followed within a few seconds by clonic movements that spread up her arm."

Seizures arising from the supplementary motor area of the mediofrontal cortex often consist of elevation of the contralateral arm and continuous or intermittent nonverbal vocalization. Seizures of limbic origin—particularly the inferomedial temporal lobe—can produce bizarre motor activity. Some limbic seizures consist of staring spells that resemble petit mal absence, although more often accompanied by primitive movements such as picking, lip smacking, or chewing (automatisms), followed by drowsiness or inattentiveness. More florid limbic seizures may produce screaming, wandering, running, laughing, or striking anyone within range; during the postictal confusional period there may be very complex behavior for which the patient has no subsequent recall. Not surprisingly, such episodes are often considered psychiatric in origin.

Myoclonus

Myoclonus is a sudden involuntary jerk of a muscle or a muscle group. Two normal varieties of myoclonus are sleep myoclonus (jerks of the trunk, neck, or limbs while nodding off) and hiccups (myoclonic jerks of the diaphragm). There are many kinds of pathological myoclonus. Epileptic myoclonus includes benign myoclonic epilepsy of child-hood, a condition easily treated and likely to remit spontaneously, and infantile spasms, consisting of flexion or extension myoclonic jerks of the trunk, associated with mental retardation and generalized tonic-clonic seizures. Myoclonus is an early symptom in subacute sclerosing panencephalitis (caused by the rubeola virus and progressing to de-mentia and death within a few years) and a late symptom in Creutzfeldt-Jacob disease (caused by a transmissible prion protein and associated with pyramidal and extrapyrami-dal signs, dementia, and death within a few months). It is an early sign in symptomatic renal failure. Myoclonus is a prominent fea-ture of many hereditary degenerative disor-ders, for example, glucocerebrosidase defi-ciency (Gaucher disease) and the mito-chondrial DNA mutation that results in myoclonic epilepsy with ragged red [mus-cle] fibers (MERRF). Following shock or suc-cessful resuscitation from cardiac arrest there is often widespread myoclonus trig-gered by movement (action myoclonus). Structural lesions of the spinal cord can pro-duce myoclonus involving only muscles in-nervated by motor neurons at the level of the lesion (segmental myoclonus).

SEE CASE 37 | p. 183

"Attempting suicide with barbiturates, a 37-year-old woman has a cardiorespiratory arrest for about 20 minutes."

Tetanus

The tetanospasms seen in tetanus—painful sustained muscle contractions without loss of consciousness—are a type of spinal sei-zure, resulting from repetitive firing of dis-inhibited lower motor neurons.

SEE CASE 27 | p. 155

"A 46-year-old woman has been a parenteral heroin abuser for over 25 years; access to veins has long been lost, and she injects the drug sub-cutaneously (skin popping)."

Tremor

The defining features of a tremor are that it is involuntary and it oscillates. It can be regu-lar or irregular, distal or proximal (including the face, tongue, or larynx), and intermittent or continuous. There are three basic types of tremor: sustention, intention, and rest. Nor-mal physiological (sustention) tremor is ob-served in the fingers of the outstretched arms; its detection is enhanced by laying a piece of paper over the extended fingers. It usually has an irregular rhythm of about 10 Hz and is accentuated by nervousness. An exaggerated form of this type of tremor is seen with thyrotoxicosis, alcohol withdrawal, and metabolic disturbances such as renal or liver failure. So-called essential tremor, an often hereditary disorder of unknown cause in otherwise healthy individuals, has more variable frequency—usually slower.

A lesion of a cerebellar hemisphere or its major outflow tract, the superior cere-bellar peduncle, causes intention tremor, which is usually coarse, regular in rhythm, and, as noted above, demonstrated on fin-ger-to-nose and heel-to-shin testing. Pa-tients with multiple sclerosis are particu-larly likely to have an intention tremor of the trunk and neck when walking (tituba-tion—see above). Whether damage to the red nucleus causes intention tremor is im-possible to say, for lesions in the red nu-cleus invariably damage crossing cerebellar outflow projections as well. Some investi-gators believe that when the red nucleus is damaged the tremor occurs both at rest and with intention. Also problematic is the wing-beating tremor of Wilson disease, a hereditary disorder of copper metabolism. Large amplitude flapping occurs as the fin-ger approaches the nose, and the arm may flail about in a manner suggesting co-exist-ing chorea (see later). Central nervous sys-tem damage in Wilson disease is wide-spread, and so it is usually unclear what combination of cerebellar and basal ganglia disturbance is responsible for a particular abnormal movement.

The tremor of Parkinson disease has a

regular rhythm of about 5 Hz and is present at rest (although it dampens with full relaxation and disappears during sleep). It usually decreases or disappears with voluntary movement. It may be mild and restricted to the thumb and index finger or coarsely involve proximal joints, including the neck or jaw. Parkinsonian tremor often consists of to-and-fro movements of the thumb across the fingertips, and a flexion dystonia (see later) of the metacarpophalyngeal joints, giving the tremor a pill-rolling quality. Some investigators believe that the cogwheeling phenomenon (see above) so common in Parkinsonian patients actually represents subclinical tremor.

SEE CASE 35 | *p. 176*

"A 63-year-old man notices a rhythmic tremor of his right hand and wrist that over the next several months becomes increasingly coarse."

Asterixis

In contrast to myoclonus, which is an active muscle contraction, asterixis is a brief electrically silent relaxation of a contracted muscle (negative myclonus). It can be demonstrated by having patients hold their arms out with wrists and fingers extended. Every few seconds the wrists and fingers drop and then quickly return to their previous position. Asterixis is most often observed in patients with either renal or hepatic failure.

Chorea

Chorea (the Greek word means *dance*) consists of abrupt but smooth involuntary movements of the limbs, face, or tongue. The movements may have a stereotypic repetitiveness (as in the grimacing of Huntington disease or in the tongue protrusions and retractions of neuroleptic-induced tardive dyskinesia) or may appear quite random, with no two successive movements the same. They may seem semipurposeful in their complexity, particularly when an experienced patient learns to blend a choreic movement into a voluntary movement. Mild chorea can suggest nervous fidgeting. Choreic movements are continuous but increase with intention or anxiety, are dampened with relaxation, and are absent during sleep. Chorea can be identified by asking the patient to hold the arms above the head with palms facing forward or to protrude the tongue. When chorea is present, neither position can be maintained. Subtler signs include respiratory irregularity and hyperextension of the fingers when the arms are held out in pronation The many causes of chorea include Huntington and other heredodegenerative diseases, rheumatic fever (Sydenham chorea), drug toxicity (particularly neuroleptic agents and L-DOPA), and lupus erythematosus.

SEE CASE 75 | *p. 272*

"Over the past year a 45-year-old lawyer has had a change in personality."

Athetosis

Athetosis has many of the same features as chorea but is slower, characteristically producing continuous writhing movements of the fingers, hands, feet, or face. When both choreic and athetotic movements are seen, the disturbance is called *choreoathetosis*. Athetosis can be a severe but isolated consequence of fetal or perinatal birth injury (one form of cerebral palsy).

Dystonia

Dystonia resembles athetosis, but differs in that abnormal postures tend to be held for a time. Common variants are rotation and tilting of the lower spine (tortipelvis) or neck (torticollis). Involvement of the tongue, pharynx, or larynx causes dysphagia, dysarthria, or aphonia. Dystonic forced eye closure is called blepharospasm. A striking feature of some dystonias is their dependence on posture; when the patient lies supine the movements may dramatically decrease, presumably the result of altered vestibular imput to the basal ganglia. With torticollis a remarkable feature is the ability of patients to keep their heads from turning simply by touching their chins without applying counterforce. Dystonia can be the result of drug toxicity, for example, as either an acute or a chronic side effect of neuroleptics. It is also a prominent feature of a number of hereditary diseases.

Ballism

Ballism (or, when unilateral, hemiballism) is a proximal continuous flinging movement of the arm; it can be viewed as a severe form of chorea. Ballism is particularly associated with acute lesions of the subthalamic nucleus (most often occlusive or hemorrhagic stroke).

SEE CASE 36 | p. 181

"A 60-year-old hypertensive woman suddenly cannot control her arm."

Tics

Tics are repetitive, stereotypic movements that although involuntary are accompanied by an irresistible compulsion. They most often involve the face, with blinking, grimacing, smiling, pursing the lips, or licking. In Tourette syndrome there may be vocalizations, ranging from brief grunts or barks to shouted obscenities. Some investigators place tics on a continuum with obsessive-compulsive disorder.

SEE CASE 76 | p. 274

"Since the age of 7, a 20-year-old man has suffered involuntary movements and vocalizations."

Fasciculations

Fasciculations are spontaneous contractions of muscle fibers innervated by a single motor neuron (a motor unit). By contrast, fibrillations are spontaneous contractions of individual muscle fibers. Fibrillations, which cannot be seen and can be identified only by electrodiagnostic testing, usually indicate denervation. Fasciculations, although insufficient to move a joint, can be seen or palpated as worm-like movements beneath the skin. When widespread, and particularly when associated with weakness and atrophy, they strongly suggest a motor neuron disease such as amyotrophic lateral sclerosis. Several subtypes of fasciculation are referred to collectively as *myokimia*. Common in fatigued but otherwise normal individuals, the movements in one type are coarse, slow, prolonged, focal, and transient and are often located in the thigh or upper arm; in another type, also associated with fatigue, fine ripplings are felt in the upper or lower eyelids. More serious is facial myokimia, in which continuous flickering contractions of the muscles on one side of the face appear suddenly; the cause is often a brain stem lesion such as infarction, multiple sclerosis, or a pontine glioma.

Hemifacial Spasm

In hemifacial spasm, not to be confused with facial myokimia, abrupt contractions of the muscles on one side of the face occur repetitively and randomly. Sometimes there is evidence of synkinesis, as with recovered Bell palsy. (See section on the Facial Nerve, Chapter 3.) Of unknown cause, hemifacial spasm might be a motor counterpart to the spontaneous trigeminal nerve discharges of trigeminal neuralgia. (See section on the Trigeminal Nerve, Chapter 3.)

Cramps

Cramps are involuntary, sustained, and often painful contractions of muscles, common in normal people after muscle overuse. They can be relieved by the oral administration of quinine sulfate, which decreases the excitability of motor end-plates. Cramps are associated with diseases at different levels of the neuraxis but are particularly common as an early feature of motor neuron disease.

Opisthotonus

Opisthotonus is marked hyperextension of the neck and spine. It occurs in severe meningitis and in tetanus.

Rigor

Unlike fasciculations, shivering involves entire muscles and occurs in bursts. A mechanism for generating heat, it accompanies the rising phase of a fever.

5

The Sensory Examination:
Boundaries and Comparisons Are Crucial

▶ Two Systems: A Brief Anatomical Review

A proper sensory examination requires knowledge of the skin areas supplied by individual dorsal roots (dermatomes) and peripheral nerves (Figure 5–1) as well as awareness of the ascending sensory pathways of the spinal cord, brain stem, and forebrain (Figures 5–2 and 5–3).

There are two major sensory systems, each of which has first-order neurons in the dorsal root ganglia. The dorsal column-medial lemniscus system mediates touch (superficial, deep, and vibratory) through a variety of encapsulated mechanoreceptors and mediates proprioception (static and dynamic) through joint mechanoreceptors and muscle stretch receptors. Its fibers are thickly myelinated and fast conducting.

Entering the spinal cord through the dorsal roots, fibers of the dorsal column-medial lemniscus system ascend in the dorsal columns; those coming from the legs are displaced medially as they ascend. Dorsal column fibers synapse in the medulla at the gracile (leg) and cuneate (arm) nuclei, axons of which decussate and project to the ventral posterior lateral nucleus of the thalamus, which in turn projects to the parietal lobe (Figure 5–4).

The anterolateral system, comprising the spinoreticular, spinomesencephalic, and spinothalamic tracts, mediates temperature (cold and warm), pain (fast and slow), and less discriminative touch through bare nerve endings. Its fibers are thinly myelinated or unmyelinated and slow conducting.

Fibers of the anterolateral system enter the spinal cord and ascend or descend one or two segments before synapsing in the dorsal horn. Second-order projections then cross in the ventral commissure and ascend in the lateral columns adjacent to the ventral horns; those coming from the legs are displaced laterally as they ascend. Synapses then occur in the brain stem reticular formation (spinoreticular tract), midbrain tectum (spinomesencephalic tract), and ventral posterior lateral nucleus of the thalamus adjacent to the area that receives the medial lemniscus (spinothalamic tract). Other projections of the spinothalamic tract are to the thalamic intralaminar nuclei. Projections of this system from the thalamus include the parietal lobe (probably essential for stimulus localization and recognition) and limbic and frontal lobe structures (probably mediating affective response) (see Figure 5–4). Reflex responses to stimuli carried by the anterolateral system include arousal (the reticular formation), head and eye turning (the colliculi), and modulation of pain (a descending pathway that passes through the midbrain periaqueductal gray).

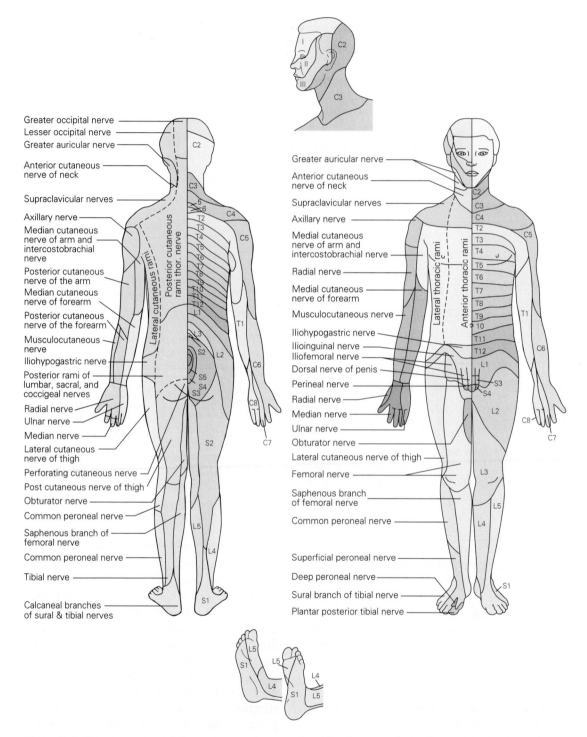

Figure 5–1. Sensory segmental dermatomes and areas of peripheral nerve supply. Considerable variation exists. (Reproduced with permission from Kandel ER, Schwartz JH, Jessell TM. 1999. *Principles of Neural Science*, 4th ed. New York: McGraw-Hill.)

Dorsal column–medial lemniscus system

Anterolateral system

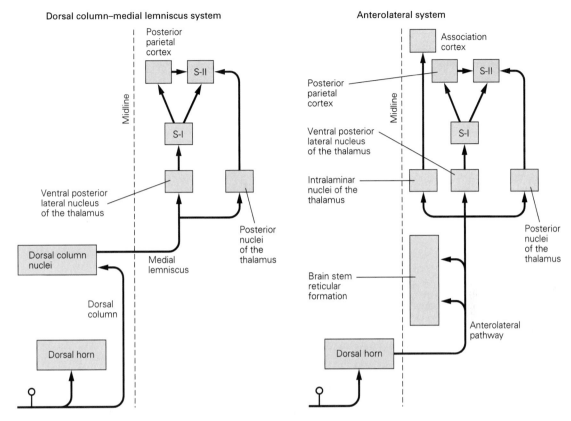

Figure 5–2. Diagram of the major ascending somatic sensory systems. The dorsal column-medial lemniscus system, mediating proprioception and discriminative tactile sensation, decussates after its first synapse in the dorsal column nuclei of the medulla. The anterolateral system, mediating pain and temperature sensation, and, to a lesser degree, tactile sensation, decussates after its first synapse in the dorsal horn of the spinal cord. S-I, primary sensory cortex; S-II, secondary sensory cortex. (Reproduced with permission from Kandel ER, Schwartz JH, Jessell TM. 1991. *Principles of Neural Science*, 3rd ed. Norwalk, CT: Appleton & Lange.)

▶ The Examination: Systems and Modalities

The sensory examination assesses different modalities in each of the two ascending systems.

Pain

Two principles—comparisons and boundaries—are used to assess the sensation of pain. With eyes closed, patients are pricked more than once with a clean unused pin (a single pinprick may not be appreciated as pain) and then asked if they can feel anything and, if so, what. If sharpness is re-

ported in one area, its degree and quality are compared to its degree and quality in other areas: left versus right, distal versus proximal, lower trunk versus upper trunk, and areas inside or outside a dermatome or a peripheral nerve territory. Such comparisons are crucial for detecting subtle abnormalities; the stimulus may be felt as sharp everywhere but less sharp over a particular area or may have a burning, electrical, or other peculiar quality. Defining the boundaries of abnormal sensation is also essential. For example, unilaterally decreased sensation over the medial calf could signify a lesion involving either the fourth lumbar root or the femoral nerve; finding additional sensory loss over

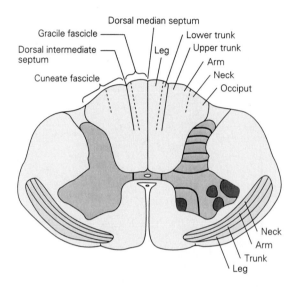

Figure 5–3. Somatotopic organization of the dorsal columns and the anterolateral system of the spinal cord. In the anterolateral system fibers representing the leg are closest to the surface of the cord. (Reproduced with permission from Martin JH. 1996. *Neuroanatomy Text and Atlas,* 2nd ed. Stamford, CT: Appleton & Lange.)

the rest of the femoral nerve territory would indicate the femoral nerve was involved. Bilaterally decreased sensation over the feet could signify either peripheral neuropathy with distal sensory loss or spinal cord disease (myelopathy) at a midlumbar level; finding additional sensory loss over the back of the legs and perianally would identify the lesion as probably myelopathic.

Decreased pain sensation is called *hypalgesia*. The subjective sense that a painful stimulus is sharper or more disagreeable than normal is called *hyperalgesia* or *hyperpathia*. Both types of abnormalities can occur with either peripheral or central lesions and can coexist within the same area.

Deep slow pain is assessed by squeezing muscles or tendons. In some peripheral neuropathies, thinly myelinated fibers mediating pinprick are more affected than unmyelinated fibers mediating deep pain. Conversely, in tabes dorsalis deep pain may be impaired although pinprick feels normal. Excessive muscle tenderness can result from local inflammatory disorders such as polymyositis, polymyalgia rheumatica, or thrombophlebitis.

Touch and Temperature

The same principles—comparisons and boundaries—apply to testing touch and temperature sensation. Rubbing the skin with the fingertips will stimulate both superficial and deep receptors for touch; superficial touch can be more selectively tested with a wisp of cotton. Temperature can be tested with a cold object such as a tuning fork. Decreased touch sensation is called *hypesthesia*. Altered (and usually unpleasant) touch sensation is called *dysesthesia*. Frank pain produced by a nonnoxious stimulus is called *allodynia*.

Proprioception

Proprioception has two components. First is awareness of the location of part of the body in space (position sense). As discussed above, dysfunction of this ability is sometimes identified when coordination is tested with the patient's eyes closed. Additional maneuvers include having the patient, with eyes closed, touch the index finger of one hand with the index finger of the other after the target finger has been moved about in

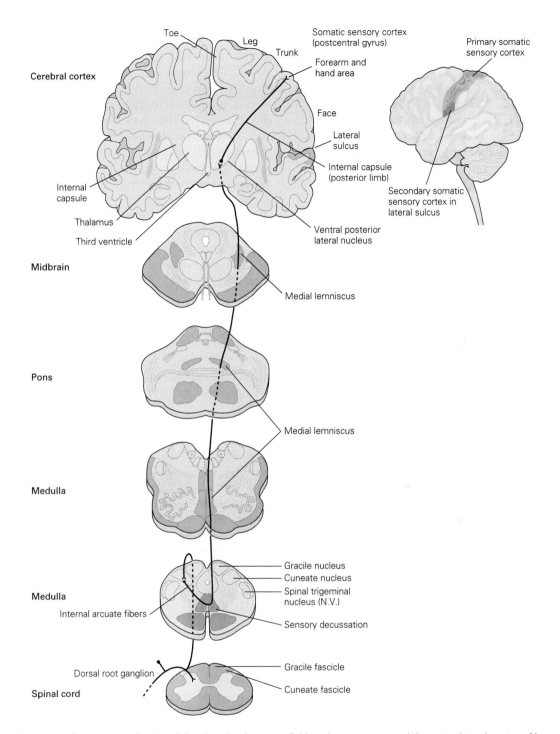

Figure 5–4. General organization of the dorsal column-medial lemniscus system and the anterolateral system. Neurons of the dorsal root ganglia conveying proprioception and discriminative touch synapse onto neurons of the dorsal column (gracile and cuneate) nuclei of the medulla, which cross and synapse onto neurons of the ventral posterior lateral nucleus of the thalamus, which synapse onto neurons of the parietal cortex. Neurons of the dorsal root ganglia conveying pain and temperature synapse onto neurons in the dorsal horn, axons of which cross and ascend. Those of the spinothalamic tract synapse onto neurons of the ventral posterior lateral nucleus of the thalamus, which project both to the parietal cortex and to the limbic system. (Reproduced with permission from Kandel ER, Schwartz JH, Jessell TM. 1991. *Principles of Neural Science,* 3rd ed. Norwalk, CT: Appleton & Lange. Adapted with permission from Carpenter MB, Sutin J. 1983. *Human Neuroanatomy,* 8th ed. Baltimore, MD: Williams & Wilkins.)

space. Second, and more routinely tested, is sense of passive movement. With the patient's eyes closed, a thumb, finger, or toe is moved passively up and down and the patient indicates if the movement is felt and in what direction. (Careful instructions and even a practice run with the eyes open are sometimes necessary.) Normally even tiny excursions are identified; cranking the joint through wide arcs will not identify mild abnormalities. If the most distal joints are impaired, the test proceeds to more proximal joints. A patient with severe proprioceptive loss in an upper extremity may have, even with eyes open, continuous involuntary movements of the outstretched hand or fingers (pseudoathetosis).

Vibration

Vibratory sense is tested with a 128-Hz tuning fork over bony prominences such as the big toe, ankle maleolus, knee, or iliac crest. Comparing different spinous processes of the vertebrae can sometimes identify impairment below a particular level, suggestive of myelopathy. Quantitative comparisons of different areas are made by having patients indicate when they can no longer feel the vibration and then determining if it is still felt elsewhere. Vibratory sense is lost early in the course of some peripheral neuropathies, including those associated with alcoholism and diabetes mellitus, and in spinal cord disorders, particularly those principally affecting myelin, such as multiple sclerosis and cobalamin deficiency. Reduced vibratory sensation in the feet or ankles is common in otherwise normal people over 65 years of age.

Discriminative or Cortical Sensation

There are a number of tests for cortical sensation. Double simultaneous stimulation consists of touching first one, then the other, side of the face, limbs, or trunk, and then touching both sides simultaneously. Failure to feel the stimulus on one side when it is accompanied by stimulation of the opposite side—*extinction*—suggests a lesion in the con-

tralateral parietal lobe. (Such patients often have other signs of hemineglect. See section on Agnosia.) Two-point discrimination varies with body region; it is most sensitive—a few millimeters—in the fingertips, lips, and tongue. Because the objective is to stimulate discriminative touch receptors, blunt, not sharp, points should be used. *Graphesthesia* is the recognition of numbers or letters written with a blunt point on the skin, usually of the palm. *Localization* is the ability to identify where on the body a stimulus is located. *Stereognosis* is the ability to recognize an object from its size and shape. Commonly employed objects are paper clips, safety pins, keys, and coins. As with other sensory testing, abnormalities may be evident only when left–right comparisons are made. Normal differences in sensitivity mean that comparisons of stereognosis or two-point discrimination between arms and legs or proximal and distal limbs are meaningless.

Impairment on these tests suggests a parietal cortical lesion only if primary touch sensation is intact. Moreover, mild peripheral lesions can selectively affect discriminative sensation. An unfortunate example is the diabetic patient, blind from diabetic retinopathy, who cannot learn Braille because of peripheral neuropathy and loss of two-point discrimination.

▶ Patterns of Sensory Impairment

The anatomical pathways of the sensory system explain the various patterns of impairment encountered clinically.

Total Unilateral (Including Facial) Loss of All Sensory Modalities

This pattern indicates a lesion involving both the dorsal column-medial lemniscus system and the anterolateral system at the level of the upper brain stem or thalamus. A comparable lesion above the thalamus would more likely cause severe impairment of proprioceptive and discriminative modalities with relative sparing of pain, touch, and temperature sensation, which might simply be described as having an altered quality or be difficult for the patient to localize. Unilateral loss of pain and temperature with preservation of proprioception, as well as dissociation in the opposite direction, can result from smaller lesions in the upper brain stem or thalamus. Unilateral severe hyperalgesia and dysesthesia are often the result of thalamic lesions.

SEE CASE 3 | p. 95

"A 62-year-old hypertensive woman abruptly develops numbness and a pins-and-needles sensation over her left arm, leg, and trunk."

SEE CASE 4 | p. 96

"During an altercation with a friend, a 27-year-old man is struck on the right side of his head with a baseball bat and rendered unconscious."

Loss of Pain and Temperature Sensation on One Side of Face and Opposite Side of Body

This pattern indicates a lesion of the lateral medulla involving the spinal trigeminal tract and nucleus and the ascending anterolateral system.

SEE CASE 50 | p. 210

"A 65-year-old hypertensive man suddenly experiences occipital headache, vertigo, nausea, vomiting, and burning pain in his left face and forehead."

Bilateral Loss of All Sensation Below a Definite Level Over the Trunk

This pattern indicates a lesion of the spinal cord. Because in most people the lower end of the spinal cord (the conus medullaris) is at the level of the first lumbar vertebrae, a spinal cord segment is not necessarily at the level of its equivalently named vertebra. High cervical segments do correspond to

their equivalent vertebra, but the C8 spinal segment is opposite the C7 vertebra, the T6 segment is opposite the T3 vertebra, and lumbar and sacral segments are opposite vertebrae T11 through L1. There may be a short zone of dysesthesia or hyperalgesia at the upper level of myelopathic sensory loss. Defining the lower end of the sensory loss provides a clue as to whether the lesion is extrinsic or intrinsic to the cord. Loss of pain sensation that includes sacral dermatomes indicates an extraparenchymal compressive lesion (such as an extradural metastasis) affecting the outer ascending fibers of the anterolateral system. Preserved sacral sensation (sacral sparing) indicates an intraparenchymal lesion (such as a glioma) that has not yet expanded enough to affect these outer fibers. Sensory loss restricted to sacral dermatomes (saddle anesthesia) could be the result of a lesion in either the lower cauda equina or the conus medullaris. Bladder and bowel control are usually impaired, but strength, sensation, and reflexes in the legs may be normal. A severe injury to the upper cauda equina (such as from a bullet) can produce sensory loss involving only lumbar and sacral dermatomes. During the course of an ascending polyneuropathy such as Guillain-Barré syndrome there may be an apparent truncal sensory level, but it is not likely to be as definite, nor the sensory loss as severe, as with a spinal cord lesion.

Bilateral Loss of Pain and Temperature Sensation Below a Definite Level, Weakness and Impaired Proprioception on Opposite Side

This pattern indicates hemisection of the spinal cord (Brown-Séquard syndrome). The lesion is on the side of the weakness and proprioceptive loss, for the anterolateral system mediating pain and temperature sensation has already crossed close to its level of entry. Resulting from lesions such as trauma, multiple sclerosis, or extrinsic compression by a neoplasm, the Brown-Séquard syndrome is often incomplete, for example, affecting pain and temperature sensation and strength but sparing proprioception. If a single lesion can be presumed, the Brown-Séquard syndrome means the lesion must be myelopathic. Conversely, a single lesion producing weakness and loss of pain and temperature sensation on the same side can be peripheral (nerve roots, brachial or lumbosacral plexus, or peripheral nerves) or within the brain stem or forebrain, but it cannot be in the spinal cord.

SEE CASE 45 | p. 199

"For several months a 37-year-old man has had midthoracic back pain, low-grade fevers, chills, night sweats, and weight loss."

Bilateral Loss of Pain and Temperature Sensation Over Several Segments, Normal Sensation Above and Below, Intact Proprioceptive and Discriminative Sensation

This pattern indicates a lesion in the center of the spinal cord interrupting bilaterally crossing fibers from the dorsal horns en route to forming the ascending projections of the anterolateral system. If the lesion extends into the anterior horns, there is atrophic weakness over the same segments; if the lesion extends into the lateral and dorsal columns, there will be spastic weakness and proprioceptive loss as well. Causes of such a central cord syndrome include trauma with hematomyelia, gliomatous tumors, and, in particular, syringomyelia. If the lesion is within the upper cervical cord, there will be a shawl-like area of pain and temperature loss; if the lesion is within the lower cervical cord, the sensory loss will affect both hands.

SEE CASE 47 | p. 203

"A 31-year-old woman notes decreased sensation in her left hand after sustaining a painless burn."

Bilateral Loss of Pain and Temperature Sensation Below a Definite Level, Intact Proprioceptive and Discriminative Sensation

This pattern indicates a lesion of the anterior spinal cord (anterior cord syndrome). Causative lesions include traumatic protrusion of an intervertebral disk and infarction in the territory of the anterior spinal artery. (The dorsal columns are supplied by two or more posterior cerebral arteries.) Below the lesion weakness usually accompanies loss of sensation.

SEE CASE 49 | p. 208

"A 62-year-old man with a 3-year history of retrosternal pain on exertion is found to have an aortic aneurysm next to the eighth and ninth thoracic vertebrae."

Bilaterally Impaired Sensation Affecting Hands and Feet

This pattern suggests peripheral neuropathy (glove and stocking anesthesia). The sensory modalities affected vary with the underlying disease. For example, in alcoholic/nutritional polyneuropathy vibratory sensation and pain sensation are impaired early, whereas proprioception is affected much later. Disordered axonal transport accounts for the distal location of the sensory loss (and weakness) in some peripheral neuropathies, and since most people's legs are longer than their arms, the feet are usually affected first. Disagreeable or painful paresthesia, dysesthesia, and hyperalgesia are sometimes more distressing to the patient than numbness.

SEE CASE 1 | p. 89

"During a routine examination a 30-year-old man is found to have diabetes mellitus."

Although peripheral neuropathy can be predominantly sensory (or motor), it is usually, to some degree, mixed. (Electrodiagnostic testing may be necessary to identify the motor involvement.) Purely sensory symptoms and signs raise the possibility of a disease process localized to dorsal root ganglia (neuronopathy).

SEE CASE 2 | *p. 93*

"A 57-year-old man experiences spontaneous sharp pains in his legs, and over the next several months the pain becomes increasingly severe and lancinating in quality."

In diseases that cause both peripheral neuropathy and myelopathy, for example, cobalamin deficiency, it may be difficult to determine whether sensory loss in the legs, particularly proprioceptive, has a neuropathic or myelopathic basis.

SEE CASE 48 | *p. 205*

"A 68-year-old man develops pins-and-needles sensation in both feet, and over the next year the paresthesias spread to his ankles and fingers."

Sensory Loss of All Modalities Confined to One Part of Body

This pattern suggests a sensory nerve root or peripheral nerve lesion, and awareness of specific root and nerve cutaneous representations will usually distinguish the two. Lesions involving the brachial or lumbosacral plexus (such as trauma, infiltration by carcinoma, or immunologically mediated brachial plexitis) cause more complex patterns of sensory loss. Peripheral nerve lesions, whether traumatic, compressive, or vascular, seldom affect sensory fibers alone, but isolated sensory loss is not unusual with root lesions such as compression from vertebral osteoarthritis or a herniated intervertebral disk. The tuberculoid form of leprosy affects small branches of sensory nerves, resulting in scattered patches of sensory loss that do not conform to recognized peripheral nerve territories. Moreover, because of normally overlapping territories, lesions af-

fecting a single root or nerve often produce areas of numbness considerably smaller than anatomic boundaries would predict.

SEE CASE 41 | *p. 193*

"For several months an 82-year-old man has had increasing difficulty controlling his right hand in tasks such as writing and buttoning."

SEE CASE 44 | *p. 198*

"For several years a 35-year-old man has had intermittent low back pain precipitated by abrupt bending or twisting and lasting 2 or 3 days."

Trophic Changes

Peripheral nerve lesions can affect autonomic as well as sensory (or motor) fibers, resulting in trophic changes in the skin (and, radiographically, bone demineralization).

SEE CASE 43 | *p. 195*

"Two days after sustaining a gunshot wound to his right upper arm, a 22-year-old man develops pain in his right hand, which over the next several months increases in intensity."

Malingering and Conversion (Hysteria)

Malingered or hysterical sensory loss is common. Indications that the sensory loss is being simulated include impaired sensation in an area that does not conform to a known anatomical pattern; loss confined to one entire limb; suggestibility and inconsistent margins; absence of disability that would be expected to accompany the sensory loss, for example, normal coordination in an arm with absent proprioception; normal vibratory sensation just off the midline over the forehead, chin, or sternum, with a sharp drop-off as soon as the fork crosses the midline to the other side; and additional impairments that would not be expected to accompany unilateral sensory loss, for example, reduced vision in the ipsilateral eye (as opposed to homonymous hemianopia—see section on the Optic Nerve, Chapter 3) or deafness in the ipsilateral ear. Occasionally, patients can be tricked by maneuvers such as being turned over, at which time the sensory loss changes sides, or being instructed to say "yes" each time they feel a stimulus and "no" each time they do not. However, it is important to recognize that simulated sensory loss does not necessarily mean that all the patient's symptoms and signs are bogus. For example, hemiparesis following a stroke may cause the patient to expect additional abnormalities; splitting of the tuning fork at the forehead is not unusual in such patients.

6

Reflexes:
Remember the Afferent Limb

▶ Is All Nervous System Activity Reflexive?

The simplest human reflex, elicited by rapidly stretching a muscle, is called the tendon (or deep tendon or muscle stretch) reflex. The afferent end is the muscle spindle (Figure 6–1), and the sensory pathway is monosynaptically linked to motor neurons, resulting in contraction of the stretched muscle (Figure 6–2). Depending on your concept of free will, the most complicated motor behaviors, and even thinking itself, might be considered reflexic, with internal or external stimuli triggering an exceedingly complex reflex arc that ultimately produces an effecter response. We previously focused on such free will reflexes. In this part of the neurological examination, we focus on monosynaptic tendon reflexes and polysynaptic superficial reflexes of a simple, stereotypic nature.

▶ Tendon Reflexes

All striated skeletal muscles have spindles and therefore will reflexly contract when stretched. Except in acute situations such as spinal shock (see section on Muscle Tone, Chapter 4), tendon reflexes are usually abnormally brisk with upper-motor-neuron lesions and decreased or absent with lesions that interrupt the reflex arc. Possible sites of interruption include the peripheral sensory

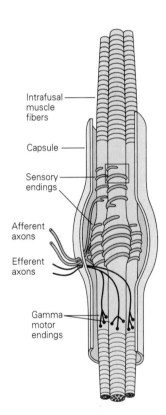

Intrafusal muscle fibers

Capsule

Sensory endings

Afferent axons

Efferent axons

Gamma motor endings

Figure 6–1. Muscle spindles contain specialized intrafusal muscle fibers, central regions of which are not contractile. Sensory endings spiraling around the central regions of intrafusal fibers fire when the intrafusal fibers are stretched. Gamma motor neurons innervate the contractile polar regions of the intrafusal fibers, and contraction of the polar regions stretches the central region from both ends. The result is a hypertonic muscle or a brisk stretch reflex. (Reproduced with permission from Kandel ER, Schwartz JH, Jessell TM. 1999. *Principles of Neural Science*, 4th ed. New York: McGraw-Hill. Adapted with permission from Hulliger M. 1984. The mammalian muscle spindle and its central control. *Rev Physiol Biochem Pharmacol* 101:1.)

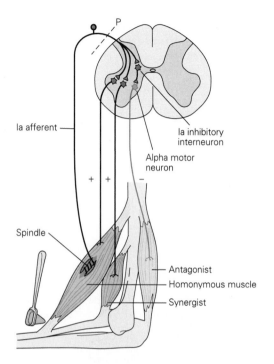

Table 6–1. Grading tendon reflexes.

Grade	Tendon reflex
0	Absent
1	Reduced
2	Normal
3	Brisk without clonus
4	Transient clonus
5	Sustained clonus

Figure 6–2. Stretch reflexes are mediated by monosynaptic pathways. When a muscle is stretched, Ia afferent fibers from muscle spindles increase their firing rate, exciting alpha motor neurons that innervate the same (homonymous) muscle as well as synergist muscles. They also excite inhibitory interneurons, thereby inhibiting motor neurons that innervate antagonist muscles. The net effect is to counteract the stretch. [Reproduced with permission from Kandel ER, Schwartz JH, Jessell TM. 1999. *Principles of Neural Science*, 4th ed. New York: McGraw-Hill. Adapted with permission from Liddell EGT, Sherrington C. 1924. Reflexes in response to stretch (myotatic reflexes). *Proc R Soc Lond B Biol Sci* 96:212.]

nerve (eg, peripheral sensory neuropathy), the dorsal root ganglion (eg, tabes dorsalis), the sensory nerve root (eg, compression by a herniated intervertebral disk), the motor neuron (for example, poliomyelitis), the peripheral motor nerve (eg, Guillain-Barré peripheral motor neuropathy), the neuromuscular junction (eg, the Lambert-Eaton syndrome), or the muscle (eg, long-standing muscular dystrophy). A standard scale defines the briskness of a reflex (Table 6–1).

Tendon reflexes are elicited with a percussion hammer, and clinical neurologists have differing but usually strongly held views as to which type of hammer is superior. The muscle is stretched by tapping the tendon; if the muscle belly is tapped, a denervated muscle will contract as a result of a direct effect on the muscle.

As with much of the neurological examination, comparisons are essential—right versus left, distal versus proximal, legs versus arms, and limbs versus jaw. Diffusely decreased or increased tendon reflexes—even clonus—can be normal and mean very little out of context. Apparently reduced or absent reflexes can often be obtained with reinforcement; as the tendon of an arm is being tapped, the patient clenches the fist of the other arm, or as the tendon of a leg is being tapped, the patient grabs the flexed fingers of one hand with the flexed fingers of the other and pulls sharply (the Jendrassek maneuver).

There are two types of prolonged reflexes. With cerebellar lesions, particularly if there is coexisting corticospinal tract disease, a tapped patellar tendon causes the knee to extend with a large amplitude and then to oscillate back and forth for several excursions (pendular reflexes). With hypothyroidism there is a strikingly delayed relaxation phase of tendon reflexes as a result of local decreased elasticity in the myxedematous muscle.

The Hoffman reflex consists of flexion of the thumb and other fingers when the patient's middle finger is flicked downward. It is a stretch reflex and not in itself pathological, signifying no more than a brisk reflex with spread.

An inverted or paradoxical reflex consists of an absent tendon reflex with simultaneous contraction of its antagonist, for example, triceps contraction on attempting to elicit a biceps jerk. The mechanism in this instance could be a spinal cord lesion—either intraparenchymal or extraparenchymal—at the fifth cervical segment (eg, a herniated intervertebral disk) causing lower-motor-neuron or motor root impairment. Concomitant corticospinal tract injury would result in hyperactive tendon reflexes below the lesion, and if the sensory limb of the reflex arc is still intact, reflex spread from the stretched biceps produces contraction of the triceps but not of the biceps.

With corticospinal tract lesions it is not unusual to observe hyperactive tendon reflexes in a limb that does not appear hypertonic when moved slowly and passively, probably because the stimulus eliciting the tendon reflex stretches muscle spindles rapidly, exciting dynamic mechanoreceptors. A rapid stretch also simultaneously stimulates a large number of spindles, and as a result of central convergence, divergence, and temporal and spatial summation, motor neurons receive a more powerful input.

▶ Superficial Reflexes

The best known eponym in clinical neurology is the *Babinski response,* described a century ago. As the patient lies with the knee slightly flexed and the thigh externally rotated, the outer sole of the foot is firmly stroked with a blunt point (such as a key or the handle of a reflex hammer) that moves distally along the fifth metatarsal bone and then curves medially over the metatarsal heads. A normal response consists of flexion of the great toe at the metatarsophalyngeal joint, usually accompanied by flexion of the other toes. An abnormal response—the Babinski response or extensor plantar response—consists of extension of the big toe at the metatarsophalyngeal joint and extension and separation (fanning) of the other

toes. Physiologically, ankle and toe extension are actually flexion (dorsiflexion), and the Babinski response, which signifies corticospinal tract dysfunction, can be considered part of a polysynaptic flexor withdrawal response released by the pyramidal lesion (Figure 6–3). It is therefore not unusual for ankle dorsiflexion and even knee or hip flexion to accompany the toe dorsiflexion, and indeed with spastic paraplegia resulting from severe spinal cord injury, the response may consist of full flexion at all lower extremity joints, accompanied by bladder and bowel evacuation.

When strength is preserved, stroking the sole often produces voluntary withdrawal, and the response is then difficult to interpret. Voluntary movements can be decreased by stroking the lateral side of the foot rather than the sole, and equivocal movements sometimes become clearer when the maneuver is repeated with the knee extended. A variety of alternative stimuli, each with its own eponym, include running the knuckles along the shin, squeezing the calf muscle or the Achilles tendon, and pricking the dorsum of the big toe with a pin.

The Babinski response signifies corticospinal tract dysfunction, but not necessarily due to a structural lesion. It is observed in metabolic encephalopathies, including hepatic coma, uremia, and hypoglycemia. Even in the presence of corticospinal tract damage, a Babinski response will not be present if there is coexisting interruption of the reflex arc, either sensory (posterior tibial nerve or S1 root) or motor (peroneal nerve or L4 and L5 roots). The corticospinal tract is not fully myelinated at birth, and so a Babinski response is normal during the first few months of life.

The abdominal reflex is obtained by lightly stroking each quadrant of the abdomen with a blunt point. A normal response consists of contraction of the abdominal muscles beneath the quadrant being stroked. An absent reflex may be due to corticospinal tract lesions above the segment being stimulated or to interruption of the reflex arc (segments T6 to L1) at either the sen-

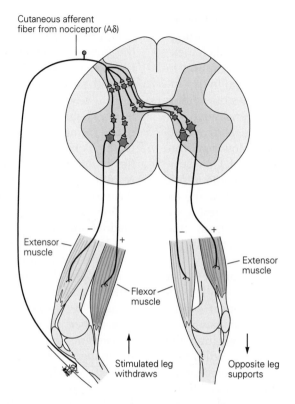

Figure 6–3. Flexion (and crossed extension) reflexes are mediated by polysynaptic pathways. A noxious stimulus activates motor neurons supplying ipsilateral flexor muscles and inhibits (through inhibitory interneurons) antagonist muscles in the same limb. Simultaneously, motor neurons supplying contralateral extensor muscles are excited, providing support during withdrawal of the limb. [Reproduced with permission from Kandel ER, Schwartz JH, Jessell TM. 1999. *Principles of Neural Science*, 4th ed. New York: McGraw-Hill. Adapted with permission from Schmidt RF. 1983. Motor systems. In: Schmidt RF, Thews G (eds), Biederman-Thorson MA (transl): *Human Physiology.* Berlin: Springer-Verlag, pp. 81–110.]

sory end (eg, severe herpes zoster) or the motor end (eg, abdominal surgery). Abdominal reflexes are often unobtainable in the obese or the very anxious. When they are absent because of corticospinal tract dysfunction, there is often coexisting hyperactivity of abdominal muscle stretch reflexes.

A normal cremasteric reflex consists of retraction of the ipsilateral testicle and scrotum when the inner upper thigh is stroked. A normal anal reflex consists of contraction of the external anal sphincter when the perianal skin is lightly scratched with a pin (anal wink). A normal bulbocavernosus reflex consists of contraction of the bulbospongiosis muscle at the base of the penis in response to pinching the glans penis. Like the

abdominal reflex, the cremasteric and the anal and bulbocavernosus reflexes will be absent as a result of either a lesion interrupting the reflex arc (involving segments L1 and L2 for the cremasteric reflex and either the pudendal nerves; sacral roots 2, 3, and 4; or the conus medullaris for the anal and bulbocavernosus reflexes) or a lesion affecting the corticospinal tracts.

▶ Other Reflexes

A number of reflexes present in newborns disappear during the first few months of life. These include the grasp reflex (the fingers involuntarily grip the examiner's fingers and hold on tight), the snout reflex (the lips purse when tapped), the rooting reflex (the mouth moves toward whichever side is being stroked), and the sucking reflex. These reflexes are sometimes observed in patients with frontal lobe damage, and are then referred to as frontal release signs, implying release from suprasegmental inhibitory control. Their mechanism is not really as well-understood as that term suggests, and they are sometimes seen in otherwise normal elderly people. Related phenomena include the palmomental reflex (contraction of the mentalis muscle as the thenar eminence is firmly stroked) and forced groping (involuntary movement of the hand toward the stimulus as the patient's palm or fingers are stroked).

Myerson's sign consists of repetitive blinking or blepharospasm as the glabella is lightly tapped. It is commonly observed in patients with Parkinson disease, but like frontal release signs is neither specific nor sensitive.

7

Examination of the Comatose Patient

▶ Definitions and Initial Assessment

Consciousness is awareness of oneself and one's environment; it requires both arousal and mental content. The anatomic substrate for arousal is the reticular activating system of the brain stem and thalamus; the anatomic substrate for mental content is the cerebrum. Impaired consciousness thus follows either small brain stem lesions or large bilateral cerebral lesions. Temporary loss of consciousness can follow sudden severe lesions within a single cerebral hemisphere, for example, intracerebral hemorrhage. The mechanism is a poorly understood transsynaptic functional suppression of the opposite hemisphere referred to as *diaschisis* and reflected in decreased blood flow, oxygen uptake, and glucose metabolism. Prolonged or permanent loss of consciousness, however, indicates damage—structural or metabolic—either to the cerebral hemispheres bilaterally or to the reticular activating system.

Coma is a state of unconsciousness that clinically differs from syncope in being sustained and from sleep in being less readily reversed. Whereas cerebral oxygen uptake is reduced in coma, it is normal during sleep and actually increases during the rapid eye movement (REM) phase. Coma, moreover, reflcts inhibition or destruction of brain circuits, whereas sleep involves activation of circuits that are normally suppressed during wakefulness.

SEE CASE 61 | p. 235

"A 50-year-old woman begins having attacks of daytime sleepiness."

SEE CASE 62 | p. 239

"A 52-year-old man begins having nocturnal insomnia, impotence, and loss of libido."

Clinically, coma is defined by the neurological examination, particularly by responses to external stimuli. As noted in Chapter 2, terms such as stupor, obtundation, and lethargy indicate different points along a continuum from coma to alertness, but such terms are not precisely defined, and it is therefore appropriate to record the minimal stimulus required to elicit a response and the nature of that response (eg, "The patient responds to her name being shouted by briefly opening her eyes and mumbling incomprehensibly, but she does not look at the examiner or follow commands."). The actual level of consciousness is sometimes difficult to determine, for example, in patients with catatonia, severe depression, or akinesia plus aphasia. A patient receiving a neuromuscular blocking drug such as curare might be fully alert, but to an examiner the alertness would be masked by total paralysis.

Delirium refers to severe inattentiveness, often with abnormal mental content and agitation. It can presage or alternate with obtundation, stupor, or coma.

Assessment of a comatose patient begins with the identification and treatment of any immediately life-threatening condition such as hemorrhage, shock, cardiac arrhythmia, airway obstruction, or apnea. If the diagnosis is uncertain, blood is drawn for glucose determination and glucose is administered intravenously, accompanied by thiamine. (Thiamine is a cofactor for a number of enzymes involved in glucose metabolism; in a thiamine-deficient patient— usually an alcoholic—glucose administration can precipitate Wernicke-Korsakoff encephalopathy by depleting critical thiamine stores in the brain.) If opioid overdose is a possibility, an opioid antagonist such as naloxone is given. If trauma is suspected, cervical fracture and damage to internal organs must be excluded.

A history is obtained from whoever accompanies the patient, including ambulance drivers and police. A previously healthy adult who collapses while playing tennis raises diagnostic considerations different from those raised by a known hypothyroid adult who, missing for several days, is found on the floor of her apartment. The general physical examination often provides important clues. For example, the skin, nails, and mucous membranes might reflect anemia (pallor), hypoxia (cyanosis), carbon monoxide poisoning (cherry redness), liver failure (jaundice), kidney failure (uremic frost), hypoadrenalism (hyperpigmentation), shock (cold clamminess), dehydration (decreased turgor), coagulopathy (petechiae or purpura), prolonged immobility (decubitus ulcers), or trauma. The optic fundi might suggest increased intracranial pressure (papilledema), hypertension (hemorrhages, exudates, and arteriolar narrowing), diabetes mellitus (microaneurysms and exudates), endocarditis (Roth spots—large exudates with a central hemorrhage), tuberculosis (granulomas), or subarachnoid hemorrhage (subhyaloid hemorrhages). Fever could indicate infection or heat stroke; hypothermia could indicate exposure to cold, hypoglycemia, hypothyroidism, or sepsis. Asymmetry of pulses might reflect dissecting aneurysm. Urinary or fecal incontinence could be the result of an unwitnessed seizure, particularly in a patient who recovers consciousness spontaneously. Fractures of the base of the skull produce ecchymosis behind the ear (Battle sign) or periorbitally (raccoon sign); when they communicate with the subarachnoid space, they cause cerebrospinal fluid otorrhea or rhinorrhea (and, eventually, bacterial meningitis). Resistance to passive neck flexion but not to turning suggests meningitis, subarachnoid hemorrhage, or herniation of the cerebellar tonsils through the foramen magnum. Resistance to movement in any direction is more typical of bone or joint disease (including fracture—the neck should be immobilized until history or radiography unequivocally excludes cervical injury).

▶ Focusing on the Neurological Evaluation

In a classic monograph, Plum and Posner (*The Diagnosis of Stupor and Coma,* 3rd edition. F.A. Davis, 1980) divided the causes of coma into three categories: supratentorial structural lesions, infratentorial structural lesions, and diffuse or metabolic disorders. They further emphasized that in the great majority of cases, the clinician can determine which of these three types of coma is present by focusing the neurological examination on four areas: (1) spontaneous movements and motor responses to stimuli, (2) the respiratory pattern, (3) the pupils, and (4) eye movements.

Limb Movement

The motor examination begins with observation of spontaneous movements, asymmetry of which could signify focal seizures or hemiparesis. Motor responses to stimuli can be appropriate, inappropriate, or absent. Appropriate responses range from correctly following verbal commands to fending off or withdrawing from a noxious stimulus (such as pressing on the supraorbital bone or sternum, pinching the neck or limbs, and squeezing a muscle, tendon, or nailbed). Inappropriate responses include provoked myoclonus or seizures as well as so-called decorticate and decerebrate rigidity (Figure 7–1). Usually occurring in response to a noxious stimulus, *decorticate rigidity* consists of arm flexion and leg extension, and *decerebrate rigidity* consists of extension of arms as well as legs. Internal rotation of the shoulders accompanies these responses, a useful feature in distinguishing them from purposeful movements. Anatomically and physiologically, decorticate and decerebrate rigidity are misleading terms. Coined by Sherrington, decorticate rigidity referred to sustained forelimb flexion and hindlimb extension in cats whose mesencephalons had been transected between the superior and inferior colliculi; decerebrate rigidity referred to sustained extension of all four limbs following brain stem transection caudal to the inferior colliculus.

The terms decorticate and decerebrate do not really reflect Sherrington's surgical sites. Moreover, stuporous or comatose humans who demonstrate these responses are usually not hypertonic; flexion or extension occurs in response to a stimulus and disappears when the stimulus is removed. When flexion or extension occurs spontaneously, alternative interpretations should be considered (eg, a tonic seizure) or an unrecognized stimulus should be sought (eg, an obstructed airway). Flexor and extensor posturing are more appropriate terms for these clinical phenomena.

Such postures most often occur with cerebral hemispheric disease, including metabolic encephalopathy; they can also follow upper brain stem lesions, including damage secondary to transtentorial herniation. Flexor posturing generally indicates a more rostral lesion (and a better prognosis) than does extensor posturing, but the pattern of response may vary with the site of stimulation (eg, sternal versus nailbed pressure), and one arm may exhibit flexion and the other arm may exhibit extension. With the descending brain stem damage that accompanies transtentorial herniation (rostrocaudal deterioration), flexor posturing may be succeeded by extensor posturing, in turn progressing to leg flexion, and finally to flaccid unresponsiveness. (Lack of motor response to any stimulus could also, of course, reflect limb paralysis from either central or peripheral lesions—eg, cervical trauma or Guillain-Barré polyneuropathy.)

Respiration

Cheyne-Stokes respiration consists of periods of hyperventilation alternating with apnea; a gradual crescendo–decrescendo pattern marks the transition between the two phases (Figure 7–2). The hyperpneic phase is usually longer than the apneic phase, and so arterial pH and pCO_2 tend to reflect respiratory alkalosis. During the apneic phase there may be decreased responsiveness, reduced muscle tone, and miosis. Cheyne-Stokes respiration occurs with bilateral cerebral hemispheric disease, including metabolic encephalopathy (particularly hypoxia). It can be a feature of impending or early transtentorial herniation, but it usually signifies that the patient is not in imminent danger; emergency endotrachial intubation would not be mandated by the presence of Cheyne-Stokes respiration.

Sustained hyperventilation in a stuporous or comatose patient is usually secondary to a readily identifiable drive such as metabolic acidosis (Kussmaul breathing) or pulmonary disease. Hyperventilation is also a feature of hepatic encephalopathy and of aspirin poisoning and other drug toxicities; in such situations arterial pH and pCO_2 usually demonstrate variable combinations of metabolic acidosis and respiratory alkalosis. Rare but more ominous is *central neurogenic hyperventilation*, sometimes a consequence of rostral brain stem lesions, including damage incurred during transtentorial herniation; in such patients respiratory alkalosis can be severe enough to lower blood levels of ionized calcium, producing tetany.

Ataxic respiration is irregularly irregular and indicates pontine or medullary injury.

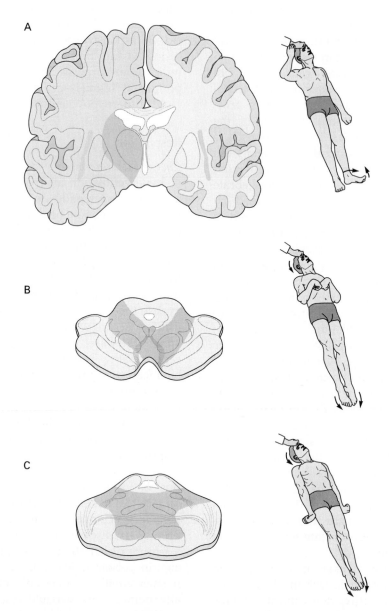

Figure 7–1. Motor responses to noxious stimulation, in this case at the supraorbital ridge. **A.** In a patient with right cerebral damage (metabolic encephalopathy), the stimulus produces voluntary movement of the right arm, which attempts to remove the stimulus. The paralyzed left arm does not move, and the paralyzed left leg lies externally rotated. **B.** In a patient with damage to the diencephalon or rostral midbrain, the stimulus produces flexion and internal rotation of the arms and extension of the legs (decorticate posturing). **C.** In a patient with more caudal midbrain or rostral pontine damage, the stimulus produces extension of all four limbs (although the wrists and fingers remain flexed) (decerebrate posturing). (Reproduced with permission from Kandel ER, Schwartz JH, Jessell TM. 1999. *Principles of Neural Science,* 4th ed. New York: McGraw-Hill.)

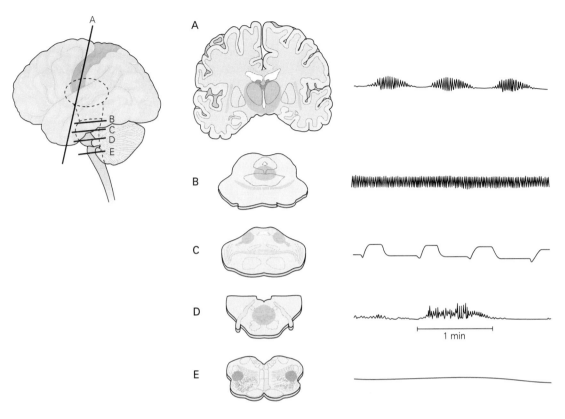

Figure 7–2. Abnormal respiratory patterns. **A.** Cheyne-Stokes respiration. **B.** Hyperventilation. **C.** Apneustic respiration. **D.** Ataxic respiration. **E.** Apnea. (Reproduced with permission from Kandel ER, Schwartz JH, Jessell TM. 1999. *Principles of Neural Science*, 4th ed. New York: McGraw-Hill.)

Sometimes the irregular breathing alternates with periods of apnea, which, unlike the apnea of Cheyne-Stokes respiration, begins and ends abruptly (cluster breathing, also referred to as short-cycle Cheyne-Stokes respiration). Ataxic or cluster breathing is an emergency mandating immediate endotracheal intubation, for sustained apnea can ensue at any time. If transtentorial herniation has progressed to the point of producing ataxic respiration, full functional recovery is unlikely.

Apneustic breathing, consisting of inspiratory pauses, is associated with pontine lesions, particularly infarction. It is infrequently encountered in metabolic encephalopathy or during the course of transtentorial herniation.

The phrenic nerve to the diaphragm arises from spinal cord segments C3 to C5. Rostral to this level are separate anatomic pathways for voluntary (as during speaking or singing) and involuntary (automatic) breathing. Lower brain stem lesions can produce a dramatic dissociation referred to as Ondine's curse, in which automatic respirations are lost but voluntary respirations are preserved; as the patient becomes less alert, fatal apnea can ensue.

Other ominous respiratory signs are end expiratory pushing (like coughing) and fishmouthing (jaw opening with each inspiration). Stertorous breathing is inspiratory noise, an indication of airway obstruction.

Pupils

As with awake patients, during coma pupillary abnormalities may reflect a disturbance of the sympathetic system, the parasympathetic system, or both (Figure 7–3) (see Chapter 3). Many normal people have slightly unequal pupils (anisocoria), but in a comatose patient anisocoria is presumed to be abnormal until proven otherwise. Parasympathetic lesions (eg, pressure on the oculomotor nerve by transtentorial herniation of a temporal lobe or by an internal carotid artery aneurysm) cause pupillary dilatation and unreactivity to light. Sympathetic lesions (eg, lateral medullary infarction or compression of the superior cervical ganglion by lung cancer) cause miosis with preserved reactivity to light. With large pontine hemorrhages the pupils are

pinpoint, and such extreme miosis makes it difficult to discern light reactivity; transection of descending intraparenchymal sympathetic pathways is an obvious explanation for the miosis, but because miosis of this degree is not encountered in Horner syndrome caused by lesions at other points along the sympathetic pathway, it has been proposed that pontine hemorrhage produces additional disinhibition of the Edinger-Westphal nucleus by destroying an inhibitory region of the pontine reticular formation.

Combined parasympathetic and sympathetic lesions produce midposition pupils unreactive to light, and the midbrain tegmentum is where the parasympathetic and sympathetic pathways pass closest to one another. Damage to the midbrain could be direct, for example, infarction secondary

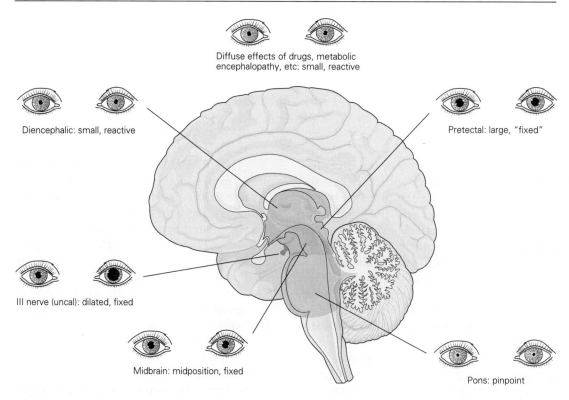

Figure 7–3. Pupillary abnormalities encountered in comatose patients. (Reproduced with permission from Kandel ER, Schwartz JH, Jessell TM. 1999. *Principles of Neural Science*, 4th ed. New York: McGraw-Hill.)

to embolic occlusion of the top of the basilar artery as it branches into the two posterior cerebral arteries. Alternatively, the midbrain could be secondarily damaged by a lesion originating elsewhere, for example, rostral extension of a pontine hemorrhage or midbrain compression during the course of transtentorial herniation. A history, serial examinations, or an image such as a computerized tomographic (CT) scan might be necessary to determine whether the problem began rostral or caudal to the midbrain or within it.

Pupillary inequality can also be local in origin, the result, for example, of iritis with lens adhesions, iris trauma during cataract surgery, or pilocarpine eye drops for glaucoma. As noted in Chapter 3, an afferent lesion (such as optic nerve trauma) will cause an afferent pupillary defect but not anisocoria.

In general, metabolic disease does not cause unequal or unreactive pupils except terminally. Exceptions include anticholinergic drugs (atropine and scopolamine, as well as some antidepressant and antiparkinsonian drugs and the rarely used sedative glutethimide) and anoxic-ischemic brain damage (in which case pupillary unreactivity lasting more than a few hours carries a poor prognosis).

Hypothermia and severe barbiturate intoxication can each produce not only unreactive pupils but loss of all brain stem reflexes, mimicking brain death (see below). Bilateral or unilateral pupillary dilatation and unreactivity can accompany (or briefly outlast) a seizure. With opioid overdose, the pupils are pinpoint and, as with pontine hemorrhage, reactivity may require a very bright light and a magnifying glass to detect. Opioids do not directly block the light reflex, but by producing apnea and anoxic-ischemic brain damage, overdose can indirectly result in mydriasis and pupillary unreactivity.

Eyelids and Eye Movements

Eye closure requires the facial nerve, and so closed eyelids or blinking in a comatose pa-

tient indicate that the lower pons is intact. Blinking can occur with or without purposeful limb movements. As in awake patients, in comatose patients eyes conjugately deviated away from paretic limbs indicate a destructive cerebral lesion on the side toward which the eyes are deviated; eyes conjugately deviated toward paretic limbs indicate either a destructive brain stem lesion or an irritative cerebral lesion (ie, a seizure) contralateral to the direction of gaze.

Conjugate gaze away from the side of the lesion is also encountered infrequently in thalamic hemorrhage—so-called wrong-way gaze. The explanation is unclear. Projections from the frontal eye fields to the pontine centers for lateral gaze (the paramedian pontine reticular formation—PPRF) cross in the lower midbrain, well below a thalamic lesion, which therefore should result in ipsilateral conjugate eye deviation similar to that produced by lesions in the frontal eye fields. Partial seizures probably explain some—but not all—cases of thalamic wrong-way gaze.

Downward deviation of the eyes (sunsetting) follows damage to the rostral interstitial nucleus of the median longitudinal fasciculus in the midbrain or to its connections through the posterior commissure to the oculomotor nerve nuclei. The damage can be direct, as with midbrain infarction or neoplasm, or indirect, as with caudal extension of a thalamic hemorrhage or extrinsic compression by a strategically placed neoplasm such as a pinealoma. Such patients often have unreactive pupils (Parinaud syndrome). Downward deviation of the eyes also occurs in metabolic coma, particularly barbiturate poisoning. During a major motor seizure the eyes may be deviated upward, followed by postictal downward deviation.

Eyes horizontally disconjugate at rest may indicate paresis of the medial or lateral rectus muscles, internuclear ophthalmoplegia, or preexisting tropia or phoria (see Chapter 3). A lesion causing horizontal disconjugate gaze could involve the brain stem, the cranial nerves innervating the extraocular muscles, or the muscles themselves. Lateral deviation of one eye secondary to medial rectus palsy occurs with transtentorial herniation and oculomotor nerve compression (in which case the pupil will very likely be larger on the side of the outwardly deviated eye). Medial deviation of one eye secondary to lateral rectus palsy occurs with structural lesions within the brain stem, along the course of the abducens nerve, or within the orbit. By a mechanism not well understood, lateral rectus palsy is sometimes a false localizing sign secondary to raised intracranial pressure in the absence of compartmental shifts—for example, in pseudotumor cerebri. The vulnerability of the abducens nerve in such a setting has been attributed to the length of its course along the base of the brain.

Eyes vertically disconjugate at rest may indicate paresis of the superior or inferior rectus muscles, the superior or inferior oblique muscles, skew deviation, or preexisting tropia or phoria.

Spontaneous eye movements can be appropriate or inappropriate. Eyes that slowly rove from side to side indicate not only that brain stem areas subserving such movements are intact, but also that the patient is not awake, for such movements cannot be made voluntarily unless the eyes are pursuing or fixating on a target. Rapid jerky saccadic eye movements, on the other hand, suggest wakefulness. Saccadic eye movements can briefly replace slow eye movements when a patient is aroused by a noxious stimulus; their presence does not necessarily imply malingering.

Inappropriate eye movements identified by simple inspection include ocular bobbing, which can be unilateral or bilateral, in either case signifying pontine dysfunction. When bobbing is bilateral, the lesion can be either intrinsic to the pons, as with infarction, or secondary to metabolic encephalopathy, to extrinsic pontine compression (eg, from a cerebellar hemorrhage), or to pontine damage during the course of transtentorial herniation. Unilateral bobbing is more suggestive of a primary pontine event. Other inappropriate eye movements include ping

pong gaze and convergence or retractatory nystagmus (see Chapter 3). Horizontal or vertical nystagmus is rare during coma.

Following inspection the examination proceeds to testing eye movement reflexes. If cervical injury has been excluded, oculocephalic testing (the so-called doll's eye maneuver) is performed by passively turning the patient's head from side to side. Unless fixated on a target, an awake subject's eyes will simply turn with the head. The eyes of a stuporous or comatose patient whose reflex arc is intact (vestibular afferents connecting in the brain stem to efferents that innervate the extrinsic eye muscles) will move conjugately in the opposite direction (Figure 7–4). If the oculocephalic maneuver produces an absent or equivocal response, a more vigorous stimulus is produced by irrigating each ear with 30 to 100 mL of ice water. As noted earlier, in an awake patient a normal response includes nystagmus and vertigo. In a comatose patient whose head is elevated 30° and whose reflex arc is intact, there will be deviation of the eyes, usually lasting several minutes, conjugately toward the stimulated side. Simultaneous bilateral irrigation produces vertical deviation, downward after cold water and upward after warm water.

Appropriate ocular deviation during oculocephalic or caloric testing signifies that the patient has depressed alertness and that the reflex arc is intact. (As with other stimuli, however, these maneuvers can themselves produce brief arousal.) Oculocephalic and caloric testing can identify gaze palsies and individual muscle palsies. (Cerebral gaze paresis can often be overcome by these maneuvers, for the reflex arc is intact; however, brain stem gaze palsy and individual muscle paresis are usually not overcome by vestibular stimulation.) An absent response could be due to labyrinthine destruction (eg, from surgery for Ménière disease) or disease in the orbits (eg, progressive external ophthalmoplegia), but in a stuporous or comatose patient an absent response usually signifies brain stem damage. Severe metabolic coma can obliterate spontaneous and reflexic eye movements, but with the ex-

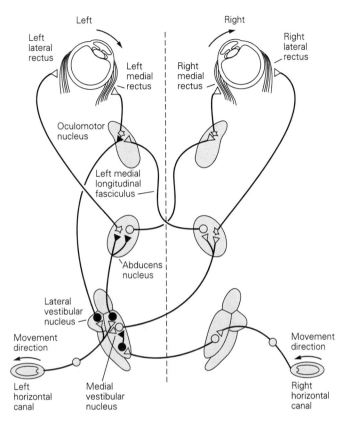

Figure 7–4. The vestibuloocular reflex begins with stimulation of peripheral vestibular receptors, either by head turning or by exposure of a semicircular canal to warm or cold temperature. The reflex is mediated through the lateral and medial vestibular nuclei, the abducens nucleus, and, via the medial longitudinal fasciculus, the contralateral oculomotor nucleus. Filled neurons represent inhibitory connections and unfilled neurons represent excitatory connections. (Reproduced with permission from Kandel ER, Schwartz JH, Jessell TM. 1991. *Principles of Neural Science,* 3rd ed. Norwalk, CT: Appleton & Lange.)

ception of certain drugs (particularly barbiturates and the anticonvulsant phenytoin), eye movements are preserved early in metabolic encephalopathy. As with unreactive pupils, their absence several hours after anoxic-ischemic brain damage is an ominous sign.

SEE CASE 58 | p. 229

"While rollerblading, an 18-year-old boy is rendered briefly unconscious after falling."

▶ Distinguishing Types of Coma

Coma from Supratentorial Structural Lesions

As previously noted, structural lesions above the tentorium can cause coma as a result of bilateral cerebral destruction, acute severe unilateral cerebral damage with contralateral functional disruption (diaschisis), or cerebral herniation, either laterally beneath the falx cerebri or transtentorially from the middle to the posterior fossa. With lateral or downward cerebral herniation, coma is the result of damage to the ascending reticular activating system in the thalamus and midbrain. Studies with computerized tomography indicate that with cerebral hemispheric mass lesions early decreased alertness correlates more with lateral brain displacement than with transtentorial herniation. Eventually, if the process is not halted, downward herniation ensues. The constellation of signs that follows depends on whether the supratentorial mass is located laterally (eg, a subdural hematoma over the cerebral convexity) or medially (eg, a thalamic hemorrhage).

In lateral herniation (also called uncal herniation—the uncus is the anterior part of the hippocampus) there is early compression of the oculomotor nerve by the inferomedial temporal lobe, with ipsilateral pupillary enlargement. If the process develops slowly, alertness may persist in the presence of anisocoria, but by the time there is full pupillary dilatation and loss of light reactivity, consciousness rapidly deteriorates and eye movements are affected. Horizontal impairment is more obvious than vertical impairment; limitation of adduction, attributable to oculomotor nerve compression, may produce an outward turning of the eye, but if there is additional limitation of abduction, attributable to the false localizing effect of increased intracranial pressure, the eye may remain in midposition. The contralateral eye is soon involved, and there is progression of respiratory abnormalities (eg, Cheyne-Stokes respirations, followed by hyperventilation, ataxic breathing, and then apnea) and posturing (eg, flexion of the arms and extension of the legs, followed by extension of all four limbs, then flexion of the legs, and then unresponsiveness even to noxious stimuli). In addition to damaging neural structures, midbrain compression obliterates the aqueduct of Sylvius, causing an obstructive hydrocephalus that accentuates rostrocaudal pressure differences and accelerates transtentorial herniation. The posterior cerebral arteries (which pass from the posterior to the middle fossa across the tentorial edge) are also sometimes compressed; the result is occipital lobe infarction.

In medial (central) herniation there is early impaired consciousness, for the reticular activating system is affected from the outset. The pupils initially may be normal or even small (perhaps from involvement of descending sympathetic pathways within the hypothalamus or upper midbrain). Pupillary and eye movement abnormalities tend to progress bilaterally, and early involvement of descending sympathetic pathways means that unreactive pupils are more likely to be midposition than fully dilated. Respiratory abnormalities and posturing progress as in lateral herniation, and the result is the same: unresponsiveness to any stimulus, unreactive pupils, ophthalmoplegia, and apnea.

During the course of transtentorial herniation there may be, unexpectedly, hemiparesis ipsilateral to the supratentorial lesion; the reason is lateral displacement of the midbrain by the herniating temporal lobe, with compression of the contralateral corticospinal tract against the tentorial edge. The corticospinal tract does not cross until the lower medulla, and so the resulting hemiparesis is ipsilateral to the supratentorial mass. Less often, lateral displacement compresses the contralateral oculomotor nerve; as a consequence, the contralateral pupil is sometimes dilated before the ipsilateral pupil.

Coma From Infratentorial Structural Lesions

Structural lesions below the tentorium— within the posterior fossa—cause coma by directly damaging the reticular activating system or, if they are extraparenchymal or within the cerebellum, by compressing it. Mass lesions can produce upward transtentorial herniation with oculomotor palsy and midbrain compression. More often posterior fossa lesions cause herniation of the inferiorly located cerebellar tonsils through the foramen magnum. Coma in such a setting is indirect, the result of respiratory and circulatory collapse, for the reticular formation at the level of the medulla does not contribute to arousal.

Metabolic Coma

Altered mentation and respiratory abnormalities tend to occur early with metabolic, diffuse, or multifocal encephalopathy; often there is tremor, asterixis, or myoclonus (see Chapter 4). There may be diffuse rigidity, frontal release reflexes (snout, suck, grasp), and flexor or extensor posturing. With the exception of anticholinergic intoxication and anoxic-ischemic brain damage, the pupils remain reactive. The eyes may be deviated downward, but lateral deviation or disconjugate eye movements are not indicative of a metabolic disturbance. Although lateralizing neurological signs should suggest a unilateral structural lesion, metabolic disorders—particularly hyperglycemia and hypoglycemia—can cause both focal seizures and hemiparesis.

▶ Differentiating From Coma

Malingering, Conversion, and Catatonia

Malingering, conversion, and catatonia apply to subjects who at first appear to be comatose but are not. By definition, *malingering* indicates conscious willful feigning of symptoms and signs, whereas *conversion* (hysteria) indicates symptoms and signs that have no actual neurological (or organic) basis but rather reflect psychological disturbances of which the patient is not consciously aware. Whether or not this distinction has neurobehavioral validity, malingered and hysterical coma are clinically identical. The eyes are usually closed, and when the lids are passively raised and then released, they do not descend smoothly as in someone who is not awake but rather close abruptly or jerkily. Lightly stroking the eyelashes produces lid fluttering. The eyes do not rove smoothly but rather move in jerky saccades. The oculocephalic maneuver does not produce eye movement in a direction contralateral to head turning, and caloric testing produces nystagmus, not conjugate eye deviation. Respirations are either nor-

mal or tachypneic. Limb tone is normal. Although visual threat or noxious stimuli often produce appropriate blinking or limb withdrawal, very determined patients sometimes demonstrate a remarkably stoic unresponsiveness even when their nailbeds are being crushed. The electroencephalogram (EEG) can be particularly useful when feigned unresponsiveness is suspected. It is always abnormal in true stupor or coma, demonstrating slowing, sharp waves, or both. With feigned coma, unless brain disease or a drug effect is also present, the EEG is normal.

Catatonia usually refers to a psychic state in which the patient, although awake, lies immobile, mute, and unresponsive except for a bizarre plastic rigidity of the limbs (catalepsy), which remain in whatever position they are placed. Sometimes immobility is abruptly interrupted by excitement or aggression. An infrequent feature of schizophrenic psychosis, catatonia can also be the result of acute anxiety, depression, toxic psychosis (particularly phencyclidine poisoning), and other brain diseases. Physiologically and anatomically, catatonia is probably related to abulia, a state of psychomotor bradykinesia and mutism resulting from damage to the mediofrontal lobes (see Chapter 2).

Locked-in Syndrome

Patients who are locked-in also appear comatose on casual inspection, lying immobile and not moving their limbs to command. Further examination reveals that they can voluntarily move their eyes up or down, and when these eye movements are used as coded responses to questions ("up means yes; down means no"), it becomes evident that mentation is normal. The lesion responsible for producing paralysis of all movement except upward and downward gaze is most often in the rostral basis pontis (eg, infarction, neoplasm, or demyelination secondary to central pontine myelinolysis). Destruction of descending corticobulbar and corticospinal projections eliminates voluntary movement of the jaw, face, pharynx, tongue, neck, limbs, and trunk. Lateral eye movements may or may not be affected, but involuntary respirations and alertness, which depend on tegmental structures, are preserved. So, usually, is sensation, for the tegmentally located medial lemnesci and spinothalamic tracks are also spared. Some locked-in patients are able to blink despite facial paralysis; this is because attempting to do so produces reflex inhibition of the orbicularis oculi's antagonist, the levator palpebrae, causing the lid to descend passively.

SEE CASE 31 | p. 165

"A 54-year-old, hypertensive diabetic man experiences vertigo, nausea, and vomiting, followed by weakness of all four limbs and inability to talk."

Vegetative State

The term *vegetative state* refers to isolated brain stem function after massive bilateral cerebral or diencephalic damage (Table 7–1).

Table 7–1. Criteria for determination of vegetative state.

1. No evidence of awareness of self or surroundings; reflex or spontaneous eye opening may occur
2. No communication between examiner and patient, auditory or written, that is meaningful and consistent; target stimuli not usually followed visually, but sometimes visual tracking present; no emotional response to verbal stimuli
3. No comprehensible speech or mouthing of words
4. Smiling, frowning, or crying inconsistently related to any apparent stimulus
5. Sleep–wake cycles present
6. Brain stem and spinal reflexes variable, for example, preservation of sucking, rooting, chewing, swallowing, pupillary reactivity to light, oculocephalic responses, and grasp or tendon reflexes
7. No voluntary movements or behavior, no matter how rudimentary; no motor activity suggesting learned behavior, no mimicry; withdrawal or posturing can occur with noxious stimuli
8. Usually intact blood pressure control and cardiorespiratory function; incontinence of bladder and bowel

Table 7–2. Criteria for determination of brain death.

1. Coma, unresponsive to stimuli above foramen magnum
2. Apnea off ventilator (with oxygenation) for a duration sufficient to produce hypercarbic respiratory drive (usually 10 to 20 minutes to achieve pCO_2 of 60 mm Hg)
3. Absence of cephalic reflexes, including pupillary, oculocephalic, oculovestibular (caloric), corneal, gag, sucking, swallowing, and extensor posturing; purely spinal reflexes may be present, including tendon reflexes, plantar responses, and limb flexion to noxious stimuli
4. Body temperature above 34 °C
5. Systemic circulation may be intact
6. Diagnosis known to be structural disease or irreversible metabolic disturbance; absence of drug intoxication, including ethanol, sedatives, potentially anesthetizing agents, or paralyzing drugs
7. In adults with known structural cause and without involvement of drugs or ethanol, at least 6 hours of absent brain function; for others, including those with anoxic-ischemic brain damage, at least 24 hours of observation plus negative drug screen
8. Diagnosis of brain death inappropriate in infants younger than 7 days of age; observation of at least 48 hours for infants aged 7 days to 2 months, at least 24 hours for those aged 2 months to 1 year, and at least 12 hours for those aged 1 to 5 years (24 hours if anoxic-ischemic brain damage); for older children, adult criteria apply
9. Optional confirmatory studies include the following:
   a. Electroencephalogram isoelectric for 30 minutes at maximal gain
   b. Absent brain stem–evoked responses
   c. Absent cerebral circulation demonstrated by radiographic, radioisotope, or magnetic resonance angiography

In contrast to patients in coma, vegetative patients have sleep–wake cycles, and in contrast to brain dead patients (see below), the brain stem reflexes of vegetative patients are preserved. Vegetative patients have intact cardiorespiratory function, and they make primitive responses to stimuli (including eye opening to loud noise), but although they demonstrate arousal, what is aroused is devoid of mental content. There is no evidence of inner or outer awareness—of an existing mind. Patients who survive coma usually show variable degrees of recovery within 2 to 4 weeks. Those who enter the vegetative state may recover further, even fully, or their recovery may stop at that point. Persistent vegetative state is defined as lasting at least 1 month. Further recovery is then unlikely, but exceptions have been anecdotally reported.

SEE CASE 60 | p. 233

"A 21-year-old woman is found apneic and pulseless following ingestion of sedatives combined with ethanol."

Brain Death

In contrast to a vegetative state, in which brain stem functions are preserved, *brain death* means that neither the cerebrum nor the brain stem is functioning. The only spontaneous activity is cardiovascular, apnea persists in the presence of hypercarbia, and the only reflexes present are those mediated by the spinal cord (Table 7–2). Brain death rarely lasts more than a few days; cardiovascular control centers in the medulla are eventually affected, and circulatory collapse ensues. In the United States brain death is equated with legal death. When the criteria of Table 7–2 are met, artificial ventilation and blood pressure support should be discontinued, whether organ donation is intended or not.

SEE CASE 57 | p. 227

"A 56-year-old hypertensive man collapses on the sidewalk."

II

79 Ways of Looking at the Nervous System: Case Presentations and Commentary

8

Mostly Somatosensory

▶ CASE 1

During a routine examination a 30-year-old man is found to have diabetes mellitus. Hyperglycemia is controlled with diet and oral hypoglycemic agents until he is age 48, when insulin becomes necessary. At age 49 he notes continuous unpleasant burning paresthesias in both feet, which steadily worsen over the next several years. On examination at age 53 vibratory sensation (128 Hz) is absent at the toes and reduced at the ankles. Pinprick, light touch, and cold sensation are diminished in both feet, and light touch and pinprick produce an abnormal burning sensation in the soles. Position sense is normal. Tendon reflexes are normal at the knees and absent at the ankles. Strength is normal, as is the rest of the neurological examination.

Electrodiagnostic studies reveal normal motor nerve conduction velocities and needle electromyography in his legs and arms. Sensory nerve amplitudes are moderately reduced in the peroneal and sural nerves and at the lower limit of normal in the median nerve. Sensory nerve conduction velocities are normal in the peroneal, sural, and median nerves.

Over the next several years, despite vigorous control of his hyperglycemia, there is gradual progression of sensory loss in his legs, and his fingertips begin to feel numb. By age 62 he is impotent and notices lightheadedness when he stands up quickly. Examination at this time reveals loss of vibratory sensation over his fingers, ankles, and knees. Pinprick, light touch, and cold sensation are markedly reduced below his knees and gradually become normal at mid-thigh; the same modalities are mildly reduced in his fingers. Rubbing his feet no longer produces discomfort. Position sense is mildly reduced in his toes and normal in his ankles and fingers; gait, including tandem, is normal. Tendon reflexes are absent in his legs and present in his arms. Strength is normal.

At electrodiagnostic study sensory nerve amplitudes and conduction velocities are now unobtainable in his legs. In his arms, sensory nerve amplitudes are markedly reduced and sensory nerve conduction velocities are mildly reduced. Motor nerve conduction velocities are moderately reduced in his legs and normal in his arms; needle electromyography reveals evidence of denervation in muscles below the knees.

Comment

The peripheral nervous system consists of sensory, motor, and autonomic nerves, including cranial and spinal nerve roots, sensory and autonomic ganglia, and efferent and afferent nerve endings. The physiology of peripheral nerve axons includes anterograde rapid transport (400/day) of vesicles and protein along neurotubules, mediated by the molecular motor protein kinesin; retrograde rapid transport (200 mm/day), also along neurotubules, of lysosomes and recycled membrane material (as well as exogenous material such as herpes virus, tetanus toxin, or growth factors); and, by less well-understood mechanisms, anterograde slow transport (0.2–3 mm/day) of neurofilament and neurotubule material (Figures 8–1 and 8–2). Large-diameter axons, including motor nerves and sensory A fibers mediating touch, vibration, and position sense, are myelinated; small-diameter axons are either myelinated or unmyelinated. The smallest unmyelinated fibers mediate pain and temperature sensation.

Some peripheral neuropathies are diseases of myelin (eg, the immunological disorder acute inflammatory demyelinating polyradiculoneuropathy, also known

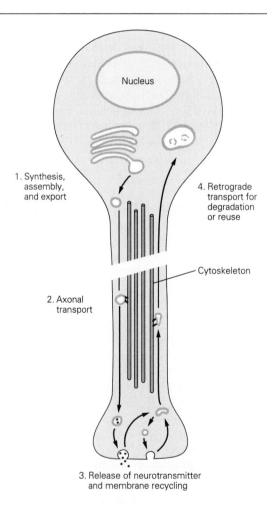

Figure 8–1. Membranous organelles synthesized in the neuron's cell body are rapidly moved by fast axonal transport to the nerve terminal. Degraded material is returned to the cell body by retrograde fast transport. In peripheral sensory neuropathies with axonal damage, impaired axonal transport causes sensory loss, which is greatest distally. (Reproduced with permission from Kandel ER, Schwartz JH, Jessell TM. 1999. *Principles of Neural Science,* 4th ed. New York: McGraw-Hill.)

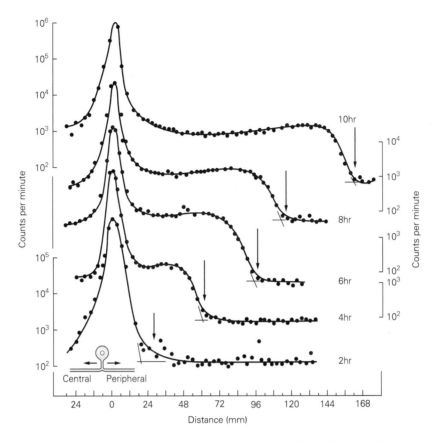

Figure 8–2. Following injection of radioactive protein into dorsal root ganglia at the level of the lumbar spinal cord, the protein is seen to move distally along the sciatic nerve. From this experiment, the rate of fast anterograde axonal transport was calculated at approximately 400 mm/day. (Reproduced with permission from Kandel ER, Schwartz JH, Jessell TM. 1999. *Principles of Neural Science*, 4th ed. New York: McGraw-Hill. Adapted with permission from Ochs S. 1972. Fast transport of materials in mammalian nerve fibers. Science 176:252.)

as Guillain-Barré syndrome—see Case 22); others are axonal disorders (eg, vincristine toxicity, which causes depolymerization of neurotubular protein). *Neuronopathies* affect motor, sensory, or autonomic neuronal cell bodies (eg, the hereditary motor neuropathies, herpes zoster neuronitis, and hereditary dysautonomia). Some peripheral neuropathies are purely sensory and others are purely motor; most are sensorimotor. Those that affect small sensory fibers often involve autonomic nerves as well. Axonal destruction results in rapid breakdown of surrounding myelin but without loss of Schwann cells, allowing axonal regeneration along Schwann cell columns. Myelin destruction results in slowing or blockage of axonal impulse conduction, but anatomic integrity of the axon is usually preserved. Peripheral neuropathy secondary to axonal damage (*axonopathy*) has diverse causes, including drugs, environmental toxins, genetic disorders, nutritional deficiency, uremia, and, as exemplified by the present patient, diabetes mellitus.

Axonal polyneuropathies characteristically produce distal (stocking-glove) weakness or sensory loss. Probably related to failure of axonal transport, degeneration begins distally, gradually advancing proximally (dying-back). Because nerves in the legs are longer than nerves in the arms, sensorimotor symptoms characteristically begin in the feet. Typical for diabetic neuropathy, this patient's symptoms were sensory and reflected involvement of both small- and large-diameter fibers. Axonal injury resulted in marked reduction in the amplitudes of potentials generated by nerve stimulation; a lesser degree of demyelination resulted in mild slowing of nerve conduction velocities. After many years there was electrodiagnostic evidence of motor nerve involvement (slowed motor nerve conduction velocities and electromyographic denervation), but strength remained normal. The patient did eventually develop impotence and postural lightheadedness, reflecting involvement of small-diameter autonomic fibers.

Diabetic polyneuropathy, which eventually affects 50% of diabetics, is probably multifactorial in origin. In experimental diabetic animals it was observed that sorbital, metabolized from glucose by aldose reductase, accumulates in peripheral nerves, where it reciprocally displaces other intraneuronal osmoles, causing, by an uncertain mechanism, depletion of Na^+–K^+-ATPase, particularly at nodes of Ranvier. The result is impaired saltatory conduction and, at electrodiagnostic study, slowing of nerve conduction velocities. This observation led to clinical trials with aldose reductase inhibitors, which, however, failed to demonstrate benefit.

Hyperglycemia also leads to nonenzymatic glycation of structural proteins, including tubulin and neurofilaments, resulting in abnormal axonal transport and distal axonal atrophy. Nonenzymatic glycation may also be responsible for microangiopathic changes observed in endoneurial blood vessels; vasculopathy, although unlikely to be the primary cause of diabetic neuropathy, may impair axonal repair and regeneration. Other observed abnormalities in diabetic nerves include reduced levels of vascular nitric oxide (a vasodilator) and of nerve-like growth factor. A possibly autoimmune microvasculitis has also been described.

Painful paresthesias in diabetic neuropathy are often lessened by tricyclic antidepressant drugs that block the reuptake of norepinephrine at synaptic nerve endings. The analgesia is independent of the drugs' antidepressant properties, and the pharmacological site of action is unknown. (In the peripheral nervous system norepinephrine is a neurotransmitter at sympathetic nerve endings. In the central nervous system norepinephrine is produced by neurons of the pontine locus coeruleus, which has widespread projections onto cortical and subcortical structures, including, presumably, pathways that subserve pain sensation.) Drugs that selectively block serotonin reuptake are ineffective in relieving painful paresthesias.

A topical agent, capsaicin (naturally present in hot peppers), relieves neuropathic pain by releasing substance P from C fibers, thereby raising heat and pain thresholds. (A potential hazard of capsaicin is traumatic or thermal injury in limbs deprived of pain or temperature sensation.)

Several anticonvulsant drugs, including phenytoin, carbamazepine, and gabapentin, also effectively reduce peripheral neuropathic pain, but by uncertain mechanisms. The anticonvulsant actions of phenytoin and carbamazepine probably depend on inhibition of neuronal sodium channels necessary for the production of action potentials. The actions of gabapentin are unclear; despite its name, it does not appear to be a GABA-mimetic drug.

SELECTED REFERENCES

Backonja M et al, for the Gabapentin Diabetic Neuropathy Study Group: Gabapentin for the symptomatic treatment of painful neuropathy in patients with diabetes mellitus: A randomized controlled trial. JAMA 1998;280:1831.

The Capsaicin Study Group: Treatment of painful diabetic neuropathy with topical capsaicin. A multicenter, double-blind, vehicle-controlled study. Arch Intern Med 1991;151:2225.

Partanen J et al: Natural history of peripheral neuropathy in patients with non-insulin-dependent diabetes mellitus. N Engl J Med 1995;333:89.

Sima AAF: Metabolic alterations of peripheral nerve in diabetes. Semin Neurol 1996;16:129.

Yagihashi S: Pathology and pathogenetic mechanisms of diabetic neuropathy. Diabetes Metab Rev 1995;11:193.

► CASE 2

A 57-year-old man experiences spontaneous sharp pains in his legs, and over the next several months the pain becomes increasingly severe and lancinating in quality. Urinary frequency then develops, with nocturia, and when he walks to the bathroom in the dark, his gait is unsteady. Attacks of stabbing abdominal pain appear, and he notes constant paresthesias—a pins-and-needles sensation—in his feet. His gait imbalance increases.

On examination his gait and stance are broad based and unsteady, and he stares at his feet as he walks. With his feet together he can barely stand unaided, and when he closes his eyes, he falls. Lying supine and attempting to move each heel along the opposite shin produces jerky and clumsy movements, and when he tries to touch the examiner's finger with his big toe, the movement is effortful with his eyes open and widely inaccurate with his eyes closed. Strength in the legs is probably normal, but the examination is limited by incoordination and difficulty sustaining individual muscle contractions. Muscle tone is normal, and there is no atrophy. The sensory examination is strikingly abnormal, with proprioception and vibratory sensation absent in his toes and ankles and reduced in his knees. Squeezing the Achilles tendon produces no pain; pinprick and temperature sensation are mildly decreased in his feet. Tendon reflexes are absent in his legs; planter responses are flexor. The rest of the neurological examination is normal except for the pupils, which are bilaterally small and unreactive to light but constrict when the patient focuses on a closely held target.

Serum Venereal Disease Research Laboratory (VDRL) and fluorescent treponemal antibody (FTA) tests are positive. Cerebrospinal fluid (CSF) contains 10 lymphocytes/mL and a protein level of 70 mg/dL; CSF VDRL is positive.

Comment

This man has *tabes dorsalis,* a form of tertiary neurosyphilis that can appear 10 years or more after an untreated primary infection. The local lesion of primary syphilis is followed by widespread dissemination of the spirochete (*Treponema pallidum*) in the blood and frequently invasion of the meninges. Symptomatic meningitis, with fever, stiff neck, and CSF pleocytosis, can occur at any time during the first year or two after the primary infection. Whether or not such neurological symptoms appear during this period, the organism is usually contained by the host's immune responses, and in the absence of antimicrobial therapy it can then lie dormant for many years. For reasons unclear, in a small proportion

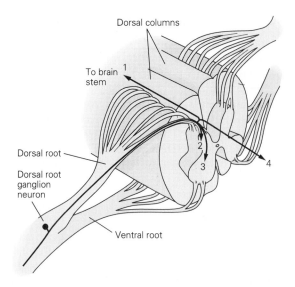

Figure 8–3. In tabes dorsalis the spirochete damages dorsal roots, with secondary degeneration of dorsal columns and dorsal root ganglia (1, fibers in the dorsal columns projecting to the cuneate and gracile nuclei of the medulla; 2 and 3, spinal gray matter; 4, additional associational connections descending to lower levels of the spinal cord). (Reproduced with permission from Kandel ER, Schwartz JH, Jessell TM. 1999. *Principles of Neural Science*, 4th ed. New York: McGraw-Hill.)

of patients the spirochete eventually produces disease in the spinal sensory nerve roots; pathologically, there is secondary degeneration of neurons in the dorsal root ganglia and, within the spinal cord, of the posterior columns (Figure 8–3).

The patient's ataxia is consequent to loss of large-diameter sensory fibers carrying static and dynamic proprioception from muscle stretch receptors and joint mechanoreceptors. When he is not looking at his feet, he has difficulty telling where they are; thus his ataxia increases when he closes his eyes (Romberg's sign). The patient also experiences the "3 Ps" of tabes dorsalis: paresthesias, pain, and polyuria. Pain, involving both the limbs and the viscera, follows damage to small sensory fibers mediating touch, pain, and temperature. Loss of larger sensory fibers contributes to the pain by producing disinhibition and overactivity of deafferented dorsal horn neurons in the spinal cord. (A similar mechanism probably accounts for the pain that follows limb amputation; to the patient, phantom limb pain seems to emanate from the limb that is no longer there.) Deafferentation also produces bladder disturbance and loss of tendon reflexes.

Like the majority of patients with tabes dorsalis, this man also has abnormal pupillary responses, referred to as Argyll Robertson pupils. The light-near dissociation is ascribed to lesions of the midbrain that interrupt the pathway mediating the light reflex while sparing the pathway subserving the near/accommodation response, but why such exquisitely focal and symmetric intraparenchymal lesions should be so frequently encountered in patients with tabes dorsalis has never been explained.

Tabes is treated with penicillin, and sometimes progression is arrested in the absence of treatment (burnt-out tabes), but ataxia and pain usually persist. Patients with longstanding disease develop Charcot joints—swollen, crepitant, and painless—a consequence of repeated articular trauma. Sometimes tabes dorsalis involves motor as well as sensory roots, resulting in weakness and atrophy. Also occasionally encountered in tabetic patients are fecal incontinence, impotence, visual loss (from involvement of the optic nerves and chiasm), and deafness (from involvement of the acoustic nerves).

People infected with the human immunodeficiency virus (HIV) are frequently coinfected with syphilis, and some investigators have described an increased frequency of neurosyphilis in such patients, with symptoms appearing unusually early and responding less predictably to treatment. Other workers have been unable to confirm such observations.

SELECTED REFERENCES

Katz DA, Berger JR, Duncan RC: Neurosyphilis. A comparative study of the effects of infection with human immunodeficiency virus. Arch Neurol 1993;50:243.
Merritt HH, Adams RD, Solomon HC: *Neurosyphilis.* Oxford University Press, 1946.
Roos KL: Neurosyphilis. Semin Neurol 1992;112:209.

► CASE 3

A 62-year-old hypertensive woman abruptly develops numbness and a pins-and-needles sensation over her left arm, leg, and trunk. Examination a few hours after the onset of symptoms reveals marked impairment on her left limbs of all sensory modalities—touch, pain, temperature, proprioception, and vibration. Strength is difficult to test because of proprioceptive loss; she is unable to control her left limbs in any coordinated activity. Tone and tendon reflexes are normal, as is facial sensation. Over the next few days there is some return of sensation, but she experiences progressively severe spontaneously burning pain in her left limbs and trunk. On examination, touching the affected side produces a highly unpleasant, diffuse, lingering, burning sensation. Pain threshold is elevated, but once it is reached, the pinprick feels sharper than normal. Pain and dysesthesia are refractory to treatment with nonopioid analgesic medications. On computerized tomographic (CT) scan there is a small infarct within the ventrobasal complex of the right thalamus involving the ventroposterior nucleus and adjacent structures.

Comment

Thalamic pain syndrome, described by Dejerine and Roussy in 1906, consists of spontaneous contralateral pain and dysesthesia, variably described as burning, aching, shooting, or "unlike any pain I've ever felt" in areas of impaired sensation (*analgesia dolorosa*). Allodynia can be striking: mild sensory stimuli, including touch, cold, or even sound, produce painful overreaction. Discomfort of this sort can follow lesions at different levels of central nociceptive pathways, not just the thalamus. In the present case the initial hemisensory loss was the result of interruption of both the spinothalamic and the dorsal column-medial lemniscus systems at the level of the ventral posterior nucleus of the thalamus. As with the pain of tabes dorsalis and phantom limb, however, deafferentation can also disinhibit neurons that participate in the processing of painful stimuli, resulting in overactivity of those neurons and spontaneous pain. The actual identity of neurons responsible for producing the thalamic pain syndrome is, however, uncertain.

Interruption of the dorsal column-medial lemniscus system accounts for the severe left-sided limb ataxia in this patient. Her preserved facial sensation means that although the lesion involves the lateral part of the ventral posterior nucleus (the terminus for sensation in the limbs and trunk), it spares the medial part (the terminus for facial sensation).

SELECTED REFERENCES

Bowsher D: Central pain: Clinical and physiological characteristics. J Neurol Neurosurg Psychiatry 1996;61:62.

Dejerine J, Roussy G: La syndrome thalamique. Rev Neurol (Paris) 1906;14:521. (Reprinted in translation in Arch Neurol 1969;20:559.)

Hayman LA, Berman SA, Hinck VC: Correlation of CT cerebral vascular territories with function: II. Posterior cerebral artery. Am J Neuroradiol 1981;2:219.

Jones A: The pain matrix and neuropathic pain. Brain 1998;121:783.

Nasreddine ZS, Saver JL: Pain after thalamic stroke: Right diencephalic predominance and clinical features in 180 patients. Neurology 1997;48:1196.

▶ CASE 4

During an altercation with a friend, a 27-year-old man is struck on the right side of his head with a baseball bat and rendered unconscious. After gradually recovering consciousness over the next half hour, he is taken to an emergency room, where he is alert and attentive but has no recollection of the argument or injury and cannot memorize new information. (For example, he is able to repeat three unrelated words but cannot recall them after 5 minutes.) Several hours later, his memory for new events has returned, but he still cannot recall the period immediately preceding or following his head injury. Examination further reveals sensory impairment of his left face and arm: touch, pinprick, and temperature sensation are mildly decreased compared to his right side, and the stimuli are inaccurately localized. Proprioception is decreased in the distal joints of the fingers on his left hand, and there is reduced two-point discrimination in his left fingertips. He is unable to identify coins with his left fingers but identifies them correctly with his right. When his face or his hands are touched bilaterally and simultaneously, he feels the stimulus only on the right. The rest of the neurological examination is normal. Computerized tomographic (CT) scan of the head reveals a patchy area of blood—ecchymosis—in the gray and white matter of the anterior right parietal convexity with a collection of blood 3 mm in thickness in the overlying subdural space.

Surgical evacuation of the subdural hematoma is deemed unnecessary, and over the next few weeks his left-sided sensory impairment improves, leaving mild residual astereognosis of his left fingers. Six months later he experiences an episode of paresthesias beginning in his left thumb and index finger, gradually spreading up his arm to his face, and clearing spontaneously after 2 or 3 minutes. CT scan of his head now shows lucency and sucal widening at the site of the ecchymosis, which, along with the subdural hematoma, has resolved. An electroencephalogram (EEG) shows intermittent focal slowing and high-voltage sharp waves over the same area.

Comment

Traumatic intraparenchymal ecchymosis—*cerebral contusion*—has damaged this patient's parietal lobe just posterior to the rolandic sulcus. This area—the primary sensory cortex—receives projections from the ventral posterior nucleus of the thalamus conveying sensory information mediated by both the spinothalamic and dorsal column-medial lemniscus systems (Figure 8–4). In contrast to the dorsal column-medial lemniscus system, however, the spinothalamic system also terminates on the intralaminar nuclei of the thalamus, which in turn has widespread cortical and limbic projections. As a consequence, a lesion restricted to the primary sensory cortex results in severe impairment of discriminative sensations such as stereognosis, but only modest impairment of affective sensations such as pain.

The brief episode of spontaeous paresthesias is a focal (or partial) seizure, in this case signifying a spontaneous firing of sensory neurons adjacent to the area of traumatic damage. Seizures can occur immediately after a blow to the head (impact seizure), within the first 1 to 2 weeks of the trauma (early posttraumatic seizures), or after a latency of weeks, months, or years. Such a delay reflects the epileptogenicity of scar tissue on adjacent viable gray matter; particularly culpable may be the presence of hemosiderin or iron, derived over time from hemoglobin. An EEG shows focal epileptiform activity, an electrical signature of increased seizure susceptibility (see Figure 11–2).

Impaired sensation and spontaneous epileptic paresthesias are examples of J. Hughlings Jackson's fundamental distinction, formulated over a century ago, between negative and positive neurological symptoms. "Epilepsy," Jackson declared in 1873, "is the name for occasional, sudden, excessive, rapid, and local

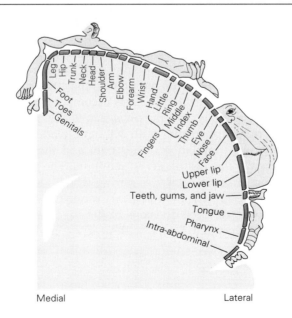

Medial   Lateral

Figure 8–4. Somatotopic organization of the primary sensory cortex produces a sensory homunculus. (Reproduced with permission from Kandel ER, Schwartz JH, Jessell TM. 1999. *Principles of Neural Science*, 4th ed. New York: McGraw-Hill.)

discharge of gray matter." [Interestingly, the first description of a focal somatosensory seizure was by Galen in the second century CE; an adolescent boy experienced paresthesias over one side of his body which felt like "a cold current of air (aura)." The term *aura*, which literally means breeze, has come to refer to any subjective warning—ie, focal discharge—of a seizure.] (See Cases 16, 71, and 72.)

The patient's transient memory disturbance, called *posttraumatic amnesia*, is probably the result of brief bilateral disruption of normal hippocampal function. In such patients the head injury has usually caused transient impairment of consciousness (*concussion*). Posttraumatic amnesia tends to clear over hours, leaving an island of permanent memory loss, both retrograde (before the injury) and anterograde (after the injury). (For other disturbances of memory, see Cases 73 and 74.)

SELECTED REFERENCES

Jackson JH: On the anatomical, physiological, and pathological investigation of the epilepsies. West Riding Lunatic Asylum Med Rep 1873;3:315.

Lennox WG, Lennox MA: *Epilepsy and Related Disorders* (2 volumes). Little, Brown & Co., 1960.

Temkin NR, Dikman SS, Winn HR: Post-traumatic seizures. Neurosurg Clin North Am 1991;2:425.

Van Ness PC, Lesser RP, Duchowny MS: Simple sensory seizures. In: Engel J, Pedley TA (eds): *Epilepsy: A Comprehensive Textbook* (pp. 533–542). Lippincott-Raven, 1998.

▶ CASE 5 _____

A 60-year-old woman develops paroxysms of sharp stabbing pain in her right malar area and upper lip, gums, and teeth. Each attack lasts a few minutes and is comparable in abruptness and severity to pain produced by a tooth being drilled. It is precipitated by brushing the teeth and by eating, so that over several weeks she has lost nearly 10 pounds. The pain never spreads beyond the region described, and between attacks she is symptom free except for fear of recurrence, which occurs many times throughout the day. Low-potency analgesics such as aspirin, acetaminophen, or codeine do not prevent the attacks.

During examination, an attack of pain is accompanied by brief convulsive movements of her face and jaw, and the physician is able to trigger the pain by lightly rubbing her right upper gum with a tongue blade. There is a delay of several seconds between stimulation of her gum and the appearance of pain, which then occurs in a volley lasting nearly a minute. The paroxysm is followed by a refractory period of several minutes during which touching the same area does not precipitate the pain. The neurological examination is otherwise normal, including sensation over all three divisions of the trigeminal nerve. She begins taking carbamazepine every few hours, with nearly complete disappearance of her pain.

Comment

This woman has *trigeminal neuralgia*. Because the paroxysms of pain often produce reactive facial movements, the condition is also known as *tic douloureux,* but the primary symptoms are strictly sensory. Jabs of searing pain most often occur in the territory of the second or third division of the trigeminal nerve; in less than

15% of cases all three divisions are eventually involved. The pain never spreads outside the trigeminal area (see Figure 3–8). A characteristic feature is the trigger zone, which can be remarkably restricted, for example, an area of the upper lip only a few millimeters wide. Also characteristic are brief refractory periods and absence of sensory loss during or after the paroxysms.

Trigeminal neuralgia-like pain can affect patients with multiple sclerosis, and autopsies in such patients demonstrate demyelinating lesions in the pons at the entry zone of the trigeminal nerve. In the far more frequent cryptogenic (cause unknown) form, trigeminal neuralgia typically begins in middle or late age, and in most cases no morphological abnormalities can be identified in the trigeminal nerve either peripherally or in its intraparenchymal course. Degenerative changes have been anecdotally reported in the trigeminal ganglion, and some cases are ascribed to compression of the proximal trigeminal nerve by tortuous arterial loops. The attacks of pain are believed to originate in discharges within the spinal trigeminal nucleus. (Consistent with a central origin, and exemplified by this patient, are the latent period of a few seconds between trigger point stimulation and the appearance of pain, continued volleys of pain after trigger point stimulation, and a refractory period of a few minutes following a painful paroxysm.) Patients respond to carbamazepine or phenytoin, which block axonal sodium conductance. These drugs are also effective anticonvulsants. Baclofen, which blocks facilitation by substance P of synaptic transmission within the spinal trigeminal nucleus and its spinal cord counterpart, the substantia gelatinosa, may be effective. (Baclofen is more often used to treat spasticity of spinal cord origin.)

Patients unresponsive to pharmacotherapy have a variety of surgical options. Destruction of the second or third division of the trigeminal nerve distal to the trigeminal ganglion can produce temporary relief, but regrowth and recurrence of pain are likely. Consistent with the idea that the pain is secondary to excessive stimulation of the spinal trigeminal nucleus, pain relief can also follow section of the occipital or greater auricular nerves, which, although not branches of the trigeminal nerve, project to the caudal spinal trigeminal nucleus. Ablation of the trigeminal ganglion or the trigeminal root will interrupt the afferent limb of the blink reflex, with the danger of corneal damage. Radiofrequency surgery to the trigeminal nerve or its branches has the advantage of destroying small-diameter pain-conducting fibers while preserving large-diameter motor fibers. An approach that spares sensory as well as motor function is posterior fossa exploration and decompression of the trigeminal nerve by overlying arteries. Compression may result from a vascular malformation, an aneurysm, or a neoplasm. It is possible that pain relief following posterior fossa surgery is the result not of decompression but of nonspecific injury to trigeminal ganglion neurons.

Trigeminal neuralgia has thus been described as having a peripheral cause and a central pathogenesis. A variety of injuries to the trigeminal nerve, root, or root entry zone result in increased firing of the nerve secondary to ectopic spike generation (and perhaps ephaptic—nonsynaptic—communication between fibers mediating pain sensation and fibers mediating touch sensation); in addition, there is reduced segmental inhibition in the spinal trigeminal nucleus. Latent herpes simplex infection in trigeminal ganglion neurons may play a contributory role. Treatment can be directed either at the peripheral lesion, for example, through nerve root decompression, or at the paroxysmally firing neurons of the spinal trigemental nucleus, for example, through the use of carbamazepine.

SELECTED REFERENCES

Fromm GH, Terrance CF, Maroon JC: Trigeminal neuralgia. Current concepts regarding etiology and pathogenesis. Arch Neurol 1984;41:1204.

Katusic S, Beard CM, Berostralh E, Kurland LT: Incidence and clinical features of trigeminal neuralgia. Rochester, Minnesota, 1945–1984. Ann Neurol 1990;27:89.

Lisney SJW: Current topics of interest in the physiology of trigeminal pain: A review. J Roy Soc Med 1983;76:292.

Sweet WH: The treatment of trigeminal neuralgia (tic doloreux). N Engl J Med 1986; 315:174.

Tenser RB: Trigeminal neuralgia. Mechanisms of treatment. Neurology 1998;51:17.

9

Mostly Visual

▶ CASE 6

For the past 6 weeks a 52-year-old man has been having spells of transient monocular visual loss. Every few days it seems as if a curtain descends over his right eye, with total loss of vision for several minutes. He has verified that only the right eye is affected by covering first one eye and then the other during the attacks. Within an hour of a typical episode, examination reveals a small yellowish refractile body at a bifurcation of an inferior retinal arteriole, obstructing distal flow. A soft, high-pitched, continuous, systolic murmur extending into diastole is present over the right anterior neck at the level of the thyroid cartilage. Physical and neurological examinations are otherwise normal.

Treated with aspirin 325 mg daily, he has one more attack 2 days later and none thereafter. Doppler ultrasonography reveals severe (90%) stenosis of the right internal carotid artery just above its origin from the common carotid artery. This finding is confirmed by carotid angiography, which further defines an ulceration on the surface of the atherosclerotic plaque. Neurosurgical consultation is obtained.

Comment

Neuroanatomy explains the location of this patient's symptoms, and vascular anatomy explains the pathophysiology. Unilateral visual loss means that the lesion involves either the optic nerve or the eye itself (see Figure 3–2). The refractile body observed on funduscopy is within an arteriolar branch of the central retinal artery, which is a branch of the ophthalmic artery. The central retinal artery and the optic nerve enter the orbit through the optic foramen. The ophthalmic artery, in turn, is the first major intracranial branch of the internal carotid artery. This patient is thus having *transient ischemic attacks* of his retina (*transient monocular blindness, amaurosis fugax*) secondary to emboli arising from thrombi on an ulcerated atherosclerotic plaque in his right internal carotid artery.

Because the internal carotid artery bifurcates into the middle and anterior cerebral arteries, patients with transient retinal ischemia often have cerebral symptoms as well, particularly hemiparesis contralateral to the affected eye.

By definition, transient ischemic attacks last less than 24 hours; in fact, most last a few minutes rather than hours. Their primary significance is prognostic, for such patients are at increased risk for both major stroke and myocardial infarction. Clinical trials have demonstrated that agents that decrease platelet aggregation (notably aspirin, ticlopidine, and clopidagrel) reduce both the frequency of attacks and the likelihood of cerebral infarction. (*Ischemia* means reduced blood supply, with or without symptoms; *infarction* means tissue death as a consequence of ischemia.) In patients who meet specific medical, neurological, and radiological criteria the treatment of choice is carotid endarterectomy—surgical removal of the atherosclerotic plaque.

SELECTED REFERENCES

Antiplatelet Trialists' Collaboration: Collaborative overview of randomized trials of antiplatelet therapy—I: Prevention of death, myocardial infarction, and stroke by prolonged antiplatelet therapy in various categories of patients. Br Med J 1994;308:81.

Caplan LC: TIAs. Neurology 1988;38:791.

North American Symptomatic Carotid Endarterectomy Trial Collaborators: Beneficial effect of carotid endarterectomy in symptomatic patients with high-grade carotid stenosis. N Engl J Med 1991;325:445.

▶ CASE 7

A 32-year-old woman awakens with impaired vision in her left eye and left retroorbital pain on eye movement. The following day her symptoms have worsened. On examination her visual acuity is 20/20 on the right and worse than 20/800 on the left; with the left eye she can detect light and finger movement in the periphery of her visual field but not centrally. Her fundi, including the optic disks, are normal. Her pupils are equal in size. When light is directed at the right eye, both pupils constrict briskly; when light is directed at the left eye, pupillary constriction in both eyes is reduced in amplitude, but the pupils remain equal in size. Physical and neurological examinations are otherwise normal. On proton density and T2-weighted magnetic resonance imaging (MRI) scans of her head there is an abnormally increased signal within her left optic nerve. The lesion is not apparent on a Tl-weighted MRI scan but becomes visible (enhanced) following intravenous injection of gadolinium. The MRI is otherwise normal.

She receives methylprednisolone (an adrenocorticosteroid) intravenously in high dosage. Over the next several weeks her vision gradually improves. Six months later her visual acuity in the left eye is 20/30, and there is mild pallor of the optic disk. Light directed into the left eye continues to produce a less vigorous pupillary constriction in both eyes compared to light directed into the right eye. On MRI scan the abnormal optic nerve signal is barely evident and no longer is enhanced with gadolinium.

Comment

The unilaterality of this patient's visual impairment places the lesion in the visual pathway anterior to the optic chiasm (see Figure 3–2). In contrast to Case 6, the examination and the MRI scan localize the lesion to the optic nerve rather than to the retina. Symptoms, signs, and MRI are consistent with a diagnosis of *optic neuritis*, a probably immune-mediated disorder characterized pathologically by inflammatory demyelination of the optic nerve. (The abnormal signal on the proton density and T2-weighted scans reflects demyelination; enhancement with gadolinium on the T1-weighted scan reflects inflammation and breakdown of the blood–brain barrier.)

The demyelinating lesion of optic neuritis tends to be deep within the nerve, affecting fibers traveling from the macular area of the retina and representing central vision; thus, visual loss usually consists of a central scotoma (or, if the area of loss extends to include the preexisting blind spot, a centrocecal scotoma). Total monocular blindness is unusual. The foveal area contains color-sensitive cones, and so mild or early optic neuritis can impair color vision while black and white vision remains normal. Because cells of the visual system are more tuned to contrast in visual information than to absolute intensity, patients with optic neuritis may have difficulty detecting subtle gradations of shading (chiaroscuro), resulting in subtle visual impairment undetectable by visual acuity testing with a Snellin chart. Patients blind in one eye lose depth perception.

When the optic nerve lesion includes the nerve head at the retina, optic disk swelling is evident on funduscopy and is distinguishable from papilledema secondary to increased intracranial pressure by the acute loss of vision. When the lesion is sufficiently posterior to the optic nerve head, as with this patient, funduscopy is initially normal.

The prognosis of optic neuritis depends on both the severity of the attack and whether the patient actually has multiple sclerosis. If the lesion is mild, axons, although demyelinated and malfunctioning, are themselves mostly undamaged; as myelin regenerates, axonal function returns. Consistent with immune-mediated inflammation, systemic corticosteriod therapy hastens recovery. Frequently encountered residua are optic atrophy (which evolves over weeks following the acute attack), decreased visual acuity, and, as with this patient, an afferent pupillary defect. More subtle residua are explained by the fact that with remyelination, nodes of Ranvier are closer together than before and therefore saltatory axonal conduction is slower. Visual evoked response testing can demonstrate delayed conduction velocity in an optic nerve even in patients whose visual acuity has returned to normal following an attack of optic neuritis.

Optic neuritis occurs as a postinfectious or postvaccination complication, but most often is without evident cause. It can occur in patients already diagnosed with multiple sclerosis, or it can represent the first manifestation of that disease (see Case 55). (Multiple sclerosis is a disease of central, not peripheral, myelin, and the optic nerve is a tract, not a peripheral nerve.) Estimates of the percentage of patients with cryptogenic optic neuritis who develop multiple sclerosis range from 15 to 85%. Not surprisingly, the likelihood is increased in patients who at the outset have additional lesions demonstrated by MRI.

SELECTED REFERENCES

Beck RW, Cleary PA, Anderson MM, et al: A randomized controlled trial of corticosteriods in the treatment of acute optic neuritis. N Engl J Med 1992;326:581.

Raine CS, Wu E: Multiple sclerosis: Remyelination in acute lesions. J Neuropathol Exp Neurol 1993;52:199.

Rizzo JF, Lessell S: Risk of developing multiple sclerosis after uncomplicated optic neuritis. A long-term prospective study. Neurology 1988;38:185.

Slamoratis S, Rosen CE, Cheng KP, et al: Visual recovery in patients with optic neuritis and visual loss to no light perception. Am J Ophthalmol 1991;111:209.

▶ CASE 8 _____

For several months a 37-year-old woman has had progressively severe bifrontal headaches. Unrelated to activity or posture, they sometimes awaken her from sleep and are incompletely relieved by acetaminophen. She then develops amenorrhea. Her physical and neurological examinations are normal except for bitemporal hemianopia affecting the upper more than the lower quadrants. The visual field impairment is more extensive when a red target is used. Magnetic resonance imaging (MRI) scan reveals enlargement of the sella turcica and extension of an intrasellar mass above the diaphragma sella, compressing the optic chiasm. Laboratory findings include abnormally reduced serum levels of growth hormone, follicle-stimulating hormone, and luteinizing hormone and a mildly elevated serum prolactin level.

Neurological consultation is obtained.

Comment

Bitemporal hemianopia localizes the lesion to the optic chiasm; the tumor is compressing the crossing fibers arising from ganglion cells of each nasal retina (see Figure 3–2). Compression is from below, and therefore the superior visual fields are affected first. (The chiasm can also be compressed from above, for example, by a craniopharyngioma or a large saccular aneurysm, in which case visual impairment will initially affect the inferior temporal quadrants.) In a typical case of pituitary tumor with suprasellar extension, visual loss, initially unrecognized by the patient, progresses into the inferior visual fields and then into the nasal fields, finally affecting visual acuity, sometimes precipitously. In some patients chiasmal compression produces bitemporal paracentral scotomas rather than a more typical bitemporal hemianopia. This is because fibers arising from the retinal fovea (serving central vision) cross in the posterior region of the chiasm and so are most vulnerable when the chiasm is compressed from behind. Such an impairment could easily be missed on gross bedside visual field examination; when a chiasmal lesion is suspected, formal visual field testing with perimetry should be performed.

A tumor compressing the chiasm from the side or arising posteriorly and compressing the optic tract can cause homonymous hemianopia. This patient also demonstrates the particular vulnerability of color vision in lesions of the optic nerve or chiasm.

The patient's headaches are caused by stretching of the diaphragma sella and other adjacent pain-sensitive structures; the headaches are frontal because these structures are innervated by the first division of the trigeminal nerve. In some patients, headaches actually decrease when the tumor finally breaks through the diaphragma sella.

Pituitary tumors are either secretory or nonsecretory. The most common endocrinologically active tumor is the prolactinoma, which causes galactorrhea (milk discharge from the breast) and amenorrhea. Other tumors produce growth hormone, resulting in acromegaly, or adrenocorticotropic hormone (ACTH), resulting in Cushing disease. Some tumors produce follicle-stimulating hormone, luteinizing hormone, or different combinations of hormones. This patient's tumor is nonsecretory. Her hypogonadism is secondary to compression of the anterior pituitary by the tumor; such hypopituitarism characteristically involves growth hormone and gonadotropins before ACTH or thyroid-stimulating hormone. Her mildly elevated prolactin level is not the result of secretion by the tumor—in such a case the level would be much higher—but rather of pituitary stalk compression and interruption of dopaminergic fibers that normally inhibit prolactin release.

Further compression within the sella causes diabetes insipidus by impairing secretion of antidiuretic hormone (ADH). Erosion of the tumor into the sphenoid sinus causes cerebrospinal fluid rhinorrhea. Lateral extension of a pituitary adenoma into the cavernous sinus can affect the third, fourth, fifth, or sixth cranial nerves. Suprasellar extension into the third ventricle can obstruct the foramen of Monro, resulting in hydrocephalus. Extension into brain parenchyma produces seizures or mental symptoms. Infrequently, a pituitary tumor is asymptomatic until it undergoes spontaneous hemorrhage (pituitary apoplexy), causing severe headache, visual loss, and progression to stupor or coma.

The treatment of *pituitary adenomas* includes a number of surgical, radiotherapeutic, and pharmacological options. With prolactinomas, the dopamine agonist bromocriptine results not only in normalization of serum prolactin levels but also in reduction in the size of the tumor. Surgical removal is most often transsphenoidally through the nasopharynx. Endocrine-deficient patients require appropriate replacement therapy, particularly of thyroid or adrenal hormones. Small asymptomatic tumors (microadenomas) do not require treatment, but periodic MRI scans and visual field examinations are necessary.

SELECTED REFERENCES

Levy A, Lightman SL: Diagnosis and management of pituitary tumours. Br Med J 1994; 308:1087.

McDonald WI: The symptomatology of tumors of the anterior visual pathways. Can J Neurol Sci 1982;9:381.

Wray SH: Neuro-ophthalmologic manifestations of pituitary and parasellar lesion. Clin Neurosurg 1977;24:86.

▶ CASE 9

A 66-year-old man with a history of childhood rheumatic fever abruptly develops difficulty seeing to the left. On examination his blood pressure is normal, but his pulse is irregularly irregular at 88/minute, and there is a diastolic murmur over his left cardiac border and apex. His only neurological abnormality is a dense left homonymous hemianopia, which on perimetry is congruent and spares the macular area. Notably absent are left hemineglect or difficulties with spatial manipulation (such as copying geometric designs). With his own glasses his visual acuity is 20/20. An opticokinetic tape produces normal nystagmus when passed in either direction across his vision. The rest of the neurological examination, including other cranial nerves, motor and sensory function, and reflexes, is normal. An electrocardiogram confirms atrial fibrillation, and an echocardiogram shows thickening and stenosis of the mitral valve. Computerized tomographic (CT) scan of his head is initially normal, but 5 days later it shows lucency without mass effect in the right occipital lobe.

Comment

Left homonymous hemianopia indicates that this lesion is in the visual pathway on the right side behind the chiasm (see Figure 3–2). Candidate locations are the optic tract, the lateral geniculate nucleus of the thalamus, the optic radiations, and the calcarine cortex of the occipital lobe. The abrupt onset and the presence of atrial fibrillation and rheumatic valvular disease make embolic infarction likely, and even without confirmatory CT findings, the likely location of the lesion would be the occipital lobe. *Optic tract infarction* is unusual—each tract is supplied by multiple small arteries arising from the circle of Willis—and the homonymous hemianopia produced by optic tract lesions is usually noncongruent. The lateral geniculate nucleus is supplied by both the anterior choroidal artery and the posterior choroidal artery; a complete homonymous hemianopia would be unlikely following occlusion of either vessel, and involvement of other structures would likely produce additional symptoms and signs. Similarly, occlusion of the middle cerebral artery proximally could destroy both the temporal and parietal divisions of the optic radiations, but in such a case there would also be motor, sensory, and either language or spatial abnormalities.

Occlusion of the occipital branch of the posterior cerebral artery, on the other hand, could damage the primary visual cortex without affecting other critical structures. The resulting homonymous hemianopia would be, as in this case, congruent. Macular sparing is explained by anastomotic blood supply to the occipital pole, where foveal vision is represented; when the posterior cerebral artery is occluded, collaterals from the middle cerebral artery take over the blood supply to this region. Also contributing to macular sparing is the fact that nearly half of the primary visual cortex is devoted to representing foveal vision (Figure 9–1). The patient's normal visual acuity is no surprise; indeed, even when there is no

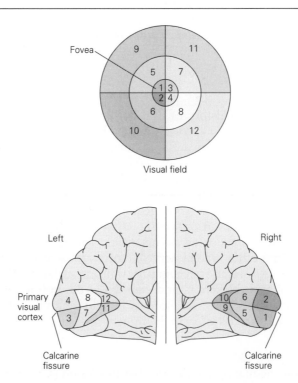

Visual field

Left
Right

Primary visual cortex

Calcarine fissure

Calcarine fissure

Figure 9–1. The primary visual cortex contains a map of the visual field, with each half of the visual field located in the contralateral hemisphere. Numbered areas of the visual field are represented by similarly numbered areas of the primary visual cortex. The upper fields are mapped below the calcarine fissure and the lower fields are mapped above it. The posterior part of the primary visual cortex—half its neural mass—is devoted to representing foveal and parafoveal vision. (Reproduced with permission from Kandel ER, Schwartz JH, Jessell TM. 1999. *Principles of Neural Science*, 4th ed. New York: McGraw-Hill.)

macular sparing, visual acuity remains normal as long as a postchiasmal lesion is unilateral. The preserved opticokinetic nystagmus is also easily explained; visual information processed by the remaining (left) occipital cortex can be relayed bilaterally to association areas where the pursuit phase of opticokinetic nystagmus is generated.

The distal location of this patient's vessel occlusion is in keeping with its embolic origin. More proximal occlusion of the posterior cerebral artery would likely have produced additional signs, including hemisensory loss (from damage to the ventral posterior nucleus of the thalamus—see Case 3), hemiballism (from damage to the subthalamic nucleus—see Case 36), disordered eye movements (from damage to the occulomotor nucleus or other midbrain areas involved in eye movement—see Case 52), or memory loss (from damage to either the inferomedial temporal lobe or the dorsomedial nucleus of the thalamus—see Cases 73 and 74).

SELECTED REFERENCES

Milandre L, Brosset C, Botti G, Khawl R: A study of 82 infarctions in the area of posterior cerebral arteries. Rev Neurol 1994;150:133.

Pessin MA, Lathi ES, Cohen MB, et al: Clinical features and mechanism of occipital infarction. Ann Neurol 1987;21:290.

► CASE 10

A 64-year-old hypertensive man suddenly loses color vision. He has no difficulty discriminating objects or identifying them, and his ability to read is unimpaired, but he feels as if he were wandering about in a black-and-white movie. Red appears black to him; blue and yellow appear almost white. The experience is most unpleasant. People seem like gray statues, and food is so unappetizing that he prefers to eat with his eyes closed. Often, there is excessive tonal contrast in what he sees, so that his visual acuity seems enhanced; on the other hand, images with subtle coloring and tonal contrast are identified with difficulty. He prefers darkened surroundings and the night.

On examination, his blood pressure is 180/110 mm Hg (sitting). His visual acuity (by Snellin chart), fundi, and visual fields (grossly and by perimetry) are normal, as is the rest of his physical and neurological examinations. Tested with color-dot Ishihara plates—a standard test for color blindness—he is unable to see any of the figures. Computerized tomographic (CT) and magnetic resonance imaging (MRI) scans show multiple small lesions (less than 5 mm) in the deep white matter of both cerebral hemispheres, suggestive of microinfarcts. Electroretinography and other laboratory studies are normal.

Comment

In the majority of cases, disturbed color vision is the result of retinal abnormalities. Congenital defects include red blindness (affecting 1% of males) and green blindness (affecting 2% of males), both sex-linked recessive genetic disorders resulting from either abnormal visual pigments or absence of pigment-specific cones. Hereditary *achromatopsia* (lack of any color vision, resulting from absence of either two or three cone types) is extremely rare. Acquired disease of the retina can also produce defective color vision; outer retinal disease tends to cause loss of short-wavelength discrimination (blue), and inner retinal disease tends to impair long-wavelength discrimination (red). This patient has developed achromatopsia without any evident retinal disease. (Electroretinography records changes in electrical potential of retinal photoreceptors after stimulation by light.)

From the retina to the cerebral cortex, visual information regarding form, location, and color is processed separately, physiologically and anatomically, and acquired selective disturbances of each have been described (Figure 9–2). The parvocellular visual system relays color information from single-opponent cells of the retina and lateral geniculate nucleus to double-opponent cells within blob zones of the primary visual cortex (V1); the parvocellular-blob system then projects to area V4 of the inferior temporooccipital lobe (where color-sensitive cells predominate), en route to its eventual termination more anteriorly in the inferior temporal cortex (where color-sensitive cells are no longer anatomically segregated). Selective damage to area V4 produces achromatopsia. If the lesion is unilateral, achromatopsia is limited to the contralateral visual hemifield; if the lesion is bilateral, as in this patient, achromatopsia occurs throughout the field of vision. The chances of two symmetric lesions destroying this area without causing additional damage are small. As a consequence, most patients with achromatopsia from such damage have additional visual or neurological impairment. For exam-

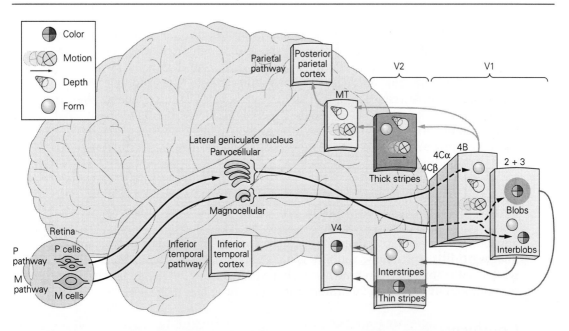

Figure 9–2. Color information is processed in the parvocellular-blob system. Retinal P cells project to parvocellular layers of the lateral geniculate nucleus of the thalamus, which project to blob zones of the primary visual cortex (V1 and V2), which project to area V4 of the inferior temporooccipital lobe and then the inferior temporal cortex. The parvocellular-interblob system, which also ultimately projects to the inferior temporal cortex, processes form. By contrast, movement, depth, and spatial information are processed by the magnocellular system, which ultimately projects to the parietal lobe. MT, middle temporal cortex. (Reproduced with permission from Kandel ER, Schwartz JH, Jessell TM. 1999. *Principles of Neural Science,* 4th ed. New York: McGraw-Hill. Adapted with permission from Van Essen DC, Gallant JL. 1994. Neural mechanisms of form and motion processing in the primate visual system. Neuron 13:1.)

ple, when the inferior occipital cortex is involved, there is loss of vision in the superior visual fields.

Hypertension, abrupt onset of symptoms, absence of evident retinal disease, and CT/MRI abnormalities suggestive of multiple small infarcts point to a cerebrovascular origin of this patient's visual disturbance. Hypertensive disease of small arteries within brain parenchyma causes small deep infarcts. When these affect noneloquent brain regions, they are asymptomatic; when, as in this case, they happen—against the odds—to affect area V4 bilaterally, the result is the strange syndrome of achromatopsia.

SELECTED REFERENCES

Masland RH: Unscrambling color vision. Science 1996;271:616.

McKeefry DJ, Zeki S: The position and topography of the human colour centre as revealed by functional magnetic resonance imaging. Brain 1997;120:2229.

Sacks O: The case of the colorblind painter. In: *An Anthropologist on Mars* (pp. 3–41). Vintage Books, 1996.

Zeki S, Marini L: Three cortical stages of colour processing in the human brain. Brain 1998;121:1669.

► CASE 11

For several years a 30-year-old woman has had headaches preceded by visual symptoms. Every few weeks she experiences a small paracentral scotoma, evident with either eye closed, that slowly expands into a C shape convex to the periphery of her vision. Shimmering angles then develop on the enlarging outer edge and become both luminous and colored as the now jagged border slowly moves toward the periphery of the involved half of the visual field. After about 20 minutes, the scintillation disappears over the horizon of peripheral vision. At this point headache appears over the contralateral occiput, rapidly becoming throbbing and severe and accompanied by nausea, vomiting, photophobia, and phonophobia. The headaches have never awakened her from sleep, and their severity is lessened by resting in a darkened room. Untreated, the headaches usually last several hours. When temporally related to emotional stress, the attacks more often follow rather than occur during the stressful period. For many years the patient's mother has had similar symptoms.

During a headache the patient appears pale and ill and there is tenderness over the scalp on the side of the headache and the ipsilateral cervical carotid artery. Between attacks her physical and neurological examinations are normal, as is a magnetic resonance imaging (MRI) scan of her head. Positron emission tomography (PET) performed during her visual symptoms reveals a strip of hypometabolism moving anteriorly from the occipital cortex at a surface rate (including sulci) of about 2–3 mm/minute.

During attacks, the headaches are minimally relieved by aspirin or acetaminophen. Oral ergotamine tartrate given at the onset of the visual symptoms, however, completely aborts the headache.

Comment

The term *classic migraine* denotes migraine headaches preceded by focal neurological symptoms. Such auras are frequently visual, and the type experienced by this patient is particularly characteristic. As the leading edge of the scintillating scotoma develops angles, like a string of connected Zs, it resembles a medieval walled town seen from the air, hence the term fortification scotoma (*teichopsia*). The origin of this visual hallucination is the occipital cortex, and as it is rarely encountered with structural lesions of the visual system such as infarction or brain tumor, teichopsia is practically pathognomonic for migraine. It has been proposed that each of the moving straight lines that together form the zig-zag pattern represents spontaneous firing of complex or hypercomplex cells within the visual cortex. Such cells are normally and selectively responsive to comparable moving borders embedded in external stimuli. (The particular sensory stimulus that results in firing of a particular sensory neuron is called the receptive field of that neuron.)

It was previously believed that migrainous auras were the result of ischemia secondary to local vasospasm and that the ensuing headache was the result of subsequent intracranial and extracranial vasodilatation. In 1944 the physiologist Leão discovered that applying potassium chloride or mechanical stimuli to mammalian cortex produced a slowly moving wave of cortical depression, preceded by a leading edge of cortical activation, over sulci and gyri at a rate of 2–3 mm/minute, precisely the rate at which a comparable wave front would travel to produce the slowly moving fortification scotomas of a migraine aura. The spreading depression hypothesis of migraine remains controversial but is supported by data from PET. If spreading depression is the initial event in classic migraine, however, its trigger is unknown. A possible clue is the observation that familial hemiplegic migraine, an autosomal dominant disorder in which attacks of migraine are accompanied by either hemiparetic aura or more prolonged hemiplegia, is associated with missense mutations of the gene for a central nervous system voltage-sensitive calcium channel. Such channelopathy (see Case 20) might be the basis for episodic cortical events resembling spreading depression.

Ergotamine drugs increase the threshold for cortical spreading depression and abort migraine attacks; their diverse actions at serotonin receptors raise the possibility that spreading depression is somehow generated by discharges from serotonergic neurons of the brain stem dorsal raphe nuclei.

The headache phase of a migraine attack, on the other hand, is the consequence of neuronal firing in the spinal trigeminal nucleus of the brain stem and is considered to have two phases. First, central transmission to the spinal trigeminal nucleus from the cortex induces pain. Second, stimulated spinal trigeminal neurons fire antidromically down their axons to nerve endings on blood vessels of the brain and meninges; this wrong-way firing causes release of vasoactive neuropeptides, which in turn induces vasodilatation, plasma protein extravasation, and release of additional substances that sensitize the nerve endings, thereby sustaining the pain. (Peptides involved in this process include substance P, neurokinin A, and calcitonin gene-related peptide.)

Triptan drugs, which include sumatriptan and related agents, are serotonin (5-hydroxytryptamine, 5-HT) agonists that act selectively at receptors of 5-$HT_{1B/1D}$ subtype. These drugs alleviate migraine headache without affecting cortical spreading depression. Triptans might nonetheless act centrally by decreasing cortical input to the spinal trigeminal nucleus. Some—but not all—triptans also act peripherally at inhibitory prejunctional 5-HT receptors located on afferent trigeminovascular nerve endings, thereby decreasing peptide release.

Nitric oxide (NO) might also play a role in migraine. Activation of the NO-cyclic GMP pathway precipitates migraine attacks in migraineurs, drugs effective in treating migraine inhibit one or more steps in the NO pathway, and substances that precipitate migraine stimulate one or more steps in the NO pathway. NO has been linked to cortical spreading depression.

Worldwide, migraine is estimated to affect roughly 5% of men and 15% of women. Future approaches to migraine treatment will be based increasingly on a specific understanding of its pathophysiology.

SELECTED REFERENCES

Goadsby PJ, Olesen J: Diagnosis and management of migraine. Br Med J 1996;312:1279.

Hans M, Luvisetto S, Williams ME, et al: Functional consequence of mutations in the human α_{1A} calcium channel subunit linked to familial hemiplegic migraine. J Neurosci 1999;19:1610.

Lashley KS: Patterns of cerebral integration indicated by the scotomas of migraine. Arch Neurol Psychiatry 1941;46:331.

Lauritzan M: Pathophysiology of the migraine aura. The spreading depression theory. Brain 1994;117:199.

Leao AAP: Spreading depression of activity in cerebral cortex. J Neurophysiol 1944;7:359.

Moskowitz MA, Macfarlane R: Neurovascular and molecular mechanisms in migraine headaches. Cerebrovasc Brain Metab Rev 1993;5:159.

Olesen J, Edvinsson L (eds): *Headache Pathogenesis*, Vol. 7. *Monoamines, Neuropeptides, Purines, and Nitric Oxide.* Lippincott-Raven, 1997.

10

Mostly Auditory or Vestibular

▶ CASE 12 _____

For over a year a 47-year-old woman has been having attacks of dizziness and tinnitus. Each episode begins with a feeling of fullness in her left ear, followed within a minute or two by left-sided hearing loss and roaring tinnitus. A few minutes later vertigo begins, with the environment appearing to spin toward her left. Rapidly increasing in severity, the vertigo is accompanied by nausea and vomiting. During attacks, which last 4–5 hours, she is unable to stand and falls toward the left. Her first few attacks were 2 or 3 weeks apart, but they have increased in frequency to one every few days. Head movement does not precipitate them, but it does aggravate the severity of vertigo once present, and during attacks vertigo is lessened by lying on her side with her left ear uppermost. In recent weeks she has noticed, while using the telephone, that her hearing is decreased on the left, yet loud noises produce subjective discomfort in that ear.

Examined during an attack, she is agitated, pale, and sweaty, lying on her side and maintaining as still a posture as possible. There is bilateral conjugate nystagmus on primary gaze, horizontal with a rotatory component, the fast phase beating toward her left. Following the attack she feels weak all over but no longer has nystagmus. Hearing is decreased on the left, with bone and air conduction equally affected; the Weber test (a 512-Hz tuning fork placed over her mid-forehead) lateralizes to the right. Audiometric testing reveals hearing loss on the left, greatest for low-pitched tones. As volume is increased, however, she reports similar subjective loudness in each ear. The left stapedial reflex threshold, determined by impedance measurements, is reduced. Caloric testing, using electronystagmographic recording, reveals a decreased response when warm or cold water is squirted onto the left tympanic membrane. Brain stem auditory evoked response (BAER) testing reveals a delay in the appearance of the first wave on the left.

Comment

Ménière disease consists of recurrent attacks of vertigo, hearing loss, and tinnitus. Patients are usually asymptomatic between attacks, but over time hearing loss becomes cumulatively persistent. Symptoms are the result of increased pressure within the endolymphatic compartment of the inner ear labyrinth, including the cochlea, saccule, utricle, and semicircular canals (see Figure 3–11). Episodic malabsorption of endolymph through the endolymphatic duct and sac cause the endolymphatic compartment to become dilated and ballooned. In some cases an underlying disease such as trauma or syphilis is identified, but most cases are cryptogenic.

Hearing loss is cochlear in type. As with any sensorineural deafness, bone and air conduction are equally affected, and the Weber test lateralizes sound to the good ear. There is also recruitment, an abnormally increased subjective sense of loudness once threshold is reached. Recruitment is objectively reflected in the abnormal impedence generated by the patient's stapedial reflex. BAERs show delay in the first wave, which is generated within the cochlea.

The patient's vertigo is the result of sudden imbalance between her left and right semicircular canals, which normally respond to angular acceleration. Vertigo is usually rotatory, as in this case, but it can resemble swaying, rolling, or pitching; patients know the problem is in the head, not simply an imbalance involving the limbs or trunk. Peripherally generated vertigo of even moderate severity is always accompanied by nystagmus, and often by nausea and vomiting. (With destructive lesions, the fast component of nystagmus is usually directed contralateral to the lesion; with irritative lesions, ipsilateral to the lesion.) During attacks movement aggravates vertigo, and patients prefer to lie with the affected ear uppermost. In some patients, usually after years of symptoms, mild movement-precipitated vertigo persists between attacks. As in this case, patients may have abnormal vestibular function on caloric testing and nystagmography yet remain asymptomatic betweeen attacks, an example of vestibular plasticity.

Patients with Ménière disease sometimes have drop attacks—sudden falls without loss of consciousness, associated with a feeling of being pulled downward. Such symptoms might be related to disturbance of the utricle or saccule, which normally respond to linear acceleration and the position of the head in relation to gravity.

The usual course of Ménière disease is resolution of attacks after months or years, at which point there is partial or incomplete deafness in the affected ear. About 10% of cases are bilateral. Antihistamine drugs lessen the severity of vertigo. The value of salt restriction (to reduce production of endolymph, which has a composition similar to that of intracellular fluid) has never been proven. Surgical approaches include labyrinthectomy and cutting the vestibular branch of the eighth cranial nerve.

SELECTED REFERENCES

Baloh RW: Neurotology. In: Joynt RJ, Griggs R (eds): *Clinical Neurology,* Vol. 3 (pp. 1–39). J.B. Lippincott, 1989.

Baloh RW, Jacobson BA, Winder T: Drop attacks with Ménière syndrome. Ann Neurol 1990;28:384.

Brandt T: Man in motion. Historical and clinical aspects of vestibular function. A review. Brain 1991;114:2159.

▶ CASE 13

For several months a 50-year-old woman has had increasing difficulty understanding what people are saying over the phone, which she customarily holds over her left ear. There is no problem with her right ear, and she has no other symptoms. On examination there is mild flattening of her left nasolabial fold, and she tends to speak out of the right side of her mouth. On tandem gait she is wobbly. Hearing, tested with a 512-Hz tuning fork, is mildly decreased on the left, whether the tuning fork is held a distance from her ear or applied to her mastoid bone, and air conduction is still present when bone conduction has ceased. When the fork is held to the middle of her forehead, the sound is louder in her right ear.

On audiometric testing there is high-frequency hearing loss on the left, with impaired speech discrimination out of proportion to pure tone impairment. There is no loudness recruitment, and continuous tones presented at threshold gradually decrease in subjective loudness (tone decay). Brain stem auditory evoked responses are abnormal on the left, with a prolonged interpeak interval between waves I and III, indicating delayed conduction between the distal eighth nerve and the lower pons. Caloric testing for vestibular function shows mild impairment on the left. Magnetic resonance imaging with Tl-weighted axial scans and gadolinium reveals an enhancing lesion 1.5 cm in diameter within the left internal auditory canal.

At surgery the tumor is an acoustic neuroma, which, with the use of microsurgical techniques, is totally removed. A month later her hearing has improved and her neurological examination is otherwise normal.

Comment

Acoustic neuromas are schwannomas that arise from the eighth cranial nerve at the cerebellopontine angle or within the internal auditory canal (Figure 10–1). Benign and encapsulated, they grow slowly at 2–10 mm/year, and although they usually arise from the vestibular portion of the nerve, initial symptoms are nearly always

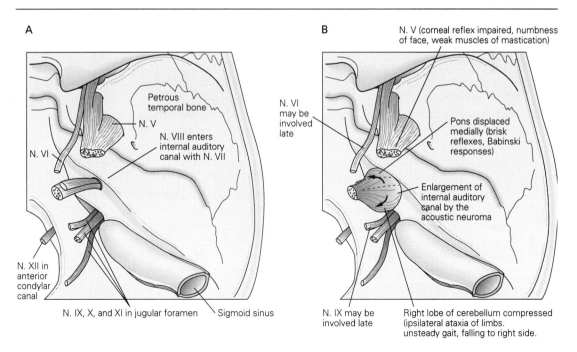

Figure 10–1. A. Inner surface of normal cerebellopontine angle (brain and cerebellum removed). **B.** Acoustic neuroma. (Reproduced with permission from Kandel ER, Schwartz JH, Jessell TM. 1991. *Principles of Neural Science*, 3rd ed. Norwalk, CT: Appleton & Lange.)

auditory. As is characteristic of lesions affecting the eighth nerve rather than the cochlea, impaired speech discrimination precedes frank deafness and may exist for months or years. Tinnitus and gait unsteadiness are commonly present by the time the patient seeks attention; less often there is headache, otalgia, facial weakness, or facial hypesthesia. Large tumors affect lower cranial nerves or cause brain stem compression with pyramidal or ipsilateral cerebellar signs. Obstruction of cerebrospinal fluid flow causes hydrocephalus, with nausea, vomiting, altered mentation, and papilledema. Probably because the tumors grow so slowly, vertigo is unusual, and when present it is less paroxysmal and severe than with Ménière disease.

Computerized tomographic and magnetic resonance imaging allows early diagnosis and treatment of acoustic neuromas. This patient's story is fortunately typical; when first seen for her hearing difficulty she had only mild signs indicating involvement of her facial nerve and the vestibular division of her acoustic nerve. Her auditory assessment revealed abnormalities characteristic of a nerve rather than a cochlear lesion, and surgery resulted in removal of the tumor without damaging the facial nerve or even producing left-sided deafness.

Bilateral acoustic neuromas appearing around the age of 20 are the principal manifestation of neurofibromatosis type 2, an autosomal dominant genetic disorder that maps to chromosome 22q12.

SELECTED REFERENCES

Glasscock ME, Hays JW, Minor LB, et al: Preservation of hearing in surgery for acoustic neuroma. J Neurosurg 1993;78:864.

Harner SG, Laws ER: Clinical findings in patients with acoustic neurinoma. Mayo Clinic Proc 1983;58:721.

Mikhael MA, Circ IS, Wolff AP: MR diagnosis of acoustic neuromas. J Comput Assist Tomogr 1987;11:232.

▶ CASE 14

A 63-year-old man suddenly develops vertigo, nausea, and vomiting and is unable to stand. There is no headache. In a hospital emergency room he is alert, attentive, and cooperative, complaining of severe dizziness aggravated by any head movement and diminished by eye closure. His pulse is irregularly irregular at a rate of 88/minute; blood pressure is 180/90 mm Hg. There is coarse horizontal nystagmus on conjugate gaze in either direction that is greater to the right. On attempting to stand, he falls to the right. Hearing is normal. There is no cerebellar dysmetria, intention tremor, or dysdiadochokinesis, and the rest of the neurological examination, including strength, sensation, and reflexes, is normal. An electrocardiogram shows atrial fibrillation.

The initial diagnostic impression is acute labyrinthitis, but magnetic resonance imaging (MRI) scan reveals probable infarction involving the inferomedial right cerebellar hemisphere, and he is admitted and treated with intravenous heparin for presumed cardioembolic stroke. Over the next 48 hours he becomes progressively obtunded and unable to move his eyes conjugately past the midline to the right. Repeat MRI scan shows increased mass effect from the infarct, with downward herniation of the cerebellar tonsils through the foramen magnum and enlargement of the third and lateral ventricles; the lower brain stem is compressed but there is no evidence of brain stem infarction. An emergency occipital craniectomy is performed, and necrotic and hemorrhagic cerebellar tissue is removed. Recovery is rapid, and a week later his neurological examination is entirely normal.

Comment

The inferomedial portion of the cerebellum is supplied by a medial branch of the posterior inferior cerebellar artery, which in this patient probably became occluded by a cardiac embolus resulting from his atrial fibrillation. This part of the cerebellum contains the flocculonodular complex, which has primarily vestibular connections (Figure 10–2). As a consequence, *infarction* produces vertigo, nausea, vomiting, and inability to stand or walk in the absence of cerebellar signs such as dysarthria, dysmetria, intention tremor, or dysdiadochokinesis. A subtle clue to the cerebellar origin of the lesion is that the fast component of the patient's nystagmus was of greatest amplitude when he looked toward the right, and he tended to fall toward the right. In destructive labyrinthine lesions, the fast com-

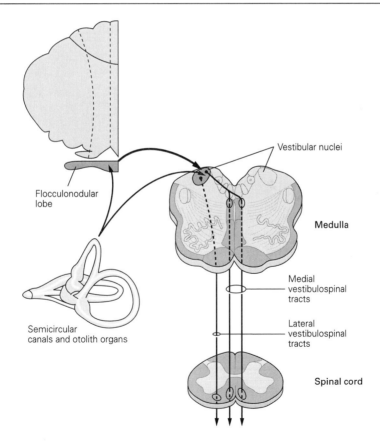

Figure 10–2. The vestibulocerebellum (flocculonodular lobe) receives input from the vestibular labyrinth and projects directly to the vestibular nuclei. Acute damage to this structure can cause vertigo suggestive of peripheral labyrinthine disease. (Reproduced with permission from Kandel ER, Schwartz JH, Jessell TM. 1991. *Principles of Neural Science*, 3rd ed. Norwalk, CT: Appleton & Lange.)

ponent of nystagmus is usually directed away from the side of the lesion and the patient tends to fall toward the side of the lesion. Vertigo and nystagmus of either origin are aggravated by movement.

Clinical deterioration in such a patient could be the result of brain stem infarction due either to reembolism or to propagation of the initial thrombus back into the posterior inferior cerebellar, vertebral, or basilar arteries. MRI revealed that the cause was increased size of the cerebellar mass, perhaps secondary to both edema and hemorrhagic transformation, with brain stem compression and obstructive hydrocephalus. Decompressive surgery (with no time to spare) resulted in complete resolution of symptoms, an example of brain tissue redundancy (noneloquence) and plasticity.

SELECTED REFERENCES

Amarenco P, Roullet E, Hommel M, et al: Infarction in the territory of the medial branch of the posterior cerebellar artery. J Neurol Neurosurg Psychiatry 1990;53:731.

Berth A, Bogousslavsky J, Regli F: The clinical and topographic spectrum of cerebellar infarcts: A clinical-magnetic resonance imaging correlation study. Ann Neurol 1993;33:451.

Norrving B, Magnusson M, Holtas S: Isolated acute vertigo in the elderly: Vestibular or vascular disease? Acta Neurol Scand 1995;91:43.

11

Mostly Olfactory

▶ CASE 15

For several months a 57-year-old woman has noticed that food seems to have less taste. She also has had intermittent midfrontal headaches. On examination there is normal taste sensation to sugar, salt, vinegar, and quinine, but smell is absent to peppermint, lemon, and coffee. Except for mildly decreased corrected visual acuity on the left, the neurological examination is normal. Magnetic resonance imaging reveals a 3-cm sharply demarcated mass occupying the olfactory grooves beneath the frontal lobe and strongly enhancing with gadolinium. A diagnosis of meningioma is confirmed at surgery; following total removal of the tumor her visual acuity on the left returns to normal, but she remains anosmic.

Comment

Meningiomas arise from arachnoidal cell clusters either within arachnoidal villi or where cranial nerves or blood vessels penetrate the dura. Comprising 20% of intracranial tumors, they are usually encapsulated and benign, and they cause symptoms by compressing adjacent structures. Approximately 10% of meningiomas are located at the olfactory cribriform and ethmoid regions, where they cause unilateral or bilateral anosmia by damaging the olfactory bulbs. As these slow-growing tumors enlarge, they compress the optic nerves or chiasm, producing visual impairment or even complete blindness. Very large olfactory meningiomas cause mental symptoms—particularly indifference or abulia—by compressing the frontal lobes or the anterior cerebral arteries (see Case 77).

Because olfactory areas of the frontal and temporal lobes are so widely distributed, lesions of frontal or temporal cortex seldom cause selective anosmia (Figure 11–1). (Subtle disturbances in olfactory discrimination, however, have been described in patients with inferomedial temporal lobe lesions; the impairment is often unilateral on the same side as the temporal lobe pathology.) Neocortical orbitofrontal olfactory areas receive projections from the piriform cortices of the temporal lobes (both directly and through the dorsomedial nucleus of the thalamus), and surgical removal of these orbitofrontal areas in animals results in impaired olfactory discrimination. These neocortical olfactory areas are too laterally placed, however, to be affected by most medially located olfactory meningiomas. More vulnerable are the olfactory bulbs and the primary olfactory fibers projecting to them from the nasal olfactory epithelium (which contains, among its several million olfactory neurons, many different G-protein-coupled odorant receptors). On the other hand, anosmia following head injury—a common occurrence—might result from shearing of olfactory fibers

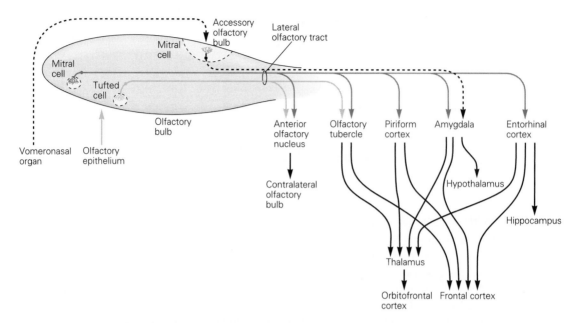

Figure 11–1. Olfactory information is transmitted to multiple regions of the olfactory cortex. This extensive distribution means that anosmia is seldom the result of cortical lesions. (Reproduced with permission from Kandel ER, Schwartz JH, Jessell TM. 1999. *Principles of Neural Science*, 4th ed. New York: McGraw-Hill.)

passing through the cribriform plate, bilateral contusion of the orbitofrontal cortex, or both.

It is not unusual for anosmia to be subjectively interpreted as altered taste. Whereas taste consists of four basic senses—sweet, salt, sour, and bitter, each with a specific receptor—over 1000 different types of olfactory receptors exist, enabling humans to distinguish thousands of odors at concentrations of a few parts per trillion. Much of what we consider subtle in what we taste, therefore, is actually what we smell.

SELECTED REFERENCES

Buck L, Axel R: A novel multigene family may encode ordorant receptors: A molecular basis for odor recognition. Cell 1991;65:175.

Cushing H: Meningiomas arising from the olfactory groove. Lancet 1927;1:1329.

Hildebrand JG, Shepherd GM: Mechanisms of olfactory discrimination: Converging evidence for common principles across phyla. Annu Rev Neurosci 1997;20:595.

Reed RR: Opening the window to odor space. Science 1998;279:193.

Savic I, Bookheimer SY, Fried I, Engel J: Olfactory bedside test. A simple approach to identify temporo-orbitofrontal dysfunction. Arch Neurol 1997;54:162.

▶ CASE 16

A 12-year-old boy suffers concussion and a skull fracture. For a few hours after the injury he displays both anterograde and retrograde amnesia. Memory then returns to normal except for inability to recall the injury and the period immediately following it. His neurological examination and computerized tomographic scan are normal.

A year later he begins having peculiar spells that occur in flurries, several times daily for a couple of days every few weeks. The attacks begin with a funny feeling in his abdomen, which rises to his chest, like a weight, and are accompanied by a sharp smell of something burning, which is most unpleasant. During and after these spells, which last 1 or 2 minutes, his mind wanders, he has difficulty concentrating, and he feels sleepy. His mother has observed a staring expression and quivering of the lips, and he often has no recall for his longer lasting spells. His neurological examination a day following an attack is normal. An electroencephalogram (EEG) during sleep reveals sharp waves emanating from the right anterior temporal lobe. A magnetic resonance imaging scan shows shrinkage of the right hippocampus on coronal section. He is prescribed carbamazapine, with reduction in the frequency of his spells.

Comment

As noted in Case 4, the clinical manifestations of a seizure depend on what part of the brain is discharging abnormally. When initial subjective symptoms are not associated with objective signs, they are referred to as *auras*. An aura is not a warning that a seizure is coming; it is a partial simple seizure, and it indicates a focal lesion.

Focal seizures consisting of olfactory hallucinations are most often associated, as in this patient, with damage to the hippocampus or uncus (hence Jackson's term uncinate seizures). The epileptic discharges accounting for the olfactory symptoms arise, however, from adjacent olfactory cortex, not the hippocampus (Figure 11–2). As noted in Case 15, there are several olfactory areas on the ventral and medial surfaces of the temporal and frontal lobes. These include the anterior olfactory nucleus, the amygdala, the olfactory tubercle, the piriform and periamygdaloid cortex, and the entorhinal cortex. In addition, the gyrus rectus of the orbitofrontal cortex has been implicated as a possible source of olfactory auras.

A hallucination of taste may accompany the olfactory symptoms, or a patient may have difficulty describing the sensation as either taste or smell. True gustatory auras are probably due to discharges from the insula. Another common aura is an unpleasant sensation in the abdomen that rises to the chest, throat, or head. Strongly associated with hippocampal scarring (mesial temporal sclerosis), abdominal auras probably also originate in either the insula or the amygdala. They may be associated with autonomic symptoms such as nausea and vomiting.

This patient's seizures sometimes progressed to staring, facial automatisms, and amnesia for the episode. Seizures consisting of focal symptoms with preserved alertness and memory are called *partial simple*. When consciousness is impaired or there is no recollection of the episode, they are called *partial complex* and probably represent spread into limbic and diencephalic structures. Both partial simple and partial complex seizures may progress further into *tonic-clonic* or *grand mal* seizures (see Case 30).

A Standard electrode placement

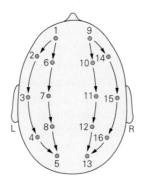

B EEG of awake human

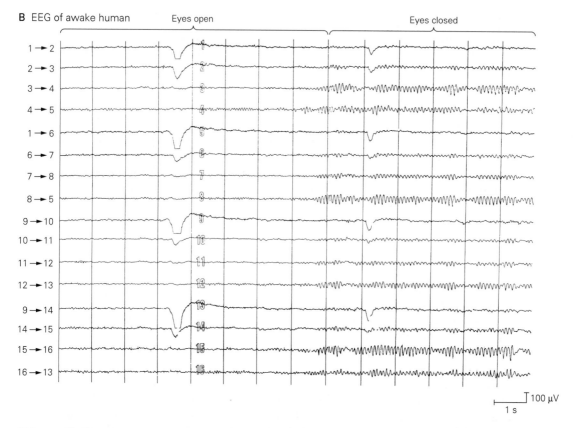

Figure 11–2. Electroencephalography (EEG). **A.** A standard set of electrode placements over the surface of the scalp. Recorded voltages are the potential differences between two electrodes. **B.** EEG activity in a normal awake subject. Vertical lines delimit 1 second. During the first 8 seconds the subject rests with eyes open, and the EEG shows rapid low-voltage (circa 20 μV) activity diffusely over the scalp (beta rhythm). During the fourth second the subject blinks, producing an artifactual high-voltage potential frontally. During the tenth second the subject's eyes close, producing another artifact, and the record now shows medium voltage sinusoidal activity at 8–10 Hz occipitally. This is alpha rhythm, thalamocortically generated and characteristic of a relaxed wakeful state. **C.** EEG activity in a subject with epilepsy. Focal sharp waves (spikes) are present in electrodes located over the right temporal lobe (enclosed in boxes) reflecting a seizure focus in that area. This paroxysmal activity arises suddenly and disrupts the normal background EEG pattern. The spikes are called interictal when no clinical seizure activity accompanies them. [Reproduced with permission from Kandel ER, Schwartz JH, Jessell TM. 1999. *Principles of Neural Science*, 4th ed. New York: McGraw-Hill. Adapted with permission from Lothman EW, Collins RC. 1990. Seizures and epilepsy. In: Pearlman AL, Collins RC (eds): *Neurobiology of Disease*. New York: Oxford University Press, pp. 276–298.]

C EEG activity in a subject with epilepsy

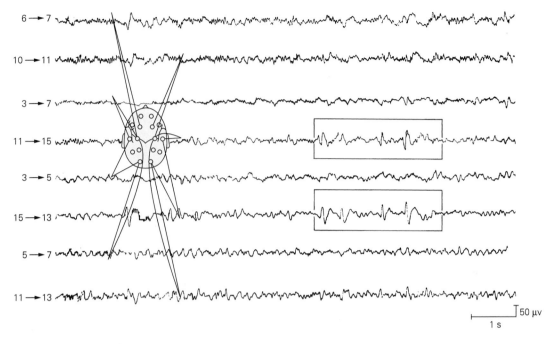

Figure 11–2. *(continued)*

SELECTED REFERENCES

Acharya V, Acharya J, Lüders H: Olfactory epileptic auras. Neurology 1998;51:56.
Lennox WG, Lennex MA: *Epilepsy and Related Disorders* (2 volumes). Little, Brown, 1960.
West SE, Doty RL: Influence of epilepsy and temporal lobe resection on olfactory function. Epilepsia 1995;36:531.

12

Mostly Motor

► CASE 17

A 15-year-old boy, weak since early childhood, has been wheelchair-bound for 3 years. Apparently normal at birth, he did not walk until 17 months of age, and he never ran normally. By age 3 toe-walking and a waddling gait were evident, and he had difficulty climbing stairs and rising from a chair without using his arms. His stance was described as broad based, with a forward pelvic tilt and compensatory lumbar lordosis. By age 12 there was obvious scoliosis, which became progressively severe after he was confined to a wheelchair. He is an only child. His parents are neurologically asymptomatic, but a maternal uncle died in his mid-20s of a progressive neuromuscular disorder.

On examination, findings include scoliosis, scapular winging, and flexion contracture of the ankles, knees, hips, and elbows. Heel-cord shortening produces an equinovarus deformity of his feet. Limb and trunk muscles are severely wasted, particularly proximally; the calf muscles (gastrocnemii) have relatively preserved bulk. He is unable to rise from a chair, to stand unsupported, or to raise his arms against gravity; his neck flexors, pectoralis major, latissimus dorsi, biceps, triceps, wrist extensors, anterior tibials, peronei, and gastrocnemii are prominently and bilaterally weak. Less weak are the muscles of his hands and feet. Facial muscles, speech, swallowing, and eye movements are normal. Tendon reflexes are absent except for a barely elicitable ankle jerk. Mentation is normal, as is sensation.

Serum creatine kinase level is 30 times normal. Nerve conduction velocities are normal. With intramuscular needle recording the electromyogram (EMG) shows no fibrillations, fasciculations, or positive waves at rest; motor unit potentials during voluntary contraction of hand and foot muscles are polyphasic and of reduced amplitude and duration (Figure 12–1). Biopsy of the gastrocnemius reveals evidence of degeneration and regeneration, hyaline fibers, and replacement by fat and connective tissue with scattered muscle fibers of variable size, some abnormally small and some abnormally large. Immunocytochemial studies indicate that dystrophin is absent from muscle surface membranes. An electrocardiogram shows increased R–S amplitude in the right precordial leads and a deep Q wave in the left precordial leads. Southern blot analysis of the patient's DNA reveals a deletion within the p21 region of the X chromosome. The

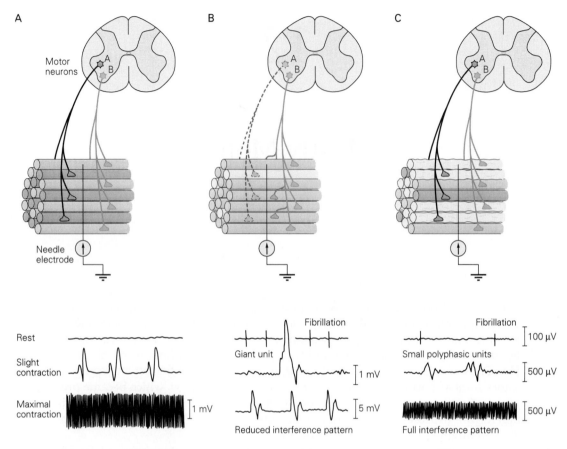

Figure 12–1. Effects of neurogenic and myopathic diseases on the motor unit as observed at electromyography (EMG). **A.** When a motor neuron fires in normal muscle, muscle fibers innervated by that motor neuron generate action potentials simultaneously, producing a compound action potential that can be recorded by a needle electrode inserted into the muscle. The muscle fibers are quiescent when the motor neuron is not firing. With maximal muscle contraction, many compound action potentials are superimposed on each other. **B.** In diseases producing denervation, motor units are lost, and maximal muscle contraction produces fewer compound action potentials. However, sprouting of preserved axons onto muscle fibers that have lost their nerve terminals produces motor units with increased numbers of muscle fibers. The result is compound action potentials with increased amplitude and duration. In addition, denervation of muscle fibers causes up-regulation of acetylcholine receptors on the muscle membrane, causing spontaneous firing of muscle fibers reflected eletromyographically as fibrillation potentials. In motor neuron disease, for example, amyotrophic lateral sclerosis, there is spontaneous firing of entire motor units—fasciculations. **C.** In myopathic disease the number of muscle fibers in each motor unit is reduced. There is no axonal sprouting, and so compound action potentials are reduced in amplitude and duration. (Reproduced with permission from Kandel ER, Schwartz JH, Jessell TM. 1999. *Principles of Neural Science,* 4th ed. New York: McGraw-Hill.)

mother's serum creatine kinase level is mildly elevated, and she is hemizygous for the deletion.

Comment
Diseases of muscle—myopathies—include inflammatory immune-mediated disorders (dermatomyositis, polymyositis, inclusion body myositis), infections (trichinosis, mycoplasma, coxsackie virus), drug toxicity (ethanol, chloroquine,

corticosteroids), endocrine disorders (hyperthyroidism, hyperparathyroidism), and many hereditary disorders. Muscular dystrophies have several characteristics. They are inherited; they cause progressive weakness; they show no evidence of denervation by clinical, histological, or EMG criteria; they do show histological evidence of muscle degeneration but no abnormal storage of a metabolic product. One of the most common progressive muscular dystrophies, first described in 1855 and affecting 1 in 3500 male births, is the X-linked disorder named after Guillaume Duchenne.

With some notable exceptions, myopathies tend to affect proximal muscles earlier and more severely than distal muscles. Waddling gait is the result of gluteus medius weakness (hip abduction), and difficulty rising from a chair or climbing stairs is the result of gluteus maximus and quadriceps weakness (hip and knee extension). To rise from a sitting position the patient puts his hands on his knees, pushes his trunk back, and then works his hands up his thighs (Gowers sign). Weakness of the abdominal and paraspinal muscles produces a forward pelvic tilt with exaggerated lordosis as a compensatory maneuver to maintain balance. Serratus anterior weakness results in scapular winging. Except for occasional mild facial weakness, cranial muscles (speech, swallowing, eye movements) are spared. Tendon reflexes are eventually lost, proportionate to wasting and weakness. Sensation is normal. Electrocardiographic changes are usually not accompanied by cardiac symptoms, but congestive heart failure sometimes develops. Investigators have described mild mental retardation.

Electromyographic abnormalities are typically myopathic. Serum creatine kinase elevations, probably secondary to sarcolemmal damage with leakage of the enzyme, are usually at least 20 times normal. Muscle biopsy shows degeneration and regeneration of muscle fibers of varying sizes with neither inflammation nor storage of a metabolic product. Replacement of muscle by fat and connective tissue is responsible for the preserved bulk of some affected muscles (pseudohypertrophy), particularly the gastrocnemius.

Duchenne muscular dystrophy is the result of a gene mutation at the p21 region of the X chromosome. The gene product, *dystrophin,* is a cytoskeletal protein located at the inner surface of the sarcolemmal membrane. Dystrophin is part of an elaborate protein complex that links actin within the muscle fiber and laminin on the muscle fiber's external surface. With 2.5 million base pairs, the dystrophin gene is the largest yet characterized in humans. In Duchenne muscular dystrophy deletions or duplications at Xp21 shift the translational reading frame such that no messenger RNA (mRNA) or dystrophin is synthesized. Absence of dystrophin probably results in membrane instability, abnormal contraction and relaxation, and eventually excessive calcium influx and fiber necrosis. Mutations that maintain the reading frame produce abnormal mRNA and dystrophin, resulting in a clinically milder myopathy called Becker muscular dystrophy. Female carriers of a single Xp21 mutation often have elevated serum creatine kinase levels but are rarely symptomatic. Mutations affecting other components of the dystrophin-associated protein complex—termed dystroglycans and sarcoglycans—result in different forms of limb-girdle muscular dystrophy (Figure 12–2).

The diagnosis of Duchenne muscular dystrophy can be made by DNA analysis, including *in utero.* There is no effective treatment, however, and the role of dystrophin in muscular physiology is still uncertain. Of two animal models, dogs lacking dystrophin are weak, but mice lacking dystrophin are not.

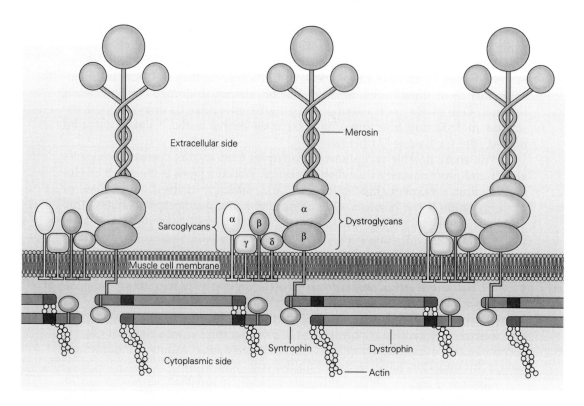

Figure 12–2. Muscle fiber membrane, showing the relationship of dystrophin to intracellular actin and extracellular sarcoglycans and dystroglycans. (Adapted with permission from Duggan DJ, Gorospe JR, Fanin M, et al. 1997. Mutations in the sarcoglycan genes in patients with myopathy. N Engl J Med 336:618.)

SELECTED REFERENCES

Brown RH: Dystrophin-associated proteins and the muscular dystrophies. Annu Rev Med 1997;48:457.

Bushby KMD: Genetic and clinical correlations of Xp21 muscular dystrophy. J Inher Metab Dis 1992;15:551.

Dubowitz V: The muscular dystrophies—clarity or chaos. N Engl J Med 1997;336:650.

Sunada Y, Campbell KP: Dystrophin-glycoprotein complex: Molecular organization and critical roles in skeletal muscle. Curr Opin Neurol 1995;8:379.

▶ CASE 18

A man in his mid-20s insidiously develops mild ptosis, which slowly progresses over the next several years. In his early 30s he notes weakness of the muscles of his lower face—he can no longer whistle. By age 40 his jaw, hands, and feet are weak, his voice has become nasal, hoarse, and monotonous, and he often chokes on food or liquids. For many years he has noticed that when he grasps an object vigorously, including handshaking, he has difficulty letting go. His father, who died accidently in his 50s, was affected by a similar illness beginning in his late 30s. A sister at age 33 has droopy eyelids.

On examination he has frontal balding, and wasting of his temporalis and masseter muscles gives his face a long lean appearance. Prominent ptosis, secondary to levator palpebrae weakness, is accompanied by a wrinkled forehead as he attempts to look upward. Eye and mouth closure are weak, and his speech is hypophonic, breathy, and nasal. His sternocleidomastoid muscles are small, and there is weakness of neck flexion. Weakness and wasting are prominent distal to the elbows and knees, and tendon reflexes are lost at the ankles and finger flexors. Tapping his thenar eminence with a reflex hammer produces a local contraction of the muscle, which then gradually relaxes. Mental status and sensation are normal, but, on ophthalmoscopic examination, refractile cataracts are seen bilaterally.

An electrocardiogram reveals right bundle branch block. Nerve conduction velocities are normal, and electromyography reveals short-duration reduced-amplitude polyphasic potentials consistent with myopathy; in addition, during relaxation there are high-frequency discharges with waxing and waning amplitude (*myotonia*). Southern blot analysis of leukocyte DNA reveals an expanded fragment on chromosome 19. With polymerase chain reaction (PCR), the expansion is shown to consist of cytosine-thymine-guanine repeats.

Comment

Whereas Duchenne muscular dystrophy primarily affects trunk and proximal limb muscles and tends to spare muscles innervated by cranial nerves, *myotonic muscular dystrophy* primarily affects distal limb and cranial muscles. The cause of these regional specificities is unknown. Myotonic muscular dystrophy is an autosomal dominant hereditary disorder; the responsible gene is located at chromosome 19q13.3, and its product is myotonin protein kinase (MT-PK). By phosphorylating specific substrates, protein kinases provide the mechanism through which many hormones, neurotransmitters, and other extracellular signals exert their physiological effects on target cells. The function of MT-PK is uncertain; it might regulate the function of sodium channels involved in muscle action potentials or of calcium channels in the sarcoplasmic reticulum (the internal membrane system that allows electrical discharges to spread rapidly throughout the muscle cell). Normally, the MT-PK gene contains a repeated trinucleotide sequence, cytosine-thymine-guanine (CTG), varying in size from 5 to 40 CTG units; myotonic muscular dystrophy patients have expansions of these repeated sequences of 50 to several thousand units, and the longer the repeat size the earlier the onset and the greater the severity of disease. Within families the repeat size often increases with each generation, accounting for *anticipation*, an earlier onset of disease in successive generations.

Short repeated elements are common in the human genome, and their expansion is responsible for a number of neurological genetic disorders, including fragile X syndrome, Friedreich ataxia, and Huntington disease. In myotonic muscular dystrophy the expanded CTG repeat is located at an untranslated region of the gene, and in contrast to some other trinucleotide repeat diseases (eg, fragile X syndrome), the mytonic muscular dystrophy gene product—MT-PK—is made. Whether it functions normally is less clear, and an alternative to decreased MT-PK function is that the expanded CTG repeat leads to increased production of a malfunctioning protein (gain of function—see Case 26). Another possibility is that the expanded CTG repeat affects the transcription or function of another protein.

A striking feature of myotonic muscular dystrophy is myotonia, delayed relaxation after a forceful contraction associated with continuous motor unit activity in the electromyogram. As with the dystrophy, the pathophysiological relationship of myotonia to decreased levels of MT-PK protein expression is unclear. Myotonia often precedes weakness in patients with mytonic muscular dystrophy, and in patients with both features, myotonia is often present in muscles (eg, tongue or finger flexors) that are not clinically weak. Infants with congenital mytonic muscular dystrophy and severe weakness may not demonstrate myotonia. Myotonia also occurs in disorders other than mytonic muscular dystrophy, including myotonia congenita, a hereditary abnormality of chloride channels mapped to chromosome 7q35. Myotonia is demonstrated by failure of a muscle to relax quickly after voluntary contraction or by focal contraction when a muscle is tapped by a reflex hammer (percussion myotonia). The latter phenomenon persists after curarization, demonstrating that it is caused by an abnormality distal to the neuromuscular junction, on the muscle surface membrane.

Frequent in mytonic muscular dystrophy, but also unexplained, are frontal balding, cataracts, testicular atrophy, and peripheral resistance to insulin. Cardiac conduction abnormalities are common and usually asymptomatic, but some patients develop congestive heart failure or die suddenly. Diaphragmatic weakness and alveolar hypoventilation predispose to chronic pulmonary infection. Gastrointestinal smooth muscle involvement produces pseudoobstruction. Behavioral abnormalities and mild mental retardation are common.

The clinical heterogeneity of mytonic muscular dystrophy is perhaps related to the fact that transcription of the gene normally results in several alternatively spliced mRNA forms that vary in different tissues and change with development. For example, during the first year of life a fetal/neonatal form of MT-PK mRNA is switched to another form. If, in fact, MT-PK dysfunction is responsible for the symptoms and signs of mytonic muscular dystrophy, this developmental switch might explain why myotonia is usually absent during infancy. The precise role of MT-PK in muscle (and other tissues) remains elusive, however.

A genetically separate disorder resembles myotonic muscular dystrophy except that limb weakness is mainly proximal. Termed myotonic muscular dystrophy type 2, this disease is linked to the long arm of chromosome 3, but as of 1999 the particular genetic fault was unknown.

SELECTED REFERENCES

Paulson HL, Fischbeck KH: Trinucleotide repeats in neurogenetic disorders. Annu Rev Neurosci 1996;19:79.

Pizzuti A, Friedman DL, Caskey CT: The mytonic muscular dystrophy gene. Arch Neurol 1993; 50:1173.

Ricker K, Grimm T, Koch MC, et al: Linkage of proximal myotonic myopathy to chromosome 3q. Neurology 1999;52:170.

Roses AD: Mytonic muscular dystrophy. In: Rosenberg RN, Prusiner SB, DiMauro S, Barchi RL (eds): *The Molecular and Genetic Basis of Neurological Disease,* 2nd edition (pp. 913–930). Butterworth-Heinemann, 1997.

► CASE 19

A 26-year-old woman notes the intermittent appearance of horizontal diplopia and bilateral ptosis. Symptoms fluctuate throughout the day but are most severe during the afternoon or evening. Ptosis is sometimes greater in the left eye and at other times is greater in the right eye. A few weeks after the appearance of these symptoms her voice becomes increasingly nasal during prolonged speaking, and soon afterward she develops difficulty swallowing both liquids and solids.

On examination there is bilateral ptosis and limitation of upward gaze, which becomes increasingly obvious as she attempts to look at the ceiling for 30 seconds. Gazing horizontally in either direction reveals bilateral medial rectus weakness, which also becomes more pronounced as lateral gaze is maintained. Less obvious is probable weakness of the left lateral and right inferior rectus muscles. Eye closure is also weak bilaterally, as is lip pursing (orbicularis oris), baring of her teeth (levator anguli oris), and jaw opening (mylohyoid). Repetition of the vowel *Ah* produces nasality, indicating failure to maintain palatal closure. There is mild weakness of neck and shoulder girdle muscles. Strength is otherwise normal, as are pupils, sensation, and tendon reflexes.

Nerve conduction velocities are normal, and electromyography (EMG) does not reveal evidence of either denervation or myopathy. Repetitive stimulation at 3 Hz produces decrement of the compound action potential by 20% of baseline, and single fiber EMG reveals increase in the intervals between discharges of muscle fibers innervated by the same motor neuron (jitter). Antibodies to acetylcholine receptor are present in her blood. Following intravenous administration of 5 mg edrophonium there is unequivocal improvement in ptosis and disconjugate eye movements lasting about 5 minutes.

Comment

Myasthenia gravis is caused by defective neuromuscular transmission secondary to antibody-mediated attack on nicotinic acetylcholine (ACh) receptors located at the muscle end-plate. A normal end-plate contains several hundred thousand ACh receptors, ligand-gated channels permeable to sodium and potassium ions (Figure 12–3). Opening of these channels by ACh produces the end-plate potential, a local depolarization of the muscle membrane. Normally, each end-plate potential produces a depolarization large enough to open adjacent voltage-gated sodium channels on the muscle membrane. When a sufficient number of voltage-gated sodium channels are opened, a muscle action potential is generated (Figure 12–4).

The polyclonal immunoglobulin G antibodies that bind to ACh receptor epitopes not only interfere with binding by acetylcholine but result in actual loss of receptors. By cross-linking receptors, antibodies to ACh receptors accelerate their internalization (endocytosis) and lysosomal hydrolysis and trigger complement-mediated lysis of the postsynaptic membrane. Neuromuscular end-plates in myasthenia gravis have an abnormally reduced density of ACh receptors, shallow and sparse junctional folds, and widened synaptic spaces. Although the amount of ACh released into the synapse is normal, the reduced density of ACh receptors makes it less likely that any single molecule of ACh will interact with an ACh receptor before being degraded by acetylcholinesterase.

The consequence of this damage is reduced amplitude of the end-plate potentials. Under resting conditions these reduced end-plate potentials can still pro-

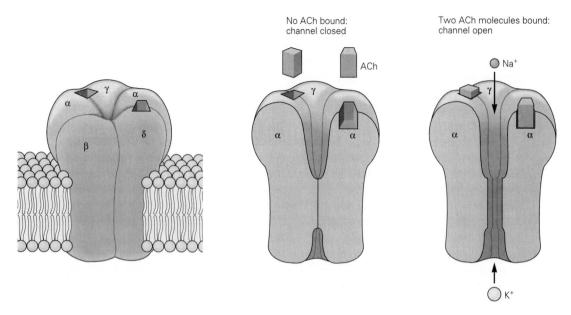

Figure 12–3. Nicotinic acetylcholine (ACh)-activated ion channels, present on the muscle end-plate region of the neuromuscular junction, produce end-plate potentials when ACh molecules bind to α-subunits. Altered conformation of the channel opens its pore, allowing Na⁺ and K⁺ to flow through the channel in the direction of their electrochemical gradients. (Reproduced with permission from Kandel ER, Schwartz JH, Jessell TM. 1999. *Principles of Neural Science*, 4th ed. New York: McGraw-Hill.)

duce muscle action potentials. During repetitive firing, however, end-plate reserve is insufficient to generate consecutive end-plate potentials large enough to trigger muscle action potentials (Figure 12–5). Inhibitors of acetylcholinesterase such as edrophonium and pyridostigmine improve neuromuscular transmission by prolonging the duration that ACh molecules remain in the synapse, thereby increasing the likelihood of their interacting with ACh receptors and raising end-plate potential amplitudes to a level capable of generating muscle action potentials.

These abnormalities are reflected electrophysiologically in reduced amplitude of spontaneous miniature end-plate potentials and of evoked end-plate potentials, decrement of the muscle compound action potential at low frequencies of repetitive stimulation, and increased jitter on single fiber EMG (Figure 12–6). They are reflected clinically in the unique features of myasthenia gravis, namely weakness that fluctuates from minute to minute, day to day, or week to week and that responds to inhibitors of acetylcholinesterase.

Myasthenia gravis affects ocular muscles initially in about 40% of cases and eventually in nearly 90% (Figure 12–7). Dysarthria, dysphagia, and weakness of eye closure, facial expression, and chewing are common, as are neck and limb weakness, but whereas weakness can be limited to cranial muscles, limb weakness rarely occurs alone. If myasthenia is limited to the ocular muscles for 2 years, it is unlikely to become generalized. Severe generalized myasthenia, on the other hand, can affect not only the diaphragm but even the external sphincters of the bladder and bowel. Cardiac and smooth muscle are spared; in particular,

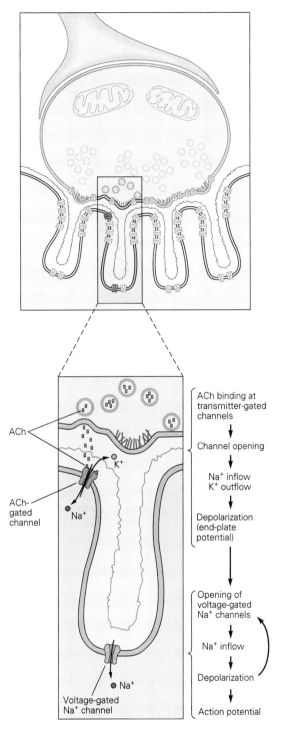

Figure 12–4. The neuromuscular junction. Acetylcholine (ACh) is stored within synaptic vesicles at presynaptic endings of motor nerves. During neuromuscular transmission calcium entry into the nerve terminal causes release of ACh into the synaptic cleft. The binding of ACh to ACh receptors at the motor end-plate opens channels permeable to both Na^+ and K^+, depolarizing the cell membrane and producing an end-plate potential. This depolarization opens adjacent voltage-gated Na^+ channels in the muscle membrane; when a sufficient number of these Na^+ channels are opened, a muscle action potential is generated. (Reproduced with permission from Kandel ER, Schwartz JH, Jessell TM. 1999. *Principles of Neural Science,* 4th ed. New York: McGraw-Hill. Adapted with permission from Alberts B, Bray D, Lewis J, et al. 1989. *Molecular Biology of the Cell,* 2nd ed. New York: Garland.)

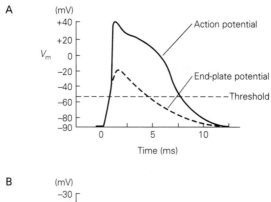

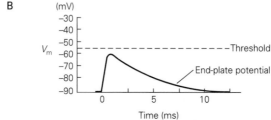

Figure 12–5. A. Under normal circumstances, stimulation of a motor axon produces an end-plate potential that, if sufficient to reach threshold, triggers a muscle action potential. **B.** Curare blocks the binding of acetylcholine (ACh) to its receptor at the muscle end-plate, preventing the end-plate potential from reaching the threshold for an action potential. In myasthenia gravis, immune-mediated damage to end-plate ACh receptors results in comparable electrophysiological abnormality and weakness. (Reproduced with permission from Kandel ER, Schwartz JH, Jessell TM. 1999. *Principles of Neural Science*, 4th ed. New York: McGraw-Hill.)

pupillary reactivity is never compromised. Myasthenic crisis refers to exacerbation of symptoms sufficient to compromise respiration so that ventilation has to be assisted mechanically.

The ultimate cause of this autoimmune disorder is unknown. Fifteen percent of adults with myasthenia have a thymoma, and, in most of the rest, the thymus is not normally involuted but rather contains multiple lymphoid follicles with germinal centers (thymic hyperplasia). Thymic myoid cells have ACh receptors, and it is believed that their proximity to thymic T cells and B cells might make them particularly vulnerable to immune attack, which would then involve similar epitopes at the neuromuscular end-plate. In most patients without thymoma, thymectomy produces sustained improvement. In those with thymoma, improvement may follow thymectomy, but less consistently than in patients without thymona.

Symptomatic treatment of myasthenia with anticholinesterase drugs such as pyridostigmine is partially effective. For patients unable to undergo thymectomy, corticosteroid or other immunosuppressive drugs are used.

About 12% of infants born to myasthenic mothers have several days or weeks of weak sucking, crying, or breathing; the cause is placental transfer of maternal ACh receptor antibodies that gradually disappear. By contrast, congenital myasthenia affects infants of asymptomatic mothers, and neither the mother nor the infant have circulating ACh receptor antibodies. This disorder, often genetic, appears to be heterogeneous in cause, with both presynaptic and postsyn-

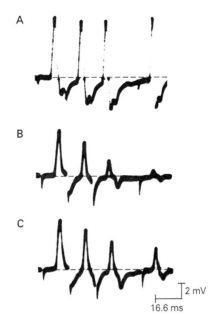

Figure 12–6. A. In a normal person, repetitive nerve stimulation at 16.6 ms intervals produces constant amplitude of muscle action potentials. **B.** In a patient with myasthenia gravis there is a rapid decrement in amplitude. **C.** Following injection of the acetylcholinesterase inhibitor neostigmine, the decrement in amplitude is partially reversed. (Reproduced with permission from Kandel ER, Schwartz JH, Jessell TM. 1999. *Principles of Neural Science,* 4th ed. New York: McGraw-Hill. Adapted with permission from Harvey AM, Lilienthal JL Jr, Talbot SA. 1941. Observations on the nature of myasthenia gravis the phenomena of facilitation and depression of neuromuscular transmission. Bull Johns Hopkins Hosp 69:547.)

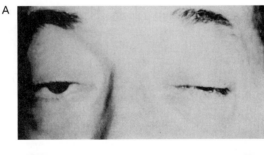

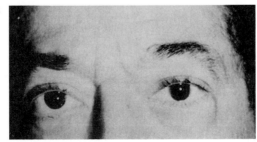

Figure 12–7. A. A patient with myasthenia gravis and severe ptosis. **B.** Following injection of the acetylcholinesterase inhibitor edrophonium, ptosis is relieved. (Reproduced with permission from Kandel ER, Schwartz JH, Jessell TM. 1999. *Principles of Neural Science,* 4th ed. New York: McGraw-Hill. Adapted with permission from Rowland LP, Hoefer PFA, Aranow H Jr. 1960. Myasthenic syndromes. Res Publ Assoc Res Nerv Ment Dis 38:548.)

aptic end-plate abnormalities that include prolonged opening of ACh receptor channels, defective structure of ACh receptor subunits, lack of end-plate acetylcholinesterase, and deficient numbers of the synaptic vesicles that contain ACh. About 15% of adult myasthenics also lack ACh receptor antibodies, and it is possible that some of them have non–immune-mediated disorders of the neuromuscular junction similar to those identified in patients with congenital myasthenia.

SELECTED REFERENCES

Drachman DB: Myasthenia gravis. N Engl J Med 1994;330:1797.

Engel AG: Myasthenic syndromes. In: Engel AG, Franzini-Armstrong C (eds): *Myology*, 2nd edition (pp. 1798–1835). McGraw-Hill, 1994.

Hohfeld R, Wekerle H: The thymus in myasthenia gravis. Neurol Clin North Am 1994;12:331.

Nichols P, Croxen R, Vincent A, et al: Mutation of the acetylcholine receptor ε-subunit promotor in congenital myasthenic syndrome. Ann Neurol 1999;45:439.

▶ CASE 20

A 7-year-old boy has had attacks of limb weakness for several months. Coming on about 15 minutes after vigorous exercise, paresis starts in his legs and lower back and spreads to his arms and shoulders but not to his cervical, cranial, or respiratory muscles. Weakness usually lasts less than an hour, and mild exercise seems to shorten the attacks, which occur every few days. On a few occasions exposure to cold has triggered weakness. Between attacks physical and neurological examinations are normal, as are serum levels of sodium and potassium. During a spontaneous attack of weakness, however, his tendon reflexes cannot be elicited, there is myotonic lid lag when he looks downward, and his serum potassium rises to 6.4 mEq/L. Between attacks electromyography (EMG) reveals high-frequency muscle fiber discharges that wax and wane in amplitude (ie, myotonia). Oral administration of potassium chloride is followed by weakness, during which serum potassium levels again rise and EMG reveals reduced amplitude and duration of some motor unit potentials plus myotonic hyperirritablity.

Following prescription of daily oral acetazolamide he experiences a marked reduction in the frequency of his attacks.

Comment

As noted in Case 19, the neuromuscular junction is a synapse with ligand-gated (directly gated) ion channels that, once activated by acetylcholine (ACh), are permeable to both sodium and potassium. By contrast, the nonjunctional muscle membrane contains separate classes of voltage-gated sodium and potassium channels activated by membrane depolarization. A muscle fiber action potential occurs when sufficient ACh has opened enough channels at the neuromuscular junction to produce an end-plate potential large enough to recruit voltage-gated channels on the adjacent muscle membrane. End-plate potentials are graded; their amplitude depends on the number of open channels, which is a function of the amount of ACh released. Action potentials are regenerative; influx of positively charged sodium ions through the sodium channel further depolarizes the membrane, opening more channels until, by continuing positive feedback, an action potential is generated. Voltage-gated sodium channels are blocked by the puffer fish toxin tetrodotoxin; ligand-gated end-plate channels are not. Myasthenia gravis is a disorder of the muscle end-plate. Hyperkalemic periodic paralysis, as exemplified by this patient, is a disorder of muscle membrane voltage-gated sodium channels.

Familial periodic paralysis is a group of genetic autosomal dominant disorders characterized by episodic limb weakness. In *hypokalemic* periodic paralysis attacks follow a period of rest or a high carbohydrate meal; weakness is often present on awakening in the morning. During an attack serum potassium levels are low and serum sodium levels are high, and attacks can be precipitated by insulin and glucose (which drive potassium into cells) and terminated by giving potassium salts. In *hyperkalemic* periodic paralysis, attacks usually occur during the day, particularly during a brief rest after vigorous exercise. They are accompanied by elevated serum potassium levels, precipitated by potassium salts, and relieved by glucose and insulin. Some patients with hyperkalemic periodic paralysis also have an unusual type of myotonia—paramyotonia congenita—often induced by cold and increased with continued muscle contraction. In both hypokalemic and hyperkalemic periodic paralysis cranial and respiratory muscles are usually spared, and in patients with either disorder daily administration of the carbonic anhydrase inhibitor acetazolamide prevents attacks.

Familial hyperkalemic periodic paralysis and paramyotonia cogenita, alone or in combination, are caused by different mutations of a gene on chromosome 17q23–25 that codes for the pore-forming α-subunit of the skeletal muscle voltage-gated sodium channel. The most frequently encountered mutations in familial hyperkalemic periodic paralysis involve a segment of the protein close to the region believed necessary for channel inactivation. Patch clamp experiments reveal abnormal sodium channel behavior in which a small percentage of channels fail to inactivate (close) during a prolonged depolarization (Figure 12–8). It is possible, therefore, that impaired inactivation of the sodium channel is responsible for both myotonia and weakness. Myotonia would occur because of persistent mild depolarization of the membrane and hyperexcitability. Weakness would occur when hyperkalemia induced by potassium intake or exercise produces further membrane depolarization (by shifting the Nernst potential for K^+), causing more sodium channels to open. Their failure to close results in membrane inexcitability and paralysis (Figure 12–9). In support of such a pathophysiological mechanism is the observation that muscle isolated from patients with hyperkalemic periodic paralysis is partially polarized at rest and that such depolarization is blocked by tetrodotoxin.

The phenotypic variation among patients with hyperkalemic periodic paralysis—different degrees of myotonia and episodic weakness—is the result of allelic heterogeneity—different mutations of the same gene on chromosome 17. Hypokalemic periodic paralysis, however, is caused by mutation of a gene on chromosome 1 encoding the L-type voltage-gated calcium channel, which, within muscle fibers, links membrane excitation to intracellular calcium release, allowing contraction (*excitation-contraction coupling*) (Figure 12–10). The pathophysiology of that disorder is less clear, and it is not readily apparent why acetazolamide, which increases potassium excretion, prevents attacks of weakness in both hypokalemic and hyperkalemic periodic paralysis.

Still another group of familial muscular diseases is caused by mutations of the skeletal muscle chloride channel gene on chromosome 7; these disorders are characterized by myotonia, usually without weakness (myotonia congenita).

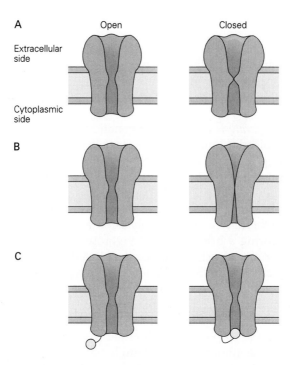

Figure 12–8. Models of ion channel gating. A channel can open and close as a result of conformational change either in one region of the channel (**A**) or along the length of the channel (**B**). In some channels a blocking particle swings into and out of the channel mouth (**C**). In hyperkalemic periodic paralysis, weakness and myotonia occur when muscle voltage-gated sodium channels fail to close properly. (Reproduced with permission from Kandel ER, Schwartz JH, Jessell TM. 1999. *Principles of Neural Science,* 4th ed. New York: McGraw-Hill.)

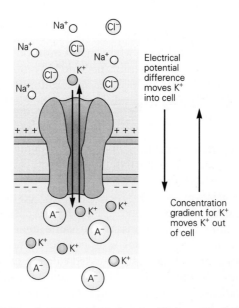

Figure 12–9. In a cell permeable to potassium, a potassium equilibrium potential will be reached when the driving force of the concentration gradient for K+ across the cell membrane, which moves K+ out of the cell, is equal to the driving force of the electrical potential across the cell membrane, which moves K+ into the cell. In hyperkalemic periodic paralysis the membrane is partially depolarized at rest; increasing extracellular K+, by shifting the Nernst potential for K+, depolarizes the membrane further, causing voltage-sensitive sodium channels to open and triggering weakness. (Reproduced with permission from Kandel ER, Schwartz JH, Jessell TM. 1999. *Principles of Neural Science,* 4th ed. New York: McGraw-Hill.)

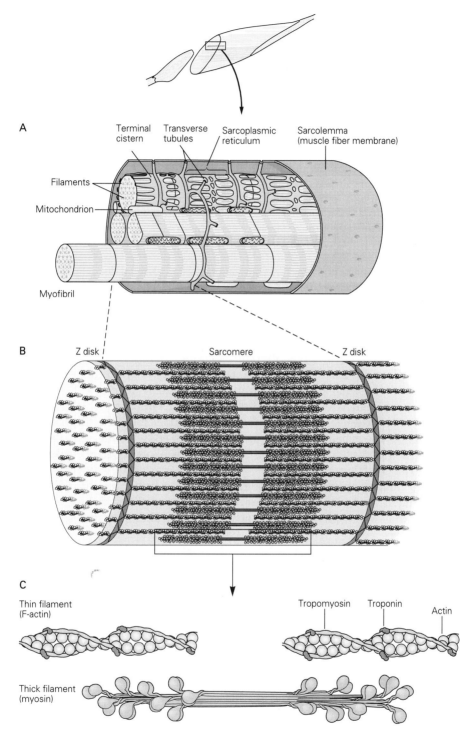

Figure 12–10. Skeletal muscle, demonstrating the structures that underlie excitation-contraction coupling. **A.** The relationship of the sarcolemma (muscle fiber membrane), the transverse tubules, the sarcoplasmic reticulum, and the myofibrils. **B.** An individual myofibril, showing light and dark bands and sarcomeres separated by thin Z disks. **C.** An individual sarcomere, showing thin actin filaments and thick myosin filaments. (Reproduced with permission from Kandel ER, Schwartz JH, Jessell TM. 1999. *Principles of Neural Science,* 4th ed. New York: McGraw-Hill. Adapted with permission from Bloom W, Fawcett DW. 1975. *A Textbook of Histology,* 10th ed. Philadelphia: Saunders and from Loeb GE, Gans C. 1986. *Electromyography for Experimentalists.* Chicago: University of Chicago Press.)

Nonneurological disorders involving sodium, potassium, or chloride channels include cystic fibrosis and the cardiac long-QT syndrome. Collectively, these diseases are appropriately termed *channelopathies.*

SELECTED REFERENCES

Ackerman MJ, Clapham DE: Ion channels—basic science and clinical disease. N Engl J Med 1997;336:1575.

Barchi RL: Ion channels and disorders of excitation in skeletal muscle. Curr Opin Neurol Neurosurg 1993;6:40.

Cannon SC: Ion-channel defects and aberrant excitability in myotonia and periodic paralysis. Trends Neurosci 1996;19:3.

Hayward LJ, Sandoval GM, Cannon SC: Defective slow inactivation of sodium channels contributes to familial periodic paralysis. Neurology 1999;52:1447.

Hudson AJ, Ebers GC, Bulman DE: The skeletal muscle sodium and chloride channel diseases. Brain 1995;118:547.

Rudel R, Ricker K, Lehmann-Horn F: Genotype-phenotype correlations in human skeletal muscle sodium channel diseases. Arch Neurol 1993;50:1241.

► CASE 21

A 54-year-old woman develops abdominal cramps, nausea, and vomiting, followed a day later by diarrhea. The next day she notes a dry mouth and dysphagia. A private physician prescribes antibiotics. She then develops diplopia and ptosis. In an emergency room 5 days after the onset of symptoms, she has a hoarse voice and repeatedly rinses her mouth with water; her tongue and pharynx are dry and red. There is bilateral ptosis, and she cannot abduct either eye. Pupils are 4 mm and do not react to light or near gaze. There is bilateral facial weakness, reduced palatal elevation, and an absent gag reflex. Her arms are moderately weak. Mentation, sensory function, and coordination are normal; tendon reflexes are barely elicitable, and plantar responses are flexor. X-ray films of the chest reveal consolidation in the right lower lobe, and a film of the abdomen shows distention of the transverse colon consistent with adynamic ileus. She receives antibiotics for pneumonia. The next day her arms and legs are weaker, ptosis is more pronounced, and there is limited eye movement in all directions of gaze. She complains of shortness of breath, and her forced vital capacity is 800 mL.

There is no improvement in strength following intravenous administration of the cholinesterase inhibitor edrophonium. Nerve conduction velocities and distal motor latencies are normal; compound muscle action potentials of the median, ulnar, and posterior tibial nerves are reduced in amplitude. Repetitive stimulation of the ulnar nerve at 3 Hz results in a mild decrement in the amplitude of the compound muscle action potential; stimulation at 30 Hz results in a marked incremental response.

She undergoes endotracheal intubation and ventilatory support, blood and stool specimens are sent for mouse injection, and she receives botulism equine trivalent antitoxin (ABE). Weakness progresses for another day, with complete external ophthalmoplegia and loss of tendon reflexes. Her strength, oral secretions, and gastrointestinal motility then gradually improve over the next 5 weeks, allowing extubation after 10 days and oral feeding after 21 days. On the eighth day of treatment blood and stool specimens are reported to contain Type B botulinum toxin.

Comment

In contrast to myasthenia gravis, which is the result of damage to the postsynaptic component of the neuromuscular junction (see Case 19), botulinum toxin impairs acetylcholine (ACh) release from presynaptic nerve endings at the endplate. The mechanism is interference with the formation of ACh vesicles and their calcium-mediated attachment to the terminal membrane. (Another disease of defective ACh release at the neuromuscular junction, the Lambert-Eaton syndrome, is the result of autoantibodies to voltage-gated calcium channels in presynaptic terminals.) Botulinum toxin is among the most potent poisons known; an amount weighing less than the weight of a period typed onto a page would kill 30 adults, and half a pound would he enough to kill every human being on earth.

Myasthenia gravis impairs cholinergic nicotinic receptors at the neuromuscular junction but spares muscarinic receptors mediating autonomic and smooth muscle function. By contrast, because botulinum toxin blocks release of ACh, it affects both nicotinic and muscarinic cholinergic transmission, and the dry mouth, unreactive pupils, ileus, and hypotension seen in this patient, although not invariant, are not unusual.

In *botulism*, repetitive stimulation of peripheral nerves at low rates of stimulation produces no change or a mild decrement in the amplitude of muscle compound action potentials, whereas high rates of stimulation produce large increments. An explanation lies in the presynaptic locus of the disease. The amount of ACh released into the synaptic cleft at the neuromuscular junction depends on both the amount of calcium entering the presynaptic nerve terminal with the arrival of the nerve action potential and the number of ACh vesicles available for release (Figure 12–11). At low rates of motor nerve firing there is little increase in the concentration of calcium within the presynaptic terminal, but the repetitive

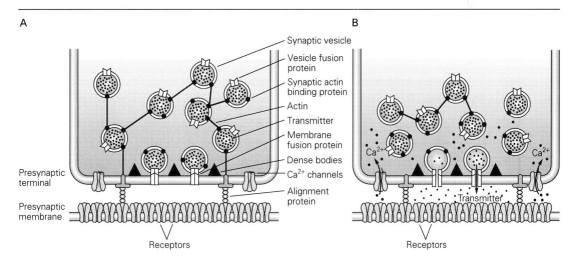

Figure 12–11. A. The neuromuscular junction in the resting state. In the nerve terminal most acetylcholine-containing vesicles are anchored to actin filaments (black bars), and voltage-gated calcium channels are closed. **B.** An action potential arriving at the nerve terminal opens the Ca^{2+} channels, and Ca^{2+} entering the cell dissolves actin filaments, allowing vesicles to move to the plasma membrane, where fusion and exocytosis occur. Botulinum toxin interferes with vesicle formation and fusion and thereby blocks neuromuscular transmission. (Reproduced with permission from Kandel ER, Schwartz JH, Jessell TM. 1991. *Principles of Neural Science*, 3rd ed. Norwalk, CT: Appleton & Lange.)

firing does deplete the already reduced stores of ACh; the result is a decrease in the amplitude of the compund muscle action potential. With high rates of stimulation, on the other hand, calcium concentration within the synaptic terminal increases to a degree sufficient to compensate briefly for the reduced ACh stores; the result is an increased amplitude of the compound muscle action potential (*posttetanic potentiation*). Response to acetylcholinesterase inhibitors in botulism is either weak or absent. Guanidine hydrochloride, a drug that facilitates release of ACh from peripheral nerve endings, is sometimes used in the treatment of botulism (or Lambert-Eaton syndrome), but its efficacy is unproven.

The diagnosis of botulism is confirmed by identification of toxin in blood and of toxin or *Clostridium botulinum* in feces. It often affects a group of people who were exposed to the same source of the poison. Treatment is intensive and often protracted. Because in severe cases the toxin actually destroys the terminal twigs of cholinergic nerve endings, necessitating terminal sprouting to form a new motor end-plate, recovery may take weeks, usually complicated by nosocomial infections.

SELECTED REFERENCES

Case records of the Massachusetts General Hospital: Botulism. N Engl J Med 1997;337: 184.

Sanders DB: Clinical neurophysiology of disorders of the neuromuscular junction. J Clin Neurophysiol 1993;10:167.

Schiavo G, Rossetto O, Benfenati F, et al: Tetanus and botulism neurotoxins are zinc proteases specific for components of the neuroexocytosis apparatus. Ann NY Acad Sci 1994;710:65.

Shapiro RL, Hatheway C, Swerdlow DL: Botulism in the United States. A clinical and epidemiologic review. Ann Intern Med 1998;129:221.

Woodrull BA, Grifin PM, McCroskey LM, et al: Clinical and laboratory comparison of botulism from toxin types A, B, and E in the United States, 1975–1988. J Infect Dis 1992;166:1281.

▶ CASE 22

Two weeks after a brief viral respiratory infection, a 62-year-old man develops mild paresthesias of his soles and achiness in his back and thighs. The following day his legs are weak, and over the next 12 hours the weakness in his legs becomes worse and spreads to his arms. In an emergency room that evening his legs have normal muscle tone and bulk, but he cannot move his toes or ankles and can barely lift either leg off the bed. His arms are moderately weak distally and severely weak proximally, and there is bilateral facial weakness. Tendon reflexes are absent in his legs and barely elicitable in his arms, and there is no plantor response. Vibratory, pinprick, and temperature sensation are mildly decreased in his feet and fingers; sensation is otherwise normal, as are his mental status and other cranial nerve functions. Vital capacity is 1.7 L (60% of predicted).

Motor nerve conduction studies show prolonged distal latencies for the facial, median, and ulnar nerves; amplitudes of compound action potentials evoked by stimulation of the median, ulnar, peroneal, and posterior tibial nerves are reduced. F-response latencies for the median and ulnar nerves are prolonged, and H-response latencies for the posterior tibial nerve/soleus muscle are unobtainable. A sural nerve sensory action potential is unobtainable, and a median nerve sensory action potential is of low amplitude. Needle electromyography (EMG) reveals a decreased amount of recruitment activity but neither positive waves nor fibrillations. The findings indicate acute, widespread, and severe sensorimotor polyneuropathy.

A course of plasmapheresis is started, but weakness progresses nearly to quadriplegia with difficulty swallowing and a fall in vital capacity to 1.1 L. He receives a tracheostomy and assisted ventilation. A week following admission, cerebrospinal fluid contains 7 lymphocytes/mL and a protein content of 120 mg/dL. For the next 4 weeks his weakness remains unchanged; it then begins to improve. A month after admission electrodiagnostic studies reveal widespread prolongation of motor conduction velocities and reduced amplitude of compound action potentials produced by proximal as compared to distal stimulation (*conduction block*). Needle EMG now reveals fibrillations and positive waves. Over the next several weeks he receives physical therapy and slowly improves. At discharge he has weakness and atrophy in his distal legs and is still diffusely areflexic.

Comment

The *Guillain-Barré syndrome* is an acute inflammatory demyelinating peripheral neuropathy of probably immunological cause. Weakness is always present. Sensory loss may be severe, mild, or absent. As in this patient, symptoms often follow a brief respiratory or gastrointestinal illness, progress rapidly over a few days or weeks, and, then, after a plateau period of usually a few weeks, gradually improve over months. Weakness of bulbar and respiratory muscles may necessitate artificial ventilation, and death can follow aspiration pneumonia or autonomic dysfunction with hypotension and cardiac arrhythmia. Recovery is often complete, but some patients are left with residual weakness, hyporeflexia, and muscle atrophy.

The earliest pathological abnormalities are perivascular and endoneurial infiltration of lymphocytes and perivenous demyelination that progresses to segmental demyelination and, if severe, axonal damage. Loss of myelin results in impaired saltatory conduction, reflected on electrodiagnostic testing by conduction block (reduced amplitude of the compound muscle action potential [CMAP] after proximal nerve stimulation compared to distal nerve stimulation) and prolonged motor nerve conduction velocities (abnormal increase in the duration between stimulating a nerve and the appearance of a CMAP) (Figures 12–12 and 12–13). In some patients the earliest damage affects the proximal nerve roots, reflected by abnormal F-waves (stimulating a motor nerve produces antidromic backfiring to its collective anterior horn cells, followed by orthodromic propagation of the impulse from these same anterior horn cells to the innervated muscle) and H-responses (stimulating sensory nerves projecting to muscle spindles produces, across a single synapse, firing of motor neurons—the electrical counterpart of the monosynaptic stretch reflex). At a time when the nerves distally may show neither conduction block nor prolonged conduction velocities, the F-wave and H-response latencies may be delayed (Figure 12–14). Finally, in severe cases there may be axonal injury, reflected electrodiagnostically by fibrillations and positive waves and, with reinnervation, polyphasic potentials of increased amplitude and duration (a result of terminal sprouting of preserved nerve terminals onto nearby denervated muscle fibers). (See Figure 12–1B.)

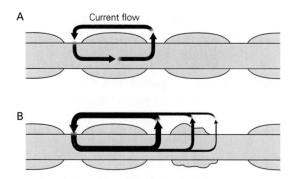

Figure 12–12. Nerve impulse conduction is impaired by demyelination. The arrows indicate current flow. **A.** The high resistance and low capacitance of myelin shunt current from one node of Ranvier to the next (saltatory conduction). **B.** With demyelination, current is lost through the damaged myelin sheath, and conduction velocity is reduced. (Reproduced with permission from Kandel ER, Schwartz JH, Jessell TM. 1999. *Principles of Neural Science,* 4th ed. New York: McGraw-Hill. Adapted with permission from Waxman S. 1982. Membranes, myelin, and the pathophysiology of multiple sclerosis. N Engl J Med 306:1529.)

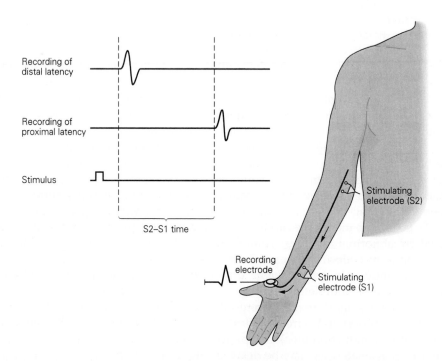

Figure 12–13. Conduction velocity of the median nerve is determined by stimulating the nerve at the elbow (S2) and wrist (S1) and recording the resulting action potentials in the thenar eminence. When the distance between the two points of stimulation is divided by the difference between the two time intervals (from stimulus to action potential), the result is the nerve's conduction velocity. (Reproduced with permission from Kandel ER, Schwartz JH, Jessell TM. 1999. *Principles of Neural Science,* 4th ed. New York: McGraw-Hill.)

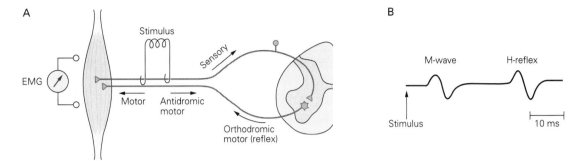

Figure 12–14. A. The anatomy underlying elicitation of the H-reflex and the M-wave. The H-reflex is evoked by electrical stimulation of afferents from primary spindle endings in mixed sensorimotor nerves. **B.** The M-wave and the H-reflex. The M-wave is the muscle action potential caused by orthodromic propagation of the volley evoked by directly stimulating the motor nerve. The H-reflex that follows is the muscle action potential produced when the evoked volley in the spindle afferents monosynaptically excites alpha motor neurons. The H-reflex is thus an electrical counterpart to the tendon stretch reflex, although it bypasses the spindle afferent endings. (Reproduced with permission from Kandel ER, Schwartz JH, Jessell TM. 1999. *Principles of Neural Science*, 4th ed. New York: McGraw-Hill.)

The cerebrospinal fluid (CSF) in Guillain-Barré syndrome characteristically shows at most a mild pleocytosis (usually less than 10 lymphocytes/dL, rarely more than 50) and an elevated protein content, but as with nerve conduction velocities, CSF abnormalities are often not present during the first few days of illness, and in some cases the CSF protein content never rises.

In animals a Guillain-Barré–like peripheral neuropathy can be produced by immunization with a particular protein, P_2, present in peripheral myelin (experimental allergic neuritis, EAN), and EAN can be transmitted by lymphocytes sensitized to myelin. The precise pathophysiology of human Guillain-Barré syndrome is less clear, but a plausible scenario is that a preceding infection stimulates an immune response to an exogenous antigen, followed by an autoimmune attack on epitopically similar antigens in myelin (molecular mimicry or innocent bystander effect). Serum from Guillain-Barré patients demyelinates peripheral nerve in culture, and circulating antibodies to different antigens, including P_2 and cerebroside, have been identified in some patients with Guillain-Barré syndrome.

A peripheral neuropathy clinically similar to Guillain-Barré syndrome, but with marked axonal degeneration and little or no demyelination, follows infection with *Campylobacter jejuni* and is associated with antibodies to ganglioside GM_1, which shares epitopes with *C jejuni* surface lipopolysaccharides. Another autoimmune neuropathy, Fisher syndrome, is characterized by gait ataxia, areflexia, and external ophthalmoplegia; in this disorder there are antibodies to the ganglioside GQ1b, which is particularly concentrated in nerve terminals innervating extraocular muscles.

Consistent with its probable immunological basis, the clinical course of Guillain-Barré syndrome is shortened by either plasmapheresis (which presumably removes offending antibodies) or infusion of human immune γ-globulin (which probably occupies myelin antigen epitopes, thereby blocking the autoimmune attack). Corticosteroids, however, are of no value. Residual weakness, greatest in patients with electrodiagnostic evidence of axonal injury, is not influenced by either plasmapheresis or immunoglobulins.

Chronic inflammatory demyelinating polyneuropathy (CIDP) refers to a peripheral neuropathy with pathological and electrodiagnostic features similar to those seen in Guillain-Barré syndrome, but with a fluctuating or progressive course over months or years. Unaccountably, this disorder, unlike Guillian-Barré syndrome, usually does respond to corticosteroids; it also responds to plasmapheresis and human immune γ-globulin.

SELECTED REFERENCES

Bolton CF: The changing concepts of Guillain-Barré syndrome. N Engl J Med 1995;333: 1415.

Hadden RDM, Cornblath DR, Hughes RAC, et al: Electrophysiological classification of Guillain-Barré syndrome: Clinical associations and outcome. Ann Neurol 1998;44:780.

Ho TW, McKhann GM, Griffin JW: Human autoimmune neuropathies. Annu Rev Neurosci 1998;21:187.

Ropper AH: The Guillain-Barré syndrome. N Engl J Med 1992;326:1130.

Steck AJ, Schaeren-Wiemers N, Hartung HP: Demyelinating inflammatory neuropathies, including Guillain-Barré syndrome. Curr Opin Neurol 1998;11:311.

The Italian Gullain-Barré Study Group: The prognosis and main prognostic indicators of Guillain-Barré syndrome. Brain 1996;119:2053.

► CASE 23

A 5-year-old boy is noted by his parents to have high arches and curled-up toes (hammer toes). Over the next few years his gait becomes awkward and clumsy; he trips easily and runs with increasing difficulty. By age 13 there is obvious weakness of his peronei, anterior tibials, and intrinsic foot muscles, and by his late teens walking requires him to lift his knees abnormally high to prevent his feet from dragging (steppage gait). Weakness of ankle plantar flexion makes it difficult to stand without continuously shifting his weight to maintain balance, and weakness of his hands makes it difficult for him to button or pick up small objects. On examination at age 24 there is atrophy of muscles below his knees, particularly the anterior tibials and peronei, and of his distal thighs. Dorsiflexion of his toes and ankles is absent (foot drop), and there is moderate weakness of gastrocnemii and his hands. Vibratory sensation and proprioception are mildly impaired in his feet. Tendon reflexes are absent throughout. Mentation and cranial nerve functions are normal.

Motor nerve conduction velocities are less than one-half of normal in his arms and legs, with distal motor latencies prolonged to three times normal. Needle electromyography shows evidence of denervation in leg and arm muscles. Sensory nerve action potentials are difficult to obtain and when present have long latency and low amplitude.

The patient's father is affected by a similar illness, which, at age 47, has rendered him wheelchair-bound. Both paternal grandparents are asymptomatic in their 70s. Genetic analysis reveals a 1.5-megabase DNA duplication in regions p11.2–p12 of chromosome 17 in the patient and his father but not in either paternal grandparent.

Comment

In 1886 Jean Martin Charcot and Pierre Marie in France and Howard Tooth in Britain described a familial form of progressive muscular atrophy that started in the feet and later spread to the hands. Sensation was affected to a lesser degree or not at all. It is now evident that *peroneal muscular atrophy* (Charcot-Marie-Tooth disease) represents a number of clinically and genetically distinct hereditary peripheral neuropathies. Type 1 is associated with markedly decreased nerve conduction velocities (reflecting demyelination) and Type 2 with normal nerve conduction velocities (reflecting primary neuronal or axonal pathology rather than demyelination). Both Type 1 and Type 2 are usually of autosomal dominant inheritance, but autosomal recessive forms of each type exist. An X-linked type, moreover, affects males more severely than females, with the result that nerve conduction velocities in males are slow (suggesting Type 1) but in females are normal or only mildly slow (suggesting Type 2). Other types have been separately classified on the basis of disease severity or association with other abnormalities such as spasticity, pigmentary retinopathy, optic atrophy, or deafness. Classification of these disorders—collectively designated *hereditary motor-sensory neuropathies* (HMSN)—has become more rational with the identification of their genetic defects.

The most common form of Type 1 HMSN (termed Type 1A) is associated with abnormality in the p11.2–p12 region of chromosome 17 (Figure 12–15). Most of these patients have a DNA duplication at that locus, resulting in overexpression of a gene coding for a peripheral myelin protein (PMP) called PMP-22. Much less often patients with the same phenotype have a point mutation in the PMP-22 gene. Spontaneous mutations and duplications of this gene are not unusual and likely account for the absence of disease in the present patient's grandparents. A hereditary peripheral neuropathy of mice (called trembler) is associated with mutations in the murine PMP-22 gene. Interestingly, in humans deletion of a 1.5-megabase region containing the PMP-22 gene produces a phenotypically different disease, *hereditary neuropathy with liability to pressure palsies*, in which weakness follows sustained pressure on peripheral nerves or the brachial plexus but with partial or complete recovery from each bout. As with HMSN Type 1A, nerve conduction velocities in this disorder are usually slow between attacks; unlike HMSN Type 1A, there is electrical conduction block (see Case 22). PMP-22 accounts for less than 5% of myelin protein, and its function is unknown. It is down-regulated following peripheral nerve injury and recovers after axonal regeneration, suggesting that axons regulate the expression of the PMP-22 gene in Schwann cells. Its low abundance makes a major structural role unlikely; PMP-22 is believed to be an adhesion molecule.

A much less common form of Type 1 HMSN (termed Type 1B) is the result of point mutations in the q22–q23 region of chromosome 1; this gene encodes a different protein, called P_O, which comprises 50% of peripheral myelin protein. A member of the immunoglobulin superfamily, P_O is believed to maintain tight compaction of myelin by linking adjacent myelin layers.

X-linked HMSN is associated with a number of point mutations at Xql3.1, which contains the gene for connexin-32, a gap junction protein. Gap junctions are small channels that connect the cytoplasm of adjacent cells, allowing passage of ions and small molecules. Connexin-32 is located at nodes of Ranvier, but its precise role in myelin physiology is uncertain; one possibility is that it allows transfer of ions and nutrients across the myelin sheath.

As in other demyelinating diseases, both peripheral (eg, Guillain-Barré neuropathy—see Case 22) and central (eg, multiple sclerosis—see Case 55), symptoms and signs correlate better with secondary axonal damage than with demyelination per se. How demyelination causes axonal loss is unclear.

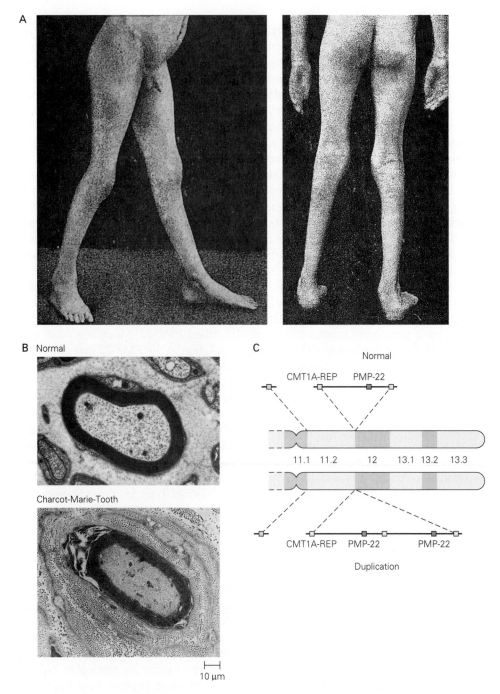

Figure 12–15. A. A patient with hereditary motor sensory neuropathy (HMSN) Type 1 (Charcot-Marie-Tooth disease), showing characteristic distal leg atrophy and foot deformity. **B.** Sural nerve biopsies from a normal subject and a patient with HMSN Type 1. The large axon in the normal nerve is ensheathed by myelin lamellae. The axon in the abnormal nerve contains collapsed lamellae and evidence of attempted myelin regeneration (onion bulbs). **C.** In HMSN Type 1, duplication of a normal 1.5-megabase region of the DNA at chromosome 17 p11.2–p12 results in overproduction of the peripheral myelin protein PMP-22. (Reproduced with permission from Kandel ER, Schwartz JH, Jessell TM. 1999. *Principles of Neural Science,* 4th ed. New York: McGraw-Hill. A. Adapted with permission from Charcot J-M, Marie P. 1886. Sur une forme particulière d'atrophie musculaire progressive, souvent familiale, débutant par les pieds et les jambes et atteignant plus tard les mains. Rev Med 6:97. B. Adapted with permission from Lupski JR, Garcia CA. 1992. Molecular genetics and neuropathology of Charcot-Marie-Tooth disease type 1A. Brain Pathol 2:337.)

Type 2 forms of HMSN, which are axonal disorders, are not associated with the genes for PMP-22, P_O, or connexin-32. Some families demonstrate linkage with the p35–p36 region of chromosome 1, and an additional locus has been mapped to chromosome 3q13–22, but the gene products are as yet unidentified. Some families with Type 2 HMSN have vocal cord paralysis and respiratory muscle weakness; chromosomal linkage has not (as of 1999) been established in this subgroup.

There is no treatment for the hereditary motor-sensory neuropathies other than braces, surgical correction of joint deformities, and physical therapy. Progression may be so indolent that over the years there is very little functional disability. In some patients (particularly the Type 2 axonal types), muscle atrophy causes the lower limbs to resemble stork legs or inverted champagne bottles.

A severe form of HMSN, traditionally referred to as Dejerine-Sottas disease, begins in infancy and is associated with either prominent peripheral nerve hypertrophy (*onion-bulbs*, from repeated demyelination and remyelination) or primary amyelination. Some families with the Dejerine-Sottas phenotype have a point mutation at the PMP-22 gene and others at the P_O gene.

SELECTED REFERENCES

Hanemann CO, Muller HW: Pathogenesis of Charcot-Marie-Tooth 1A (CMT1A) neuropathy. Trends Neurosci 1998;21:282.

Harding AE: From the syndrome of Charcot, Marie and Tooth to disorders of peripheral myelin proteins. Brain 1995;118:809.

Mendell JR: Charcot-Marie-Tooth neuropathies and related disorders. Semin Neurol 1998; 18:41.

Murakami T, Garcia CA, Reiter LT, et al: Charcot-Marie-Tooth disease and related inherited neuropathies. Medicine 1996;75:233.

Scherer S: Axonal pathology in demyelinating diseases. Ann Neurol 1999;45:6.

Suter L, Welcher AA, Snipes GJ: Progress in the molecular understanding of hereditary peripheral neuropathies reveals new insights into the biology of the peripheral nervous system. Trends Neurosci 1993;16:50.

▶ CASE 24

A 21-year-old man has noted hoarseness for 2 years, pain in the left side of his neck for several months, and slurred speech for several weeks. On examination a mass is felt in his left neck and retropharyngeal region. There is paralysis of his left palate, pharynx, and vocal cords; loss of general sensation over his left palate and pharynx; and loss of general sensation and taste over his left posterior tongue. The left palatal and gag reflexes are absent. His left sternocleidomastoid and trapezius muscles are weak and mildly atrophic. His tongue deviates to the left and has left-sided atrophy and fasciculations. The left pupil is 1 mm smaller than the right pupil and there is mild left upper and lower lid ptosis.

Computerized tomography confirms the presence of a soft tissue mass extending from the base of the skull to the third cervical vertebral body and projecting intracranially through the jugular foramen into the posterior fossa. The extracranial portion of the tumor is removed surgically and is found to be a meningioma. At a later date the intracranial portion is also removed.

A year later his neurological symptoms and signs have neither progressed nor improved.

Comment

The transverse venous sinus passes through the jugular foramen to become, in the neck, the jugular vein. Also passing through the jugular foramen are the glossopharyngeal (9), vagus (10), and spinal accessory (11) nerves (see Figure 3–14). Structural lesions in the region of the jugular foramen therefore damage all three of these lower cranial nerves, producing, as in this man, loss of general sensation over the palate and pharynx (9 and 10), loss of general sensation and taste over the posterior third of the tongue (9), paralysis of the palate, pharynx, and larynx (10), and atrophic weakness of the sternocleidomastoid and trapezius muscles (11). Together these symptoms and signs constitute the *jugular foramen syndrome*. Adjacent to the jugular foramen is the hypoglossal foramen, through which the twelfth cranial nerve exits; weakness of the tongue, with atrophy and fasciculations, is therefore often additionally present. Miosis and ptosis (Horner syndrome) occur when a tumor extends extracranially to involve the cervical sympathetic nervous system.

A variety of neoplastic and inflammatory processes, including metastatic cancer and tuberculosis, are associated with the jugular foramen syndrome. Glomus jugulare tumors, which arise from extraadrenal portions of the paraganglion chemoreceptor system, often erode the petrous bone and affect lower cranial nerves, but in the great majority of cases there is early invasion of the middle ear, with deafness, tinnitus, and a mass behind or protruding through the tympanic membrane.

SELECTED REFERENCES

Haymaker W: *Bing's Local Diagnosis in Neurological Diseases.* C.V. Mosby, 1969.

Kalovidouris A, Mancuso AA, Dillon W: A CT-clinical approach to patients with symptoms related to the V, VII, IX–XII cranial nerves and cervical sympathetics. Radiology 1984;151:671.

Thomas PK, Mathias CJ: Diseases of the ninth, tenth, eleventh, and twelfth cranial nerves. In: Dyck PJ, Thomas PK, Griffin JW, et al (eds). *Peripheral Neuropathy.* W.G. Saunders, 1993.

▶ CASE 25

A 22-year-old woman develops difficulty climbing stairs and running, and findings on examination include mild proximal weakness of her legs and arms, decreased tendon reflexes, and normal sensation. Muscular dystrophy is suspected, but electrodiagnostic studies reveal fibrillations, positive waves, and polyphasic potentials of increased duration and amplitude, indicative of denervation. Motor nerve conduction velocities and distal sensory latencies are normal. Biopsy of the quadriceps muscle also indicates denervation; many muscle fibers are reduced in size, and histochemical stains for adenosine triphosphatase and phosphorylase reveal fiber-type grouping—abnormal groups of fibers of the same histochemical type.

Over the next decade her proximal limb weakness slowly progresses, but at age 32 she is still fully ambulatory. On examination she walks with a side-to-side waddle, and there is mild-to-moderate weakness and atrophy of her pelvic and shoulder girdle muscles. Fasciculations—fleeting contractions of the muscle beneath the skin—are frequently observed. Tendon reflexes are absent. Mental status, cranial nerves, sensation, and vital capacity are normal.

Two younger brothers become similarly affected during their early 20s. Four other siblings and both of her parents are neurologically normal.

Comment

The hereditary *spinal muscular atrophies* (SMA) are defined by neuronal degeneration limited to alpha motor neurons. Although age of onset and severity vary widely, the great majority of affected families have a disorder of autosomal recessive inheritance resulting from abnormalities at the q11–q13 region of chromosome 5. A gene in this region, involved in all subtypes of SMA, codes for a protein designated survival motor neuron protein (SMNP). This protein is thought to exert a preventive action against apoptotic activity. Most patients with SMA 5q have homozygous deletions of exon 7, exon 8, or both of the SMNP genes. Another gene, located nearby, codes for a protein called neuronal apoptosis inhibitory protein (NAIP). Deletion of NAIP occurs in some cases of SMA 5q and probably contributes to clinical severity.

In the most severe form of SMA 5q, known as Werdnig-Hoffman disease, hypotonic weakness is present at birth or within the first 6 months of life and progresses to flaccid paralysis, respiratory failure, and death usually before age 2. Less severe forms of SMA 5q have onset of weakness during childhood, adolescence, or adulthood; generally, the later the onset, the more protracted the course. Later onset forms tend to produce proximal weakness affecting the legs more than the arms; in some of these families the disease limits neither social functioning nor life span. In such families it is unclear whether loss of motor units continues throughout life or whether the disease becomes static, with functional worsening the result of decompensating respiratory insufficiency, development of contractures, or inability to respond normally to the adolescent growth spurt. In any case, the varied phenotypy of SMA 5q is another example of allelic heterogeneity, similar to what is seen with the Duchenne-Becker group of muscular dystrophies (see Case 17).

Another hereditary disorder of lower motor neurons, *spinobulbar muscular atrophy* (Kennedy disease), begins in middle age with dysarthria and dysphagia, followed after a number of years by limb weakness. An X-linked recessive disorder, Kennedy disease, affects only men and is caused by expansion of a trinucleotide repeat (see Case 18) at Xq11–12, the site of the androgen receptor. Gynecomastia (breast hypertrophy) is usually present.

SELECTED REFERENCES

Dubowitz V: Chaos in classification of the spinal muscular atrophies of childhood. Neuromusc Disord 1991;1:77.
Gambardella A, Mazzei R, Toscano A, et al: Spinal muscular atrophy due to an isolated deletion of exon 8 of the telomeric survival motor neuron gene. Ann Neurol 1998;44:836.
Lannaccone ST: Spinal muscular atrophy. Semin Neurol 1998;18:19.
LaSpada AR, Wilson EM, Lubahn DB, et al: Androgen receptor gene mutation in X-linked spinal and bulbar muscular atrophy. Nature 1991;352:77.
Melki J, LeFebvre S, Burglen L, et al: De novo and inherited deletions of the 5q13 region in spinal muscular atrophies. Science 1994;264:1474.

▶ CASE 26

A 55-year-old man notices difficulty buttoning and turning keys. There is no pain, and over the next few weeks he realizes that his right hand is weak and has less muscle bulk than his left hand. Weakness then appears in his left hand and spreads to involve his entire right arm, and he experiences difficulty climbing stairs. Finger flexor cramps occur frequently, and he becomes aware of muscle twitching beneath the skin of his arms and chest. Eight months after the onset of his initial symptoms he develops slurred speech and difficulty swallowing liquids.

Examination reveals marked weakness and atrophy of his right hand, arm, and shoulder. He can barely move his fingers, which are held in a claw-like position (extension of the metacarpal-phalangeal joints and flexion of the interphalangeal joints, signifying lumbrical weakness). His thumb is held in a simian-like position (in the plane of the hand rather than at an angle to it, signifying weakness of thenar eminence muscles). Flexion and extension are weak at his right wrist and elbow, and he can raise his right arm only a few inches against gravity. Moderate weakness and atrophy are present in his left hand and arm. Leg weakness is less obvious, but he cannot step onto a chair with either leg and rises with effort onto the toes of either foot. His gait is short-stepped and stiff, and as he walks, his right arm hangs at his side without swinging. Tone is markedly increased in his legs and decreased in his right arm. Muscle twitches are continuously present over his arms, chest, and back; they are occasionally observed in his thighs and calves. Tendon reflexes are absent in his right finger flexors, 3+ in his left finger flexors, 3+ in his biceps and triceps bilaterally, and 4+ at his knees and ankles. Bilateral Babinski responses are present. His speech is nasal, he has difficulty pronouncing lingual consonants, and his tongue displays worm-like fasciculations. His palate does not move with vocalization or when touched, and his gag reflex is absent. Other cranial nerves, mental status, and sensation are normal. He has had no problem with micturition and specifically denies nocturia, frequency, urgency, or incontinence.

Motor nerve conduction velocities are normal in his legs and mildly reduced in his arms; there is no sign of conduction block. Electromyographically there is denervation, marked in his arms and moderate in his legs, with fibrillations, positive waves, and spontaneous polyphasic potentials, some with extremely prolonged duration and amplitude. Sensory latencies and amplitudes are normal.

Over the following year his weakness and atrophy progress relentlessly, and choking on food and liquids necessitates a feeding gastrostomy. Following a bout of pneumonia, his vital capacity is measured at 800 mL, and he is offered tracheostomy and ventilatory support.

Comment

This man has both lower-motor-neuron signs (weakness, atrophy, fasciculations, hypotonia, and decreased tendon reflexes) and upper-motor-neuron signs (weakness, spasticity, increased tendon reflexes, and Babinski signs) affecting his arms, legs, and cranial muscles (see Figure 4–1). Sensation is preserved. Such a combination is practically pathognomonic of *amyotrophic lateral sclerosis* (ALS), a degenerative disease of unknown cause selectively affecting upper and lower motor neurons. A key feature of the disease is the coexistence of upper- and lower-motor-neuron signs in the same muscle group, for example, as in this patient, a brisk tendon reflex in an atrophic, fasciculating biceps. When only upper-motor-neuron signs are present, the diagnosis of ALS requires electromyographic evidence of denervation. When only lower-motor-neuron signs are present, a definite diagnosis of ALS would have to await autopsy evidence of corticospinal tract involvement. Lower-motor-neuron signs limited to the arms and spasticity and hyperreflexia limited to the legs could be the result of cervical spinal cord compression. Such patients usually have sensory loss, either segmental (within the territory of one or more spinal roots) or below the level of the lesion (from involvment of the spinothalamic tracts or the dorsal columns), and the great majority have bladder symptoms. Bladder function is spared in ALS, at least until the final stage of the illness. Patients who choose ventilatory support can progress to total paralysis, their only voluntary movement consisting of eye movements (locked-in state; see Case 31).

Muscle cramps in ALS are attributed to irritability of denervated muscle. Fasciculations—brief spontaneous contraction of muscle fibers comprising a motor unit—are not specific for motor neuron disease; in fact, intermittent segmental fasciculations occur in normal people. In ALS, fasciculations are seen in weak atrophic muscles, presumably an indication that damaged motor neurons become irritable before they die.

ALS has an annual incidence of up to 2 per 100,000 population (in the United States, about 5000 new cases yearly). Because the mean duration of illness is only 3 years, the prevalence of ALS is lower (in the United States, 15,000 to 30,000 people) than that of diseases such as multiple sclerosis with comparable incidence but a more protracted course. In France the disorder is called Charcot disease, after the neurologist who did most to define it; in the United States it is called Lou Gehrig disease, after its most famous victim. ALS more often occurs in late middle age—less than 10% of cases begin before age 40—and men are affected twice as often as women.

Five to ten percent of ALS cases are familial, and in most of these cases there is autosomal dominant inheritance. Twenty percent of dominantly inherited ALS families are associated with mutations at the q21 region of chromosome 21, which contains the gene for Cu,Zn superoxide dismutase (SOD1), an enzyme that catatyzes the conversion of the superoxide anion (O_2^-) to hydrogen peroxide (which is further converted to water). This discovery led to speculation that motor neuron damage in familial, and perhaps sporadic, ALS is the consequence of SOD1 deficiency and impaired cellular defenses against oxygen and its toxic derivatives. However, transgenic mice expressing human mutated SOD1 have normal levels of wild-type mouse SODl, yet the animals develop progressive motor neuron disease. It appears that the disease in mice is the result of a toxic property of the mutant SOD1 rather than loss of SOD1 activity—in other words, a gain-of-function disorder—but the identity of this toxic property is uncertain. It has been hypothesized that mutant SOD1 has peroxidase activity that facilitates the conversion of hydrogen peroxide to toxic hydroxyl radicals, that mutant SOD1 interacts with peroxynitrate (generated by the interaction of superoxide and nitric oxide) to produce neurotoxic nitronium ions, and that mutant SOD1 triggers apoptosis. These mechanisms are not mutually exclusive.

The mean age of onset for dominantly inherited ALS is 10 years earlier than for sporadic ALS; otherwise, they are clinically indistinguishable. There are several clinically distinct forms of recessively inherited ALS, and one of these, with childhood onset, is linked to the q33 region of chromosme 2, but the gene and its product have not (as of 1999) been identified.

SOD1 mutations are only rarely present in sporadic ALS patients (as new mutations). An alternative hypothesis on the pathogenesis of sporadic ALS proposes that the selective neuronal damage is the result of glutamate excitotoxicity. Released at central excitatory synaptic nerve endings, glutamate acts on N-methyl-D-aspartate (NMDA), 2-(aminomethyl)phenylacetic acid (AMPA), and kainate receptors, allowing both sodium and calcium entry across the postsynaptic membrane. Glutamate is cleared from the synaptic cleft by glutamate transporter proteins located on both astrocytes and neurons. Experimentally, pharmacological blockade of glutamate transporters causes neuronal death, probably because excess glutamate leads to increased calcium influx, activation of oxidant-generating enzymes, and production of nitric oxide, hydroxyl radicals, and superoxide anions. Cerebrospinal fluid from ALS patients contains elevated levels of glutamate, ALS postmortem tissue demonstrates loss of glutamate transport, and aberrant forms of messenger RNA for an astrocytic glutamate transporter may be responsible for lack of this protein and the accumulation of glutamate in extracellular fluid. Knockout mice lacking the gene for the same transporter develop progressive weakness. These observations led to the use of riluzole, a drug that inhibits presynaptic release of glutamate. In controlled trials riluzole resulted in a 3 to 6 month prolongation of survival in ALS patients yet did not measurably alter progression of actual muscle strength. It was approved by the Federal Drug Administration in 1996.

Antibodies to voltage-gated calcium channels are found in some patients with sporadic ALS, as are both monoclonal and polyclonal antibodies to the neuronal ganglioside GM_1. Lymphoproliferative disease is overrepresented in ALS populations. Clinical trials with immunosuppressive agents in ALS, however, have met with failure. (By contrast, in *multifocal motor neuropathy with conduction block*, a disease that must be excluded electrodiagnostically when upper-motor-neuron signs are not evident, symptoms improve following immunosuppressive drugs or intravenous human immunoglobulin.)

Although there is no evidence for deficiency of any motor neuron growth factor in ALS, several neurotrophins have been shown to protect motor neuron cell bodies after axonal section, and a placebo-controlled clinical trial of recombinant human insulin-like growth factor I in ALS demonstrated a small but significant reduction in the progression of weakness.

SELECTED REFERENCES

Bredsen DE, Ellerby LM, Hart P, et al: Do post translational modifications of CuZnSOD lead to sporadic amyotrophic lateral sclerosis? Ann Neurol 1997;42:135.

Brown RH: Amyotrophic lateral sclerosis. Insights from genetics. Arch Neurol 1997;54:1246.

Lin CL, Bristol LA, Jin L, et al: Aberrant RNA processing in a neurodengenerative disease: The cause for absent EAAT2, a glutamate transporter, in amyotrophic lateral sclerosis. Neuron 1998;20:589.

Miller RG, Rosenberg JA, Gelinas DF, et al: Practice parameter: The case of the patient with amyotrophic lateral sclerosis (an evidence-based review). Neurology 1999;52:1311.

Rothstein JD: Excitotoxicity hypothesis. Neurology 1996;47(Suppl 2):S19.

Rowland LP: Natural history and clinical features of amyotrophic lateral sclerosis and related motor neuron diseases. In: Calne DB (ed): *Neurodegenerative Diseases*. W.B. Saunders, 1993.

Siddique T, Nishawan D, Hentati A: Molecular genetic basis of familial ALS. Neurology 1996;47(Suppl 2):S27.

▶ CASE 27

A 46-year-old woman has been a parenteral heroin abuser for over 25 years; access to veins has long been lost, and she injects the drug subcutaneously ("skin popping"). Over the course of a day she notices increasing difficulty opening her mouth, followed by inability to swallow her own saliva. In a hospital emergency room an attempt to pry her mouth open results in a chipped tooth, and she walks out. Over the next 3 days muscle stiffness spreads to her neck, back, abdomen, and limbs, and a friend brings her back to the emergency room.

On examination temperature is 100 °F, pulse is 120/minute and regular, respirations are 24/minute and regular, and blood pressure is 100/60 mm Hg. All four limbs and her abdomen are covered with scars indicative of previously infected injection sites. She is irritable but alert and attentive. Her masseter muscles are tightly contracted, preventing jaw opening, and involuntary facial muscle contraction produces partial eye closure and fixed elevation of the angles of the mouth (risus sardonicus). Her posterior neck and paraspinal muscles pull her cervical spine into hyperextension (opisthotonus), and her abdomen is board-like stiff. Her arms are held in flexion and adduction with clenched fists, and her legs are extended. While being examined, she has several paroxysms of more intense muscle spasms lasting 30–60 seconds, during which she becomes cyanotic but remains awake.

She receives tetanus toxoid, human tetanus immune globulin, penicillin G, and, with the aid of succinylcholine paralysis, emergency endotracheal intubation. As neuromuscular blockade wears off, paroxysmal muscle spasms resume, and when they fail to respond to large parenteral doses of benzodiazepines, maintenance neuromuscular blockade is begun and tracheostomy is performed.

Comment

Tetanus is caused by a toxin, tetanospasmin, produced by a bacterium, *Clostridium tetani.* The toxin, a polypeptide, prevents synaptic vesicles from fusing with cell membranes within the central nervous system and peripherally at autonomic and motor nerve endings. Central effects predominate, and particularly affected are interneurons that normally inhibit brain stem and spinal cord motor neurons. In the spinal cord these inhibitory neurons, called *Renshaw cells,* are stimulated by cholinergic collaterals from anterior horn cells; Renshaw cells project back onto the same anterior horn cells, release glycine from their nerve terminals, and bring motor neuron firing to an abrupt halt. In tetanus loss of this recurrent inhibition results in sustained firing of motor neurons (Figure 12–16). Superimposed paroxysms of more severe muscle spasms (tetanic seizures) can occur spontaneously but are often provoked by external stimuli; when they involve the larynx and muscles of respiration, they can cause fatal asphyxia. (In contrast to tetanospasmin, strychnine, from seeds of a plant native to India, blocks glycine receptors. Symptoms of strychnine poisoning—usually from accidental pesticide ingestion by children—resemble those of tetanus except that muscles are usually relaxed between paroxysmal spasms and cranial muscles are usually spared.)

Clostridium tetani is shed in mammalian feces (including human), and its spores are ubiquitous in the environment. Infected wounds, with necrosis and anaerobiosis, provide an opportunity for bacterial growth and production of

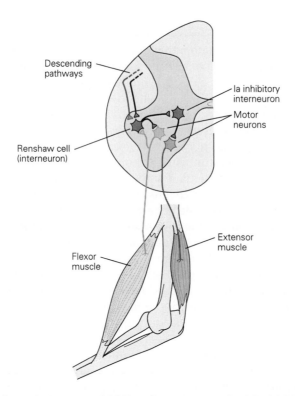

Figure 12–16. Renshaw cells produce recurrent inhibition of motor neurons (and, by inhibiting inhibitory interneurons, facilitation of motor neurons innervating antagonists of the same motor neurons). In tetanus loss of Renshaw cell inhibition causes sustained firing of motor neurons—tetanospasms. (Reproduced with permission from Kandel ER, Schwartz JH, Jessell TM. 1999. *Principles of Neural Science,* 4th ed. New York: McGraw-Hill.)

toxin, which ascends from peripheral nerve terminals to cell bodies by fast retrograde axonal transport. The toxin also spreads hematogenously to the central nervous system. When spread is largely retrograde through nerve axons, symptoms may be restricted to a single limb, truncal segment, or cranial muscle (local or cephalic tetanus), and inhibitory effects at the neuromuscular junction may result in weakness alternating with paroxysmal spasms. When spread is systemic, the result, as in this patient, is generalized tetanus, which carries a 50% fatality rate, with death resulting either from asphyxiation or autonomic instability. Tetanospasms refractory to benzodiazepines are appropriately treated with neuromuscular blockade.

A bout of tetanus does not confer immunity, and so patients receive not only human tetanus immune globulin (antitoxin) but also, in a different limb, denatured tetanospasmin (tetanus toxoid). Antitoxin does not affect toxin that has already been taken up by inhibitory interneurons; symptomatic treatment may be required for weeks.

SELECTED REFERENCES

Kefer MP: Tetanus. Am J Emerg Med 1992;10:445.
Sanford JP: Tetanus—forgotten but not gone. N Engl J Med 1995;332:812.

► CASE 28

A 53-year-old hypertensive man awakens one morning with weakness of his right arm and leg and dysarthria. On examination 2 hours later, his blood pressure is 170/100 mm Hg and his regular pulse is 88/minute. Eye closure and mouth movement are reduced on the right, but he wrinkles his brow symmetrically. His speech is slurred, with particular difficulty pronouncing posterior lingual consonants (*k* and *g*), but his tongue protrudes fully in the midline. Muscle tone in his right arm and leg is mildly decreased, and strength in these limbs is 4/5 proximally and 3/5 distally. Tendon reflexes are 3+ on the right and 2+ on the left. The left plantar response is flexor and the right is silent. Mental status is normal, including language function, as are gross visual fields, eye movements, and sensation, including proprioception and stereognosis.

Computerized tomography reveals a 1-cm-diameter lucency, consistent with infarction, just posterior to the genu of the left internal capsule. He is treated with bed rest for a few days and then progressive mobilization, physical therapy, and resumption of his antihypertensive medications. There is gradual improvement in his strength, which a month after admission is nearly normal in his right arm and leg; however, finger movements and foot tapping on the right are reduced in rate and amplitude out of proportion to demonstrable weakness. This impairment of movement results in difficulty manipulating objects with his right hand; his writing is clumsy even though there is no true agraphia or other language disturbance. When he holds his arms outstretched, with palms upward, the right arm slowly pronates and descends. When he lies prone with his knees flexed, his right leg gradually drifts out of flexion. Tendon reflexes are still hyperactive on the right, and muscle tone in his right arm and leg is now greater than on his left. He remains mildly dysarthric.

Comment

Right hemiparesis and facial weakness signify a lesion involving the corticospinal system either at the prerolandic motor cortex of the frontal lobe or in the descending corticospinal/corticobulbar tract. The lesion must be on the left above the pyramidal decussation, and because the facial weakness is on the same side as the hemiparesis, it must be rostral to the facial nucleus in the pons. Hypertension and abrupt onset of symptoms indicate stroke as the disease process, and the absence of headache or altered mentation is more consistent with infarction secondary to vessel occlusion than with hemorrhage. In most people the region of the motor cortex representing the face, arm, and hand, on the cerebral convexity, is supplied by the middle cerebral artery, whereas the region representing the leg and foot, on the medial surface of the cerebrum, is supplied by the anterior cerebral artery.

Infarction of the motor cortex extensive enough to cause weakness of the contralateral face, arm, and leg would be unlikely, as in this patient, to spare language function, eye movements, sensation, and visual fields. By contrast, as the corticobulbar/corticospinal tract descends through the genu and posterior limb of the internal capsule, its cross-sectional area becomes quite small, and occlusion of a single penetrating artery from the circle of Willis can selectively damage it.

The patient's facial weakness spares his frontalis muscle, probably because of greater bihemispheric representation of that muscle. (An everyday consequence of such bilateral representation is the difficulty most people have in rais-

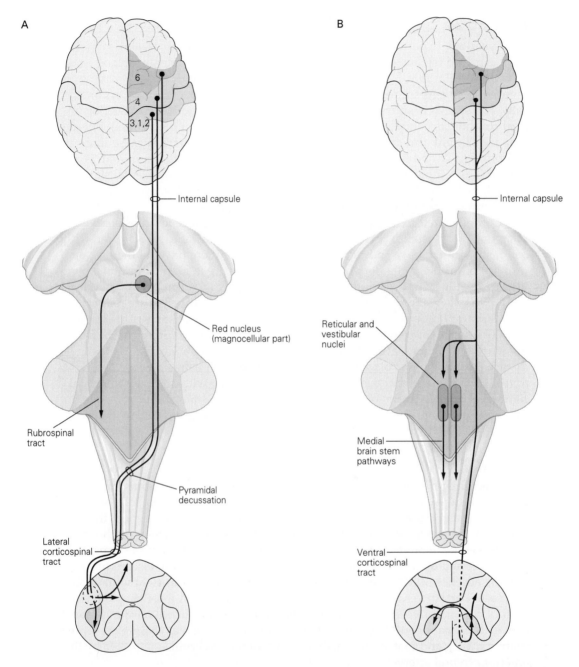

Figure 12–17. A. The lateral corticospinal tract crosses in the lower medulla and projects to spinal cord anterior horn cells that control distal muscles. In the brain stem are projections to the red nucleus (which gives rise to the crossed rubrospinal tract, a participant in motor control) and to certain cranial motor nuclei (corticobulbar projections). Fibers in the corticospinal tract that arise from the parietal lobe sensory cortex project to the dorsal column nuclei of the medulla. **B.** The uncrossed ventral corticospinal tract projects to certain cranial motor nuclei and to spinal cord anterior horn cells that control proximal muscles. The ventral corticospinal tract's terminations are bilateral, probably accounting for the observation that paraspinal muscles and muscles of the pharynx, jaw, and forehead tend to be spared in unilateral suprasegmental lesions. (Reproduced with permission from Kandel ER, Schwartz JH, Jessell TM. 1999. *Principles of Neural Science,* 4th ed. New York: McGraw-Hill.)

ing one eyebrow.) Similar bihemispheric representation probably also explains the relative sparing in most unilateral cerebral lesions of jaw, pharyngeal, and paraspinal muscles. The lateral corticospinal (pyramidal) tract crosses in the lower medulla and terminates contralaterally in areas of the spinal cord anterior horns that control distal muscles. By contrast, the ventral corticospinal tract is uncrossed and terminates bilaterally in areas of anterior horns that control proximal muscles (Figure 12–17).

This patient also demonstrates a dissociation frequently encountered with corticobulbar/corticospinal lesions, namely incoordination, with reduced rate and amplitude of movement out of proportion to weakness. Thus, he has lingual dysarthria yet is able to protrude his tongue in the midline, and although strength returns to his right hand, his movements remain slow and clumsy.

The patient's paretic limbs are initially hypotonic, with no resistance to passive movement, yet they display brisker-than-normal tendon reflexes. Different kinds of intrafusal fibers and receptors within muscle spindles, producing different responses to velocity or to absolute degree of stretch (dynamic versus static), probably account for this frequently observed dissociation (see Figure 6–1). Over days tone usually increases, eventually paralleling hyperreflexia and often accompanied by improved strength. (Persistent hypotonia is a poor prognostic sign.)

SELECTED REFERENCES

Brust JCM: Cerebral infarction. In: Rowland LP (ed): *Merritt's Textbook of Neurology,* 10th edition. Williams & Wilkins, 1999.
Davidoff RA: The pyramidal tract. Neurology 1990;40:332.
Fisher CM, Curry HB: Pure motor hemiplegia of vascular origin. Arch Neurol 1965;13:30.
Rascol A, Clanet M, Manelfe C, et al: Pure motor hemiplegia: CT study of 30 cases. Stroke 1982;13:11.

► CASE 29

A 58-year-old business executive develops slurred speech and difficulty swallowing liquids. He also complains that his vision is not normal, yet an examination reveals normal corrected visual acuity. His gait then becomes unsteady, with frequent falls, and his friends observe a peculiar emotional lability, with explosive bursts of laughter. At work he has difficulty concentrating and remembering details.

On examination, he is instructed to move his eyes; there is absence of upgaze and downgaze and limitation of horizontal gaze. Pursuing a target with his eyes results in somewhat fuller movements horizontally, but catch-up saccades are required for his eyes to keep up with the target. With an opticokinetic tape there is no movement of his eyes vertically, and horizontally there is pursuit movement in the direction of the tape but no corrective nystagmus. When he fixes on a stationary object and his head is moved passively, eye movements are full both horizontally and vertically. There is infrequent blinking, and a tendency to stare, giving him an expression of surprise. Facial muscles are contracted and stiff, producing a perpetual expressionless grimace. Speech is slurred, he has trouble swallowing his own saliva, and his tongue movements are slow and incomplete. His jaw and gag reflexes are brisk. His neck is extended and resists passive forward movement, and his gait is broad based and unsteady with a tendency to fall backward. Strength is normal but limb movements are slow, muscle tone is increased in his legs, tendon reflexes are brisk throughout, and plantar responses are extensor. On mental status testing, his responses are delayed and incomplete, and he has difficuty performing sequential tasks, but his memory is only mildly impaired. Sensory examination is normal.

Magnetic resonance imaging (MRI) reveals mild diffuse cerebral and cerebellar atrophy and more pronounced atrophy of the midbrain, particularly the superior colliculus.

Over the next few years his symptoms relentlessly progress. On examination 5 years after the onset of his illness, his speech is unintelligible and feeding is through a gastrostomy. He cannot stand or walk unaided, and both limb and truncal movements are restricted and clumsy. Willed and pursuit eye movements are absent, but passive head movement still produces eye movement, albeit incomplete, both horizontally and vertically.

Several months later he dies of pneumonia. At autopsy there is neuronal loss and gliosis of varying degrees in the cerebral cortex, diencephalon, cerebellum, and brain stem. The subthalamic nuclei, globus pallidus, superior colliculus, periaqueductal gray matter, substantia nigra, and dentate nucleus of the cerebellum are particularly affected. Neuronal loss is associated with neurofibrillary tangles that stain for tau protein.

Comment

Progressive supranuclear palsy (PSP) is a degenerative disorder that produces a characteristic combination of symptoms and signs, namely, disordered eye movements, pseudobulbar palsy, dystonia, dementia, and variable degrees of pyramidal and cerebellar dysfunction. In most cases a relentlessly progressive course leads to death, usually from aspiration, within 10 years of onset.

The earliest eye movement abnormalities are fleeting lapses in fixation (square wave jerks), inability during visual pursuit to match eye velocity to target velocity, necessitating catch-up saccades (cogwheel pursuit), and hypometric saccades. Eventually, willed saccadic movements and then pursuit movements became impossible (see Figures 3–5 and 3–6). Vertical eye movements are affected earlier and more severely than horizontal eye movements, reflecting the particular vulnerability in PSP of midbrain structures, including the rostral interstitial nucleus of the median longitudinal fasciculus, a critical way station for vertical gaze. At the same time vestibular-evoked eye movements are maintained, reflecting the preservation of the oculomotor and abducens nuclei (hence the term progressive supranuclear palsy). Some patients have difficulty voluntarily closing their eyes, yet involuntary blinking continues (apraxia of eye closure). Others have difficulty voluntarily opening their eyes. If a patient lives long enough, the oculomotor and abducens nuclei eventually become affected, and then all eye movements are absent.

Pseudobulbar palsy refers to dysarthria and dysphagia secondary to dysfunction of muscles innervated by lower brain stem cranial nerves as a result of bilateral supranuclear lesions (see Chapter 3). In contrast to true bulbar palsy, in which the tongue is atrophic and fasciculating and the gag and palatal reflexes are absent (see Cases 24 and 26), in pseudobulbar palsy the tongue is neither atrophic nor fasciculating and the gag and palatal reflexes are brisk. The patient also evidenced upper-motor-neuron involvement of his jaw and face muscles and displayed emotional incontinence, explosive laughing or crying out of proportion to his actual mood. This strange and poorly understood symptom is less common when pseudobulbar palsy is the result of PSP than when it is the result of bilateral lesions restricted to the corticobulbar/corticospinal tracts, for example, in amyotrophic lateral sclerosis or bilateral infarcts affecting corticobulbar projections within the internal capsule. It has been hypothesized that emotional responsiveness in PSP is dampened by involvement of extrapyramidal structures as well as by coexisting dementia.

An occasional early feature of PSP is dystonic hyperextension of the neck—retrocollis; if there is also inability to move the eyes vertically, there may be considerable difficulty descending stairs. Gait disturbance in PSP reflects varying combinations of axial dystonia, parkinsonism, cerebellar ataxia, and spasticity.

The dementia of PSP is characterized by slowness of thinking and speaking, an appearance of apathy, and difficulty with sequential tasks. Memory is only mildly impaired. The mental changes do not readily correlate with neuronal loss in the cerebral cortex.

Neuropathologically, there is widespread neuronal degeneration, most severe in the basal nucleus of Meynert, globus pallidus, subthalamic nucleus, superior colliculus, midbrain tegmentum, and substantia nigra. Neurofibrillary tangles (NFT) are prominent but differ from the NFTs of Alzheimer disease (AD; see Case 73), being composed of straight tubules rather than paired helical filaments. The NFTs of PSP, like those of AD, are composed of tau, a microtubule-binding protein. In each disease tau is chemically abnormal, but the abnormalities in PSP and AD are not the same, and in contrast to AD, neuritic plaques and amyloid deposits are not found in PSP.

The cause of PSP is unknown. Rarely, cases have affected family members in a fashion suggesting autosomal dominant inheritance. Other reports suggest autosomal recessive inheritance. Suggesting a genetic role, and consistent with tau pathology, is the observation that a particular intronic allele of the tau gene is overrepresented in patients with PSP.

SELECTED REFERENCES

Bennett P, Bonifati V, Bonuccelli U, et al: Direct genetic evidence for involvement of tau in progressive supranuclear palsy. Neurology 1998;51:982.

Case records of the Massachusetts General Hospital: Progressive supranuclear palsy. N Engl J Med 1997;337:549.

De Yebenes JG, Sarasa JL, Daniel SE, Lees AJ: Familial progressive supranuclear palsy. Brain 1995;118:1095.

Gearing M, Olson DA, Watts RL, Mirra SS: Progressive supranuclear palsy: Neuropathologic and clinical heterogeneity. Neurology 1994;44:1015.

Rojo A, Pernaute RS, Fontan A, et al: Clinical genetics of familial progressive supranuclear palsy. Brain 1999;122:1233.

Troost BT, Daroff RB: The ocular motor defects in progressive supranuclear palsy (PSP). Ann Neurol 1977;2:397.

► CASE 30

A previously healthy 27-year-old woman suddenly experiences tonic contractions of her left fingers, followed within a few seconds by clonic movements that spread up her arm. Over the next 30 seconds the jerking involves her arm, face, and leg. She then loses consciousness and has a minute-and-a half of bilateral symmetric jerking of all four limbs, with her eyes and head turned toward the left. Participation of the muscles of respiration produces rhythmic expectoration of blood-tinged saliva, and she is incontinent of urine. The jerking gradually decreases over 30 seconds, and she then lies motionless and flaccid, slowly regaining consciousness. Examined in an emergency room 20 minutes after the seizure, she is sleepy but responds appropriately to verbal stimuli. There is right gaze preference and mild weakness of her left face and arm. The left lateral surface of her tongue is lacerated. A soft pulsatile bruit is heard over her right eye and anterior scalp.

She receives phenytoin intravenously and is admitted. An hour later her gaze preference and left-sided weakness have cleared. An electroencephalogram (EEG) contains intermittent sharp deflections (spikes) recorded from electrodes over the right anterior scalp. Magnetic resonance imaging (MRI) reveals a 2 × 4-cm vascular malformation in the gray and white matter of the right frontal convexity anterior to the motor cortex.

Comment

This patient has what are called *Jacksonian motor seizures* (after the nineteenth-century British neurologist J. Hughlings Jackson; see Case 4). In such cases an abnormal synchronous neuronal discharge begins in the area of the motor cortex (Brodmann area 4) or premotor cortex (Brodmann area 6) representing the hand; it then spreads along the motor/premotor cortex, successively involving areas representing the arm, face, and leg (Figure 12–18). The discharge then probably

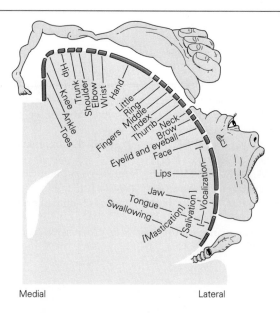

Medial   Lateral

Figure 12–18. Somatotopic organization of the motor cortex produces a motor homunculus. (Reproduced with permission from Kandel ER, Schwartz JH, Jessell TM. 1999. *Principles of Neural Science*, 4th ed. New York: McGraw-Hill.)

spreads across the corpus callosum to the opposite hemisphere and downward to integrating areas of the thalamus and the mesencephalic reticular formation. The result is conversion of her focal motor seizure into a generalized major motor (grand mal) convulsion (Figure 12–19). During the generalized seizure her head and eyes are tonically deviated to the left, reflecting discharge in the frontal eye field of her right cerebral convexity (Brodmann area 8) (see Figure 3–7).

The seizure is followed by a brief period of left-sided weakness and left gaze

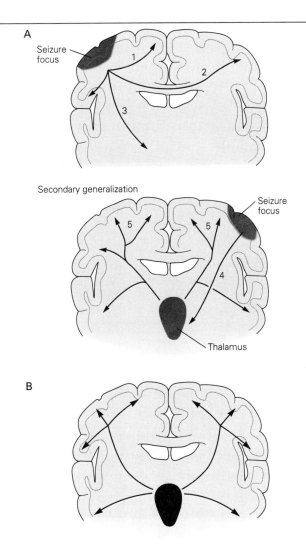

Figure 12–19. A. In a partial seizure, seizure activity can spread from a cortical focus to nearby cortex via intrahemispheric commissural fibers (**1**), to homotopic contralateral cortex via the corpus callosum (**2**), or to subcortical centers (**3**) via projections to the thalamus (**4**). Widespread thalamocortical projections then activate both cerebral hemispheres (**5**), resulting in secondary generalization of the seizure. **B.** By contrast, in primary generalized epilepsy, for example, petit mal absence or primary tonic-clonic seizures, epileptic activity begins with diffuse thalamocortical discharge. [Reproduced with permission from Kandel ER, Schwartz JH, Jessell TM. 1999. *Principles of Neural Science,* 4th ed. New York: McGraw-Hill. Adapted with permission from Lothman EW. 1993. Pathophysiology of seizures and epilepsy in the mature and immature brain: Cells, synapses and circuits. In: Dodson WE, Pollock JM (eds): *Pediatric Epilepsy: Diagnosis and Therapy.* New York: Demos Publications (pp. 1–15).]

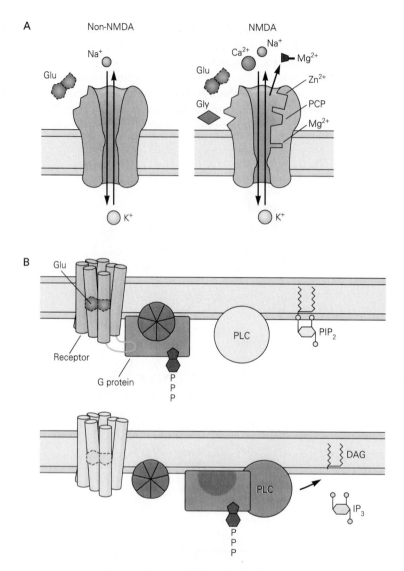

Figure 12–20. Three classes of glutamate receptors regulate excitatory synaptic activity in neurons of the brain and spinal cord. **A.** Two types of ionotropic glutamate receptors directly gate ion channels. *N*-Methyl-D-aspartate (NMDA) receptors, with binding sites for glutamate (Glu), glycine (Gly), phencyclidine (PCP), zinc, and magnesium, regulate channels permeable to Ca^{2+}, Na^+, and K^+. Two subtypes of non-NMDA receptors bind the glutamate agonists 2-(aminomethyl)phenylacetic acid or kainate and regulate channels permeable to Na^+ and K^+. **B.** Glutamate metabotropic receptors indirectly gate ion channels by activating a second messenger system. Activated G protein in turn activates the enzyme phospholipase C (PLC), which cleaves phosphatidylinositol biphosphate (PIP_2) into two second messengers, inositol triphosphate (IP_3) and diacylglycerol (DAG). These second messengers recruit various signaling pathways within the cell to modulate ion channel function as well as other cellular metabolic processes. (Reproduced with permission from Kandel ER, Schwartz JH, Jessell TM. 1999. *Principles of Neural Science,* 4th ed. New York: McGraw-Hill.)

paresis. Transient postictal focal weakness (*Todd paresis*), signifying functional un-responsiveness of neurons in the area of maximal discharge, might be the result of excessive and abnormal glutamate neurotransmission—at first producing the seizure discharges by generating excitatory postsynaptic potentials but then pro-ducing neuronal dysfunction (excitotoxicity) secondary to excessive calcium en-try. (Todd paresis is not limited to weakness; depending on the location of the seizure focus, there might be sensory loss, language dysfunction, or homony-mous hemianopia.)

The anticonvulsant drug phenytoin blocks sodium conductance, the source of dendritic fast action potentials induced by stimulation of postsynaptic gluta-mate receptors (Figure 12–20). This patient has no further clinical seizures after she receives phenytoin, yet her EEG reveals persistent electrical spikes over the right frontal convexity. (Each spike represents the synchronous discharge of un-derlying cortical neurons; each neuron's discharge consists of a brief burst of high-amplitude action potentials superimposed on a paroxysmal depolarizing shift.) Evidently, phenytoin has prevented the spread of this local discharge suffi-cient to prevent a clinical seizure but has not eliminated the focal discharge itself.

Vascular malformations are congenital and nonneoplastic, and are of five types: telangiectasia, varix, cavernous malformation, arteriovenous fistula, and venous. Their most feared complication is subarachnoid or intracerebral hemor-rhage, but they can cause symptoms, particularly headache and seizures, in the absence of obvious rupture. (Some focal seizures are probably precipitated by tiny leaks undetected by CT or MRI.) If their location permits, the definitive treat-ment of cerebral vascular malformations is surgical removal.

SELECTED REFERENCES

Commission on Classification and Terminology of the International League Against Epilepsy: Proposal for revised classification of epilepsies and epileptic syndromes. Epilepsia 1989;30:389.

Kotagal P, Lüders HO: Simple motor seizures. In: Engel J, Pedley TA (eds): *Epilepsy: A Comprehensive Textbook* (pp. 525–532). Lippincott-Raven, 1998.

Scheuer ML, Pedley TA: The evaluation and treatment of seizures. N Engl J Med 1990;323: 1468.

Wylie E, Lüders H, Morris HH, et al: The lateralizing significance of versive head and eye movements during epileptic seizures. Neurology 1986;36:606.

▶ CASE 31

A 54-year-old, hypertensive, diabetic man experiences vertigo, nausea, and vom-iting, followed by weakness of all four limbs and inability to talk. Brought to an emergency room, he lies motionless with open eyes and on casual inspection ap-pears not to be awake. He does not vocalize or move his arms, legs, mouth, or jaw spontaneously or to command. His eyes are directed conjugately forward. He does not look laterally in either direction when told to do so, and he does not follow horizontally moving objects with his eyes. There is no response to an opti-cokinetic tape moving either to the right or the left. He does, however, follow verbal instructions to blink and to look up or down, and with these actions as codes (one blink = yes; two = no) it becomes evident that he is alert and attentive with grossly preserved memory, language comprehension, and cognitive function. Respirations are 20/minute and regular but lack voluntary control. Corneal reflexes are present bilaterally, and there is normal sensation to pinprick over his face, limbs, and trunk. Hearing is intact. His limbs are flaccid with absent tendon reflexes and silent plantar responses.

Magnetic resonance imaging (MRI) reveals bilateral infarction of the basis pontis, and magnetic resonance angiography reveals occlusion of the basilar artery between the anterior inferior cerebellar and superior cerebellar arteries.

Two weeks after admission there is still no lateral eye movement to command, but cold water instilled into either ear produces conjugate deviation of the eyes toward the stimulus without nystagmus. Except for blinks there is still paralysis of the face, jaw, and tongue. He cannot swallow or cough voluntarily but does so automatically. His arms and legs, still paralyzed, are now mildly hypertonic with brisk tendon reflexes and Babinski signs. Painful stimuli to either foot produce involuntary flexion withdrawal of the leg. He is able to control his urine voluntarily but can initiate voiding only when he feels a full bladder. An electroencephalogram (EEG) shows a normal waking pattern.

Comment

This man has lost voluntary control of all muscles except those innervated by his oculomotor nerves. The cause is a brain stem infarct that transects descending corticospinal and corticobulbar fibers within the basis pontis while preserving the pontine tegmentum, which contains ascending somatic sensory and auditory pathways as well as the reticular activating system. Horizontal eye movements are absent because although the medial rectus muscle, effecting adduction, is innervated by the oculomotor nerve, its voluntary control depends on projections from the frontal eye fields (Brodmann area 8) to the pontine paramedian reticular formation. Vertical gaze, on the other hand, is mediated through structures rostral to the pons, including, within the midbrain, the rostral interstitial nucleus of the median longitudinal fasciculus and the oculomotor nucleus and nerves. (The nucleus of the trochlear nerve, which contributes to upward gaze, is in the dorsal pontine tegmentum and is therefore spared in this patient.)

Voluntary movement of muscles innervated by cranial nerves 5, 7, 9, 10, 11, and 12 are absent. His preserved blinking is a reflection of reciprocal innervation; attempting to contract his paralyzed orbicularis oculi inhibits its antagonist, the levator palpebrae, causing brief incomplete eye closure. By a similar mechanism his corneal reflexes are present. In addition there is reflexic but not voluntary swallowing and coughing, and although he breathes with normal rate and depth, he cannot override automatic breathing voluntarily (a dissociation that is the reverse of Ondine's curse; see Chapter 7).

Cold water caloric testing produces deviation of the eyes toward the stimulus, reflecting an intact reflex arc from vestibular afferents through connections within the pontine tegmentum (including the medial longitudinal fasciculus) to oculomotor and abducens nerve efferents. (Reflex abduction indicates that the pontine infarct spares the sixth nerve as it traverses the brain stem parenchyma en route to exiting.) Because the oculomotor and abducens nuclei are disconnected from the cerebrum, the patient cannot move his eyes laterally on command or follow a horizontally moving object. Loss of cerebral control also explains the absence of nystagmus during vestibular caloric testing; nystagmus is a normal feature of the reflex in awake subjects.

This patient's infarct, destroying descending corticospinal and corticobulbar projections within the basis pontis, occupies the territories of the paramedian and short circumferential branches of the occluded basilar artery. Spared is the pontine tegmentum, which receives adequate blood flow from long circumferential branches—the anterior inferior cerebellar and superior cerebellar arteries—which arise from the basilar artery below and above its occlusion. In this patient, flow through the superior cerebellar arteries depends on an intact circle of Willis, allowing blood entering the cranium through the internal carotid arteries to pass through the posterior communicating and posterior cerebral arteries to the posterior fossa.

The patient's condition—loss of all voluntary movement except blinking and vertical gaze—is termed *locked-in state*. A famous literary example is M. Noitrier de Villefort in Dumas's *The Count of Monte Christo;* following a stroke he is able to communicate only by blinking his eyes. Not surprisingly, patients described in the medical literature have varied. Some, presumably with smaller areas of infarction, have retained horizontal eye movements. Others, with tegmental involvement, have had somatic sensory loss or have progressed into coma. It is obviously a tragic error when a physician fails to recognize the locked-in state and treats as comatose someone awake and mentally intact.

SELECTED REFERENCES

Bauby J-D: *The Diving Bell and the Butterfly.* Vintage Books, 1998.

Feldman MH: Physiological observations in a chronic case of locked-in syndrome. Neurology 1971;21:459.

Katz RT, Haig AJ, Clark BB, DiPaola RJ: Long-term survival, prognosis, and life-care planning for 29 patients with chronic locked-in syndrome. Arch Phys Med Rehabil 1992;73:403.

Kemper TL, Romanul FCA: State resembling akinetic mutism in basilar artery occlusion. Neurology 1967;17:74.

Patterson JR, Grabois M: Locked-in-syndrome: A review of 139 cases. Stroke 1986;17:758.

Plum F, Posner J: *The Diagnosis of Stupor and Coma,* 3rd edition. F.A. Davis, 1980.

▶ CASE 32

A 64-year-old hypertensive man suddenly develops difficulty speaking and using his left leg and arm. Examined a few hours later, he has very limited speech, which is initiated after long pauses and consists mostly of monosyllabic replies to questions. Speech comprehension, naming, repetition, writing, and reading are normal, however. He initially does not move his left limbs either spontaneously or to command, but with much verbal prodding he demonstrates weakness of his left leg, more pronounced distally, and akinesia of his left arm; except for mild weakness of his shoulder, strength in his left arm and hand is normal.

A few days later akinesia has improved, but his left arm remains slow in initiating and executing movements, and although range of movement is normal for visually guided movements (such as touching the examiner's finger), there is reduced amplitude of complex movements based on memory (eg, pretending to use a hammer).

Two weeks later strength is normal throughout, but repetitive movements of the left arm are slow and arrhythmic. Alternating movements (such as tapping one hand with the palm and back of the other) and bilateral movements (such as making a fist with the right hand and then flexing the left elbow) are clumsy and display errors of sequencing. When tested alone, his right arm demonstrates mildly reduced velocity of movement, but the impairment is much less than on the left. Mental status, cranial nerves, and sensation are normal. Tendon reflexes are mildly hyperactive on the left, and the left planter response is less vigorously flexor than on the right.

Computerized tomography reveals infarction in the territory of the right anterior cerebral artery, anterior to the motor cortex and prominently affecting the supplementary motor area.

Comment

The *supplementary motor area* (SMA) appears to be involved with programming complex movements, particularly those requiring bimanual coordination. During isometric muscle contraction (such as pressing a spring with a finger) there is increased blood flow and metabolism in the hand area of the primary motor cortex. During more complex sequential movements (such as repetitively tapping the fingers in a short sequence, eg, 1–4–2–3, or tapping a particular rhythm) increased blood flow and metabolism spread to the SMA (Figure 12–21). During mental rehearsal of complex sequential movements (thinking about the task but not actually doing it) blood flow and metabolism increase only in the SMA.

Projecting to the primary motor cortex bilaterally, the SMA receives major projections from the basal ganglia (via the ventral anterior nucleus of the thalamus), from sensory association areas of the parietal lobe, and from prefrontal limbic areas, particularly the cingulate gyrus. Information related to external stimuli, internal motor programs, and motivation thus converges on the SMA, from which it is relayed to the primary motor cortex. By integrating these diverse inputs, the SMA plays a key role in movement planning and execution. It is particularly involved with the temporal coordination of internally generated or intended (ie, willed) movements that occur in the absence of environmental stimuli. (By contrast, the dorsal premotor cortex on the convexity of the frontal lobe appears to control externally cued movements that occur in response to visual stimuli.)

A variety of symptoms and signs are attributed to SMA damage. A problem in interpreting such observations is that the most commonly encountered lesions—vascular, neoplastic, or traumatic—often affect additional structures, including the primary motor cortex, the dorsal premotor frontal cortex, the cingulate gyrus, and the corpus callosum. Surgical corticectomy largely restricted to the SMA produces fairly consistent abnormalities, however. For a week or two postoperatively there is bilateral loss of spontaneous movement—akinesia—including facial expression. Vigorous verbal commands elicit movement of the ipsilateral limbs but only feeble or no movement of the contralateral limbs. Speech is either absent or reduced to monosyllabic replies, yet speech comprehension is preserved. The ipsilateral limbs then rather suddenly begin moving spontaneously; contralateral limb movements still require repeated commands, yet strength is bilaterally normal. Spontaneous speech then returns, although it remains sparse, and there is an apparent disinclination to use the contralateral limbs—*motor neglect*—as well as awkwardness of complex repetitive movements and bimanual sequencing tasks. Such a description fits this patient, whose additional contralateral leg weakness was likely caused by ischemia of the medial hemispheric motor cortex; the rapid recovery of strength was probably the result

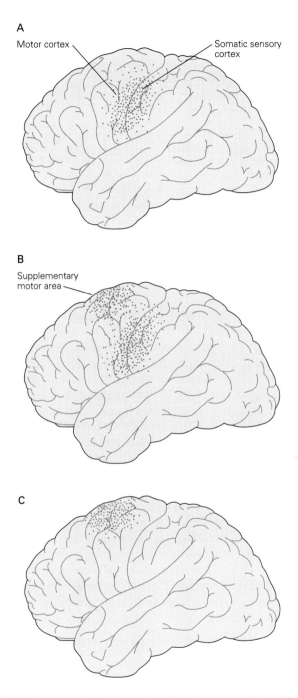

Figure 12–21. A. When a finger is pressed against a spring, there is increased blood flow in the hand areas of the primary motor and sensory cortices. **B.** During a complex sequence of finger movements, the increased blood flow extends to the supplementary motor area. **C.** During mental rehearsal of the same sequence illustrated in B, blood flow increases only in the supplementary motor area. (Blood flow, measured here with radioactive xenon, reflects underlying neuronal activity.) (Reproduced with permission from Kandel ER, Schwartz JH, Jessell TM. 1999. *Principles of Neural Science,* 4th ed. New York: McGraw-Hill.)

of collateral blood flow to that area from the posterior cerebral artery. Permanent infarction of the SMA, however, resulted in a disorder of programming, with impaired initiation of movements, bradykinesia or impersistence in sustaining them, and clumsiness in their temporal sequencing.

SELECTED REFERENCES

Brust JCM: Lesions of the supplementary motor area. In: Lüders HO (ed): *Supplementary Sensorimotor Area. Advances in Neurology,* Volume 70 (pp. 237–248). Lippincott-Raven, 1996.

Grafton ST: Cortical control of movement. Ann Neurol 1994;36:3.

Halsband U, Ito N, Tanji J, Freund H-J: The role of premotor cortex and the supplementary motor area in the temporal control of movement in man. Brain 1993;116:243.

Lüders HO: The supplementary sensorimotor area. An overview. In: Lüders HO (ed): *Supplementary Sensorimotor Area. Advances in Neurology,* Volume 70 (pp. 1–16). Lippincott-Raven, 1996.

Wise SP, Boussaoud D, Johnson PB, et al: Premotor and parietal cortex: Corticocortical connectivity and combinatorial computations. Annu Rev Neurosci 1997;20:25.

▶ CASE 33

A 50-year-old alcoholic man has had an unsteady gait for several years. His symptoms began when he was drinking up to two pints of vodka daily and progressed over several weeks. Although attempts at abstinence have been punctuated by episodic binge drinking, his gait ataxia has been largely unchanged since then.

On examination his gait is broad based and wobbly with a coarse anteroposterior truncal tremor (titubation). He cannot perform heel–toe walking (tandem gait). When he lies supine and moves either heel along the opposite shin from knee to ankle, the movements are clumsy with side-to-side tremor. Lifting either leg to touch the examiner's finger with the big toe results in overshoot (hypermetria). When he taps the floor with his foot, however, he is able to maintain a steady rhythm. His arms are normal, with neither tremor, dysmetria, nor adiadochokinesis. Mentation is normal except for mildly impaired memory; he is fully oriented to time and place but recalls only one of three unrelated words after 5 minutes. Vibratory and pinprick sensation are mildly decreased in his feet, but proprioception is normal. Tendon reflexes are reduced at the ankles and symmetrically brisk elsewhere. The rest of his neurological examination is normal.

Computerized tomography shows abnormal prominence of cerebellar sulci in the anterior superior vermis.

Comment

Alcoholic cerebellar degeneration is probably the result of nutritional deficiency. Similar cerebellar pathology is encountered in patients with thiamine deficiency and Wernicke disease (a syndrome of altered mentation, abnormal eye movements, and truncal ataxia; see Case 74), but other vitamin deficiencies or direct ethanol toxicity could be contributory. Histologically, there is loss of neurons, particularly Purkinje cells, in the cerebellar cortex; restriction of such damage to the cerebellar vermis explains the symptoms and signs.

The cerebellar vermis projects by way of the fastigial nuclei to the brain stem reticular formation, the lateral vestibular nuclei, and (via the ventrolateral nucleus of the thalamus) the primary motor cortex (Figure 12–22). Areas receiving

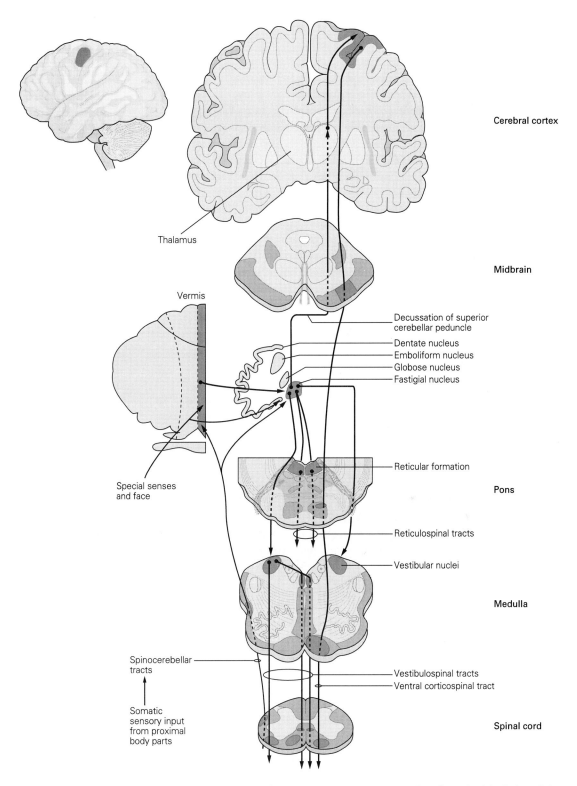

Figure 12–22. The cerebellar vermis receives input from the neck and trunk as well as from the labyrinth and the eyes. Its output, from the deep fastigial nuclei, is principally to areas of the cerebral cortex that give rise to the ventral corticospinal tract (which controls trunk and neck muscles), and to the descending reticulospinal and vestibulospinal systems (which modulate axial tone and posture). Damage to this area therefore impairs gait and stance. (Reproduced with permission from Kandel ER, Schwartz JH, Jessell TM. 1991. *Principles of Neural Science,* 3rd ed. Norwalk, CT: Appleton & Lange.)

these projections give rise to ventromedially descending systems in the brain stem and spinal cord (the reticulospinal, vestibulospinal, and ventral corticospinal tracts) that control axial and proximal limb muscles. More distal limb muscles are under the control of the intermediate and lateral regions of the cerebellar hemispheres, and within the anterior lobe of the cerebellum the arms are somatotopically represented posterior to the legs. This anatomy explains why alcoholic cerebellar degeneration, usually limited to the anterior vermis, causes ataxia of gait, stance, and proximal leg movement but spares arm and distal leg movement. Cranial cerebellar signs such as nystagmus and dysarthria are also usually absent.

This patient's memory impairment probably signifies Korsakoff syndrome, also a consequence of thiamine deficiency (see Case 74). His mild sensory impairment and decreased ankle reflexes are consistent with alcoholic/nutritional peripheral neuropathy, but normal proprioception makes it unlikely that distal sensory loss is contributing significantly to his gait ataxia.

SELECTED REFERENCES

Brust JCM: *Neurological Aspects of Substance Abuse* (pp. 190–252). Butterworth-Heinemann, 1993.

Phillips SC, Harper CG, Kril J: A quantitative histological study of the cerebellar vermis in alcoholic patients. Brain 1987;110:301.

Victor M, Adams RD, Mancall EL: A restricted form of cerebellar cortical degeneration occurring in alcoholic patients. Arch Neurol 1959;1:579.

Voogd J, Glickstein M: The anatomy of the cerebellum. Trends Neurosci 1998;21:370.

▶ CASE 34

A 16-year-old girl, who has had occasional ear infections since age 12, awakens with left postauricular pain. Over the next 3 days the pain becomes increasingly severe, and her physician, diagnosing otitis media, prescribes oral amoxicillin. Headache persists, however, and a week after the onset of symptoms she notices unsteadiness on walking and clumsiness on reaching for objects with her left hand.

On examination, her temperature, pulse, blood pressure, and respirations are normal. The left tympanic membrane is thickened and dull, and there is tenderness to percussion over the left mastoid. Her speech is mildly slurred, and bilateral left-beating nystagmus is present when she attempts to fixate gaze on a target to her left. Finger-to-nose and heel-to-shin testing reveal dysmetria and action tremor on the left, and there is irregularity in the rate and rhythm of rapid successive and alternating movements of the left limbs (adiadochokinesis). Delays are evident in initiating movement, and when the task is complex and involves multiple joints, there are errors in timing of the successive components (decomposition of movement). Her gait is broad based and cautious, with veering to the left. Tendon reflexes are normal and symmetric except for a pendular quality to the left knee jerk. Plantar reflexes are flexor; strength, sensation, and mental status are normal.

Computerized tomography reveals opacified mastoid sinuses on the left; a lesion 2 cm in diameter within the left cerebellar hemisphere displays ring enhancement following administration of contrast material and is surrounded by considerable white matter edema, resulting in distortion of the fourth ventricle. At surgery pus is drained from both the left mastoid bone and the cerebellar hemisphere. Cultures of this material are negative.

Comment

Otogenic brain abscesses most often reach the nervous system by direct extension; spread may be across infected bone (osteomyelitis) or along the walls of veins (thrombophlebitis). Both the middle ear and the cerebellum drain into the lateral (transverse) dural sinus, making the anterior superior portion of the ipsilateral cerebellar hemisphere a vulnerable site for infection in patients with otitis media.

The intermediate zone of the cerebellar hemisphere receives information from the limbs and projects, by way of the deep interposed nuclei, to the red nucleus and, via the ventrolateral nucleus of the thalamus, to the motor cortex. Areas receiving these projections give rise to ventrolaterally descending systems in the brain stem and spinal cord (the rubrospinal and lateral corticospinal tracts) that control limb muscles (Figure 12–23). The lateral zone of each cerebellar hemisphere (cerebrocerebellum) receives projections, by way of the pontine nuclei and the middle cerebellar peduncle, from the cerebral cortex and, by way of the dentate nucleus and the ventrolateral nucleus of the thalamus, projects back to motor and premotor regions of the cerebral cortex; this part of the cerebellum is particularly concerned with rapid or finely coordinated limb movements and with motor learning (Figure 12–24). In contrast to patients with cerebellar vermal lesions (see Case 33), this patient's impairment is most evident in tasks requiring dexterity of the distal limbs; signs indicative of cerebellar hemispheric damage include dysmetria, intention tremor, adiadochokinesis, and decomposition of multijoint movements. Projections from the interposed and dentate nuclei are crossed, as are the rubrospinal and lateral corticospinal tracts; such double crossing explains why the patient's cerebellar signs were ipsilateral to the side of her lesion.

The patient's otitis, by affecting her vestibular labyrinth, could have contributed to her tendency to veer leftward when walking. She did not complain of vertigo, however, and her nystagmus, present during attempted fixation on a target toward the side of the lesion, was characteristic of a cerebellar hemispheric lesion. With vestibular damage nystagmus is more often present on forward and contralateral gaze, and the fast component (often accompanied by a rotatory component) is directed away from the side of the lesion. (An abrupt change in the direction of nystagmus in a patient with otitis may be the first indication that infection has spread to the cerebellum.)

Cerebellar hemispheric damage can result in difficulty maintaining fixation of gaze; nystagmus, as in this patient, then signifies repetitive corrective saccades. Other eye movement abnormalities encountered in patients with lesions of the cerebellar hemisphere are ocular dysmetria (saccadic overshoot of a target) and catch-up saccades (saccadic intrusions during pursuit gaze, a compensation for abnormally slow pursuit velocity).

Cerebellar lesions produce different kinds of dysarthria—slurring, scanning (words broken into syllables), and explosive (involuntary interruptions and syllables of abnormally increased or decreased force). As with this patient, dysarthria is more often associated with hemispheric than with vermal lesions.

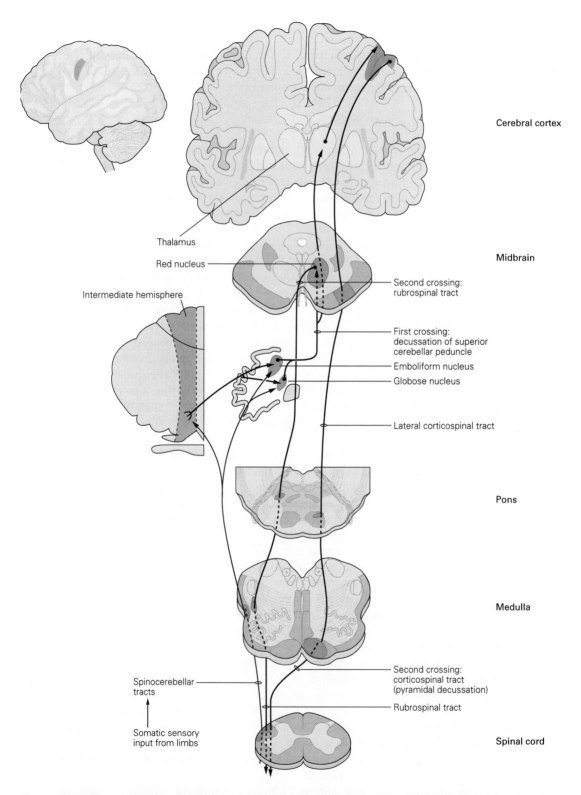

Cerebral cortex

Thalamus

Red nucleus

Midbrain

Second crossing:
rubrospinal tract

Intermediate hemisphere

First crossing:
decussation of superior
cerebellar peduncle

Emboliform nucleus

Globose nucleus

Lateral corticospinal tract

Pons

Medulla

Second crossing:
corticospinal tract
(pyramidal decussation)

Spinocerebellar
tracts

Rubrospinal tract

Somatic sensory
input from limbs

Spinal cord

Figure 12–23. The intermediate zone of the cerebellum receives information from the limbs and projects, directly or indirectly, to dorsolateral descending systems (corticospinal and rubrospinal tracks) that control ongoing limb movement. (Reproduced with permission from Kandel ER, Schwartz JH, Jessell TM. 1991. *Principles of Neural Science*, 3rd ed. Norwalk, CT: Appleton & Lange.)

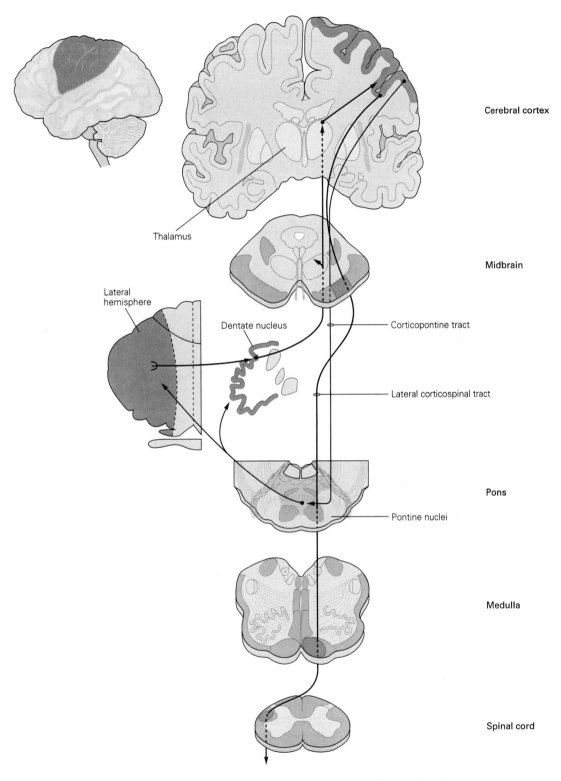

Cerebral cortex

Thalamus

Midbrain

Lateral
hemisphere

Dentate nucleus

Corticopontine tract

Lateral corticospinal tract

Pons

Pontine nuclei

Medulla

Spinal cord

Figure 12–24. The lateral zone of each cerebellar hemisphere (cerebrocerebellum) receives input, via the pontine nuclei, from the cerebral cortex and projects, via the ventrolateral nucleus of the thalamus, to the motor and premotor cerebral cortex. The cerebrocerebellum is involved with planning, initiation, and timing of limb movements. (Reproduced with permission from Kandel ER, Schwartz JH, Jessell TM. 1991. *Principles of Neural Science,* 3rd ed. Norwalk, CT: Appleton & Lange.)

SELECTED REFERENCES

Lechtenberg R, Gilman S: Speech disorders in cerebellar disease. Ann Neurol 1978;3:285.

Raymond JL, Lisberger SG, Mauk MD: The cerebellum: A neuronal learning machine? Science 1996;272:1126.

Shaw MDM, Russell JA: Cerebellar abscess: A review of 47 cases. J Neurol Neurosurg Psychiatry 1975;38:429.

Van Dellen JR, Bullock R, Postma MH: Cerebellar abscess: The impact of computed tomographic scanning. Neurosurgery 1987;21:547.

► CASE 35

A 63-year-old man notices a rhythmic tremor of his right hand and wrist that over the next several months becomes increasingly coarse. It is most obvious when he walks or when he is under stress. Although the tremor disappears during manual tasks, he finds it increasingly difficult to perform rapid coordinated movements with his right hand, particularly writing. He describes his difficulty as stiffness rather than weakness. A year later his left arm and hand have become similarly affected, and he develops a forward stoop and a tendency to shuffle when he walks. Rising from a chair becomes difficult, and he becomes increasingly unsure of his balance. His voice becomes softer and his pronunciation becomes less distinct.

On examination there is a dearth of spontaneous movement, including facial expression (masked facies, hypominia). He blinks infrequently, and his voice is soft, with reduced inflection and a tendency to run syllables together (tachyphemia). Repetitively tapping the glabellar area of his forehead produces uncontrollable blinking (Myerson's sign). As he sits, there is bilateral distal upper limb tremor, regular at 4 to 5 Hz and coarser on the right. A tendency to flex the metacarpal-phalangeal joints gives the tremor a pill-rolling quality. Less obvious tremor is present in the lips and chin. There is resistance to passive movement of his arms, legs, and neck, greater on the right, persisting throughout the range of movement, independent of velocity, and featuring rhythmic ratchet-like interruptions synchronous with his tremor (cogwheeling). Repetitive movements—alternately tapping a tabletop with the palm and back of each hand or the floor with the toes and heel of each foot—are initiated with difficulty (akinesia), performed slowly (bradykinesia), and tend to decrement in amplitude (hypokinesia). He is unable to rise from a chair without using his arms, and his gait is marked by delayed initiation, a forward stoop, absent arm swing with the forearms internally rotated (simian posture), shuffling, and involuntary acceleration, as if he were trying to catch up with his own center of gravity (festination). His upper limb tremor increases as he walks. Turning 180° requires several steps, and when he stands with his feet together, pulling him backward produces retropulsion. The rest of his examination, including mentation, sensation, and tendon and plantar reflexes, is normal.

Computerized tomography is normal. He is prescribed levodopa/carbidopa, and after 2 weeks there is improvement in all his symptoms.

Comment

Like the cerebellum, the basal ganglia participate in feedback control of the motor system. The input and output of these two systems differ, however. The cerebellum receives direct and indirect projections from sensorimotor areas of the cerebral cortex as well as from the spinal cord and brain stem, and its output is directed, via the ventrolateral nucleus of the thalamus, to motor and premotor areas of the frontal lobe. The basal ganglia receive projections from the entire cerebral cortex, and their output is directed, via the ventrolateral, ventroanterior, centromedial, and dorsomedial nuclei of the thalamus, to premotor and anterior association areas of the frontal lobe (Figure 12–25). Consistent with their different connections, the cerebellum is considered a regulator of ongoing movement, whereas the basal ganglia are more involved in the planning and execution of complex motor acts. Like the supplementary motor area (a major target of basal ganglia output), the basal ganglia appear to play little if any role in initiating stimulus-triggered movements (such as visually guided tracking tasks or catching an object unexpectedly tossed in one's direction); they play a major role, however, in the initiation of internally generated movements.

The direct and indirect pathways from the cerebral cortex through the basal ganglia and back to the cerebral cortex consist of a succession of synapses that are variably excitatory (glutamatergic) and inhibitory (γ-aminobutyric acid,

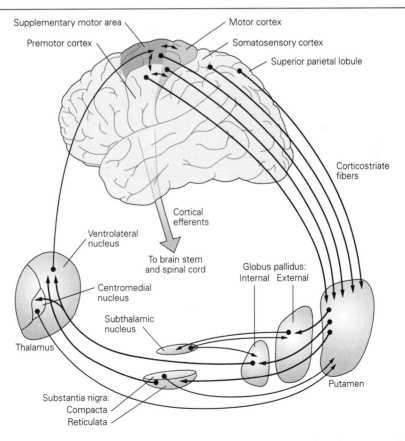

Figure 12–25. The motor circuitry of the basal ganglia comprises a feedback loop from the motor and somatosensory cerebral cortex through the basal ganglia and thalamus and back to the premotor, supplementary motor, and motor cortex. (Reproduced with permission from Kandel ER, Schwartz JH, Jessell TM. 1991. *Principles of Neural Science*, 3rd ed. Norwalk, CT: Appleton & Lange.)

[GABA]ergic); the main output of the basal ganglia—namely, the projection from the internal globus pallidus to the thalamus—is inhibitory (Figure 12–26). Activation of the direct pathway via excitatory (glutamatergic) input from the cortex to the striatum causes inhibition (via GABA) of tonically active inhibitory GABAergic neurons in the internal globus pallidus and therefore disinhibition of their projection targets in the thalamus. The result is increased excitatory (glutamatergic) output from the thalamus back to the cerebral cortex. By contrast, activation of the indirect pathway, which includes inhibitory (GABAergic) projections from the external globus pallidus to the subthalamic nucleus and excitatory (glutamatergic) projections from the subthalamic nucleus to the internal globus pallidus, increases inhibition to the thalamus, with reduced firing of thalamocortical projections. In normal individuals, then, the direct pathway provides a positive feedback on movements initiated in the cerebral cortex, and the indirect pathway provides a negative feedback on such movements. The supposition is that the direct pathway enhances desired movements, whereas the indirect pathway inhibits undesired movements.

Both the direct and the indirect pathways are modulated by dopaminergic projections from the pars compacta of the substantia nigra to the striatum (caudate and putamen); dopamine excites the direct pathway (via D_1 receptors) and inhibits the indirect pathway (via D_2 receptors). The ultimate effect of dopamine is therefore to increase firing of excitatory projections from the thalamus to the cortex.

Parkinson disease is defined neuropathologically by nerve cell loss in the sub-

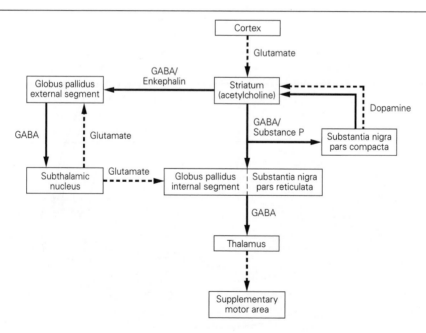

Figure 12–26. There are two different pathways through the basal ganglia. A direct route goes from the striatum through the globus pallidus internal segment (GPi)/substantia nigra pars reticulata (SNr) to the thalamus. An indirect route goes from the striatum through the globus pallidus external segment (GPe), subthalamic nucleus, and GPi/SNr to the thalamus. Black arrows indicate inhibitory projections; white arrows indicate excitatory projections. (Reproduced with permission from Kandel ER, Schwartz JH, Jessell TM. 1991. *Principles of Neural Science*, 3rd ed. Norwalk, CT: Appleton & Lange.)

stantia nigra and the presence of Lewy bodies, intracytoplasmic inclusions containing filamentous material. Neuronal loss is also present in other brain areas, including the nucleus basalis of Meynert, the locus coeruleus, the brain stem raphe nuclei, and the dorsal motor nucleus of the vagus. As a result of substantia nigra degeneration there is secondary loss of striatal dopamine. Loss of dopaminergic input ultimately results in increased output of the internal globus pallidus/substantia nigra pars reticulata to the thalamus and therefore decreased output of the thalamus to the motor cortex (Figure 12–27). The consequence is disordered movement.

The term *parkinsonism* refers to the symptoms and signs that occur in varying combinations in this disease: tremor at rest, rigidity, akinesia/bradykinesia, flexed posture, and loss of postural reflexes. Similar clinical features are encountered not only in Parkinson disease (idiopathic parkinson ism) but in a variety of other circumstances, including encephalitis, use of dopamine-blocking antipsychotic drugs, and a number of sporadic and hereditary degenerative diseases.

In the 1980s parenteral heroin abusers given a synthetic substitute contaminated with 1-methyl-4-phenyl-1,2,3,6-tetrahydropyridine (MPTP) developed severe irreversible parkinsonism, and animal studies subsequently showed that MPTP is metabolized by monoamine oxidase to 1-methyl-4-phenylpyridinium (MPP^+), which is taken up by dopaminergic neurons of the substantia nigra. MPP^+ damages complex I of the mitochondrial electron transport system, leading to accumulation of free radicals, activation of neuronal nitric oxide synthase, production of peroxynitrite, and neuronal death. Complex I activity is also reduced in the substantia nigra of patients with Parkinson disease, but the cause of the damage is unknown.

Members of several kindreds with autosomal dominant familial Parkinson disease have a missense mutation on chromosome 4q21–q23 for a gene encoding a protein called α-synuclein. The function of this protein is unknown (as of 1999), but it is an abundant brain protein concentrated in nerve terminals. Although the great majority of cases of Parkinson disease are not familial, Lewy bodies from both sporadic and familial cases are strongly immunoreactive for α-synuclein. It has been proposed that missense mutations of the α-synuclein gene (at least two have been described) cause the protein to aggregate into filaments, which, analogous to β-amyloid in Alzheimer disease (see Case 73), are neurotoxic.

In another form of familial Parkinson disease, autosomal recessive juvenile parkinsonism, there are deletional mutations or point mutations of a gene coding for a protein called *parkin*. The function of this protein is also unknown.

Parkinson disease is treated with levodopa, which, unlike dopamine, crosses the blood–brain barrier and is taken up by the remaining dopaminergic neurons of the substantia nigra and converted to dopamine. Levodopa is usually combined with carbidopa, which inhibits peripheral dopa-decarboxylase and thereby reduces the systemic side effects (nausea and vomiting) caused by levodopa metabolites. Other drugs available for the treatment of Parkinson disease include direct dopamine agonists such as bromocriptine and pergolide, the indirect dopaminergic agent amantadine (which also reduces glutamate neurotransmission at *N*-methyl-D-aspartate receptors), and inhibitors of cathechol-*o*-methyltransferase, an enzyme that methylates both levodopa and dopamine. Anticholinergic drugs such as trihexyphenidyl and benztropine also produce symptomatic improvement, presumably by dampening the activity of striatal cholinergic neurons that have been disinhibited by loss of their dopaminergic in-

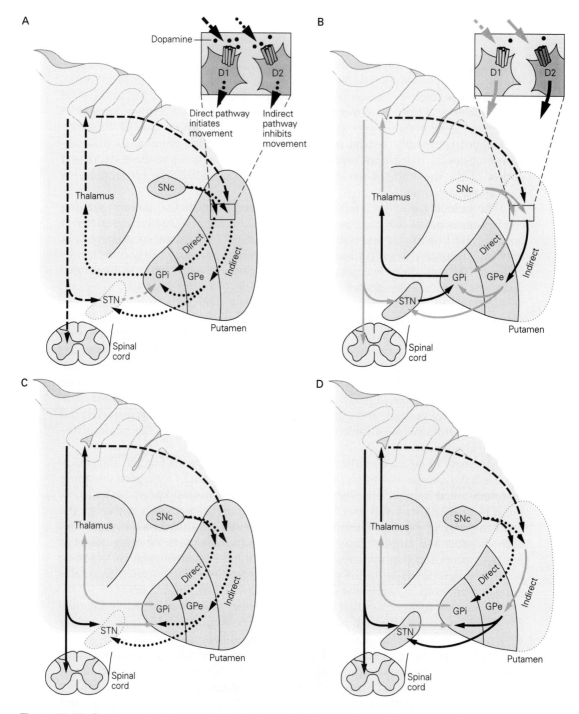

Figure 12–27. Basal ganglia-thalamocortical circuitry under (**A**) normal conditions and in (**B**) Parkinson disease, (**C**) hemiballism, and (**D**) chorea. In (**A**) inhibitory connections are shown as dotted arrows and excitatory connections as dashed arrows. Degeneration of the nigrostriatal dopamine pathway in Parkinson disease leads to differential changes in the direct and indirect striatopallidal pathways, indicated by changes in the appearance of the connecting arrows. Solid black arrows indicate increased neuronal activity and solid gray arrows indicate decreased neuronal activity. The result is increased output of the basal ganglia to the thalamus, decreased output of the thalamus to the motor cortex, and, clinically, bradykinesia. In hemiballism, damage to the subthalamic nucleus and in chorea damage to the putamen result in decreased output of the basal ganglia to the thalamus, increased output of the thalamus to the motor cortex, and, clinically, abnormal movement. GPe, external segment of the globus pallidus; GPi, internal segment of the globus pallidus; SNc, substantia nigra pars compacta; STN, subthalamic nucleus. (Reproduced with permission from Kandel ER, Schwartz JH, Jessell TM. 1999. *Principles of Neural Science,* 4th ed. New York: McGraw-Hill.)

put. Studies of MPTP-induced parkinsonism in animals suggest that excitatory amino acid antagonists or neuronal nitric oxide synthase inhibitors might be useful in the treatment of Parkinson disease.

The hypothesis that an exogenous or endogenous toxin comparable to MPTP might be involved in Parkinson disease and the observation that MPTP is converted to MPP[+] by monoamine oxidase (MAO) led to clinical trials with the MAO-B inhibitor selegiline (deprenyl). Symptomatic relief was observed, but the drug's efficacy was probably the result of reduced dopamine metabolism rather than an effect on the basic disease process.

An understanding of basal ganglia anatomy has led to surgical interventions in Parkinson disease. Following cerebral implantation of fetal substantia nigra neurons, their dopamine-containing nerve endings make synaptic contact with appropriate striatal targets, and some patients receiving such therapy demonstrate modest improvement in symptoms and signs. Alternatively, ablation of the internal globus pallidus results in restoration of thalamocortical excitation, and jamming of the subthalamic nucleus by electrically stimulating it reduces excitation of the internal globus pallidus, with a similar net effect.

Unlike MPTP poisoning, which is highly selective for dopaminergic neurons in the substantia nigra, Parkinson disease also affects nonnigral dopaminergic projections to the frontal cortex and to limbic structures such as the nucleus accumbens; there is also loss of noradrenergic neurons in the locus coeruleus and serotonergic neurons in the brain stem raphe nuclei. Damage to nonnigral pathways probably contributes to the cognitive abnormalities often observed in patients with Parkinson disease.

SELECTED REFERENCES

Beal MF: Excitotoxicity and nitric oxide in Parkinson's disease pathogenesis. Ann Neurol 1998;44(Suppl 1):S110.

Clayton DF, George JM: The synucleins: A family of proteins involved in synaptic function, plasticity, neurodegeneration and disease. Trends Neurosci 1998;21:249.

Freed CR, Breeze RE, Greene PE, et al: Double-blind controlled trial of human embryonic dopamine cell transplants in advanced Parkinson's disease: Study design, surgical strategy, patient demographics and pathological outcome. Neurology 1999;52(Suppl 2):A272.

Gerfen CR: Dopamine receptor function in the basal ganglia. Clin Neuropharmacol 1995;18:S162.

Kitada T, Asakawa S, Hattori N, et al: Mutations in the Parkin gene cause autosomal recessive juvenile parkinsonism. Nature 1998;392:605.

Lang AE, Lozano AM: Parkinson's disease. Parts 1 and 2. N Engl J Med 1998;339:1130.

Limousin P, Pollak P, Benazzouz A, et al: Effect on parkinsonian signs and symptoms of bilateral subthalamic nucleus stimulation. Lancet 1996;345:91.

Obeso JA, Rodriguez MC, DeLong MR: Basal ganglia pathophysiology: A critical review. Adv Neurol 1997;74:3.

Olanow CW, Tatton WG: Etiology and pathogensis of Parkinson's disease. Annu Rev Neurosci 1999;22:123.

Polymeropoulos MH, Higgins JJ, Golbe LI, et al: Mapping of a gene for Parkinson's disease to chromosome 4q21–q23. Science 1996;274:1197.

▶ CASE 36

A 60-year-old hypertensive woman suddenly cannot control her arm. On examination an hour later there are rapid, irregular, continuous, involuntary movements of her left arm and, to a lesser degree, her left leg. The arm movements are most severe proximally, causing the limb to be flung aimlessly about. She is able voluntarily to suppress the movements, but only for 5 or 10 seconds at a time. Her face and right limbs are unaffected. Within the limits of testing no other neurological abnormalities are present.

Computerized tomographic scan reveals a 1 × 2-cm hemorrhage in the region of the right subthalamic nucleus.

During hospitalization her abnormal movements decrease when she is relaxed and disappear during sleep. As she receives gradually increasing doses of haloperidol, the movements are substantially reduced.

Comment

The subthalamic nucleus, part of the basal ganglia's indirect pathway, receives inhibitory (GABAergic) projections from the external segment of the globus pallidus and sends excitatory (glutamatergic) projections to both the internal and external segments of the globus pallidus (see Figure 12–26). As noted in Case 35, projections from the pallidal internal segment to the thalamus are inhibitory, and projections from the thalamus to motor areas of the frontal cortex are excitatory. Subthalamic nucleus damage therefore results in decreased firing of pallidal neurons and increased firing of both thalamic neurons and frontal motor area neurons (see Figure 12–27). The result is involuntary movement.

Chorea, from the Greek word for *dance,* refers to rapid, irregular, smooth, involuntary movements. It has diverse causes, including hereditary disorders such as neuroacanthocytosis and Huntington disease (see Case 75), autoimmune diseases such as poststreptococcal rheumatic fever (Sydenham chorea) and systemic lupus erythematosus, side effects of drugs such as levodopa (a direct toxic side effect) and dopamine-blocking antipsychotic agents (a withdrawal phenomenon), encephalitis, stroke, and neoplasm. Depending on etiology, chorea can be proximal or distal and unilateral or bilateral, and it can affect the face and tongue. When it is unilateral and florrid, producing flinging or flailing movements of the arm, it is called *hemiballism* (from the Greek word for *throwing*).

Hemiballism is the major symptom of either occlusive or hemorrhagic stroke affecting the contralateral subthalamic nucleus. In studies with primates, ablation of at least 20% of the subthalamic nucleus or of its efferent projections produces hemiballism. Similar abnormal movements have also followed small infarcts in the contralateral caudate nucleus or putamen, and in this setting an explanation is more difficult, for the striatum has a complex architecture, with multiple cell types and neurochemically specialized subregions (striosomes).

Hemiballism following stroke in either location usually improves with dopamine blocking agents such as haloperidol. There is also usually spontaneous improvement over weeks or months, and so the drug should be periodically discontinued to determine if it is still necessary. In patients with intractable hemiballism, surgical ablation of the disinhibited ventrolateral thalamic nucleus can reduce symptoms.

SELECTED REFERENCES

Chesselet MF, Delfs JMD, DeLong MR: Basal ganglia and movement disorders: An update. Trends Neurosci 1996;19:417.

Hamada I, DeLong MR: Excitotoxic acid lesions of the primate subthalamic nucleus result in reduced pallidal neuronal activity during active holding. J Neurophysiol 1992; 68:1859.

Provenzale JM, Glass JP: Hemiballismus: CT and MR findings. J Comp Assist Tomogr 1995;19:537.

Wichmann T, DeLong MR: Functional and pathological models of the basal ganglia. Curr Opinion Neurobiol 1996;6:751.

▶ CASE 37

Attempting suicide with barbiturates, a 37-year-old woman has a cardiorespiratory arrest for about 20 minutes. Regaining consciousness 24 hours later, she displays arrhythmic jerking of her limbs and cranial muscles on any attempted movement. The muscle jerks are greater distally than proximally and occur only in the limb being moved; continuing repetitively throughout the range of movement, they resemble a coarse irregular intention tremor. The jerks are also precipitated by passive joint movement. Similar jerking of cranial muscles renders her speech unintelligible. On two occasions she has a major motor seizure, and there is diffuse muscular rigidity, bradykinesia, and bilateral grasp reflexes.

Electroencephalography (EEG) demonstrates bilateral, synchronous sharp waves that are most evident at, and sometimes confined to, the vertex. Simultaneous EEG and electromyography (EMG) reveal that the EEG spikes can be triggered by finger tapping and that they are followed, 53 ms after the stimulus, by EMG potentials associated with jerking of forearm muscles. Median nerve stimulation produces an abnormally large cortical somatosensory evoked potential. Therapy with either 5-hydroxytryptophan or clonazepam results in moderate improvement of her abnormal movements.

Comment

Myoclonus, defined as a sudden involuntary jerk of a muscle or a muscle group, has diverse patterns and causes. It can be focal (only a limited set of muscles is affected), multifocal (focal jerks occur in different parts of the body), or generalized (most of the body is involved in each jerk). Myoclonus can be a normal physiological occurrence, for example, sleep jerks and hiccups, or it can be a manifestation of many different diseases, including epileptic disorders (infantile spasms), storage diseases (GM_2 gangliosidosis or Tay-Sachs disease), spinocerebellar degenerations (Friedreich ataxia), basal ganglia degeneration (Wilson disease), viral encephalitis (herpes simplex), prion disease (Creutzfeldt-Jacob disease), metabolic disorders (uremia), and toxicity (β-lactam antibiotics). Myoclonus triggered by movement is often encountered in patients who have survived cardiac arrest.

The myoclonus exhibited by this patient is termed *cortical reflex myoclonus*. In addition to the monosynaptic stretch reflex, which is mediated at the level of the spinal cord, a long loop stretch reflex is mediated through the cerebral cortex; proprioceptive and other sensory information is conveyed to the parietal somatosensory cortex (where it produces the somatosensory evoked potential, SEP) and then via corticocortical connections to the frontal motor cortex, a feedback system for motor control. In this patient, anoxic-ischemic damage has somehow disinhibited the parietal cortex. As a result, somatosensory stimuli produce an enlarged SEP, excessive firing into the motor cortex, and multifocal myoclonic jerks. Consistent with such an interpretation, the interval from tapping her finger to the appearance of a myoclonic jerk—53 ms—corresponds to the expected duration of the long-latency stretch reflex.

A physiologically different kind of myoclonus, also encountered in cardiac arrest survivors, is termed *reticular reflex myoclonus*. Here there is no increase in the SEP, and when EEG and EMG are performed together, cortical spikes, if they are seen at all, follow, rather than precede, the EMG discharges and myoclonic jerks. Moreover, if cranial muscles are involved, their myoclonic jerks occur in a caudal-to-rostral order, in contrast to what is seen in cortical reflex myoclonus. The initial discharge therefore originates in the lower brain stem, probably the medullary reticular formation. Whereas muscle jerks in cortical reflex myoclonus are usually multifocal and distal, in reticular reflex myoclonus they are usually generalized and proximal.

The precise neurochemical basis of postanoxic myoclonus is unknown. Damage to serotonin systems is implicated by the frequent findings of low cerebrospinal fluid levels of the serotonin metabolite 5-hydroxyindoleacetic acid and symptomatic response to the serotonin precursor, 5-hydroxytryptophan. Also effective in such patients are the benzodiazepine clonazepam and the anticonvulsant valproic acid. Benzodiazepines occupy stereospecific receptors on the GABA-benzodiazepine macromolecular complex; by allosterically influencing GABA receptor binding, they increase the frequency of chloride channel opening (see Figure 15–2). Valproic acid inhibits the enzyme succinic semialdehyde dehydrogenase, resulting in increased levels of GABA. GABAergic nerve terminals inhibit serotonergic neurons of the brain stem raphe nuclei, but whether it is through these systems that clonazepam and valproic acid exert their antimyoclonus effects is uncertain.

SELECTED REFERENCES

Brown P, Ridding MC, Werhaus KJ, et al: Abnormalities of the balance between inhibition and excitation in the motor cortex of patients with cortical myoclonus. Brain 1996;119:309.

Chadwick D, Hallett M, Harris R, et al: Clinical, biochemical, and physiological features distinguishing myoclonus responsive to 5-hydroxytryptophan, tryptophan with a monoamine oxidase inhibitor, and clonazepam. Brain 1977;100:455.

Hallett M, Chadwick D, Marsden CD: Cortical reflex myoclonus. Neurology 1979;29:1107.

Lance JW, Adams RD: The syndrome of intention or action myoclonus as a sequal to hypoxic encephalopathy. Brain 1963;87:111.

13

Mostly Autonomic

▶ CASE 38

Following a year of impotence and nocturnal urinary frequency, a 57-year-old man experiences blurred vision during exercise. Over the next several months his symptoms increase; when he stands for more than a few minutes or walks a few hundred yards, he experiences constriction of his visual fields and loss of color perception followed by lightheadedness and diffuse weakness. If he does not then sit down, he loses consciousness. Neither pallor nor sweating precedes syncope. Over the next year he develops slowly progressive facial immobility and bradykinesia but neither tremor, ataxia, nor dysarthria.

On examination there is reduced facial expression and spontaneous blinking, and his limbs are mildly bradykinetic and rigid. When he is supine, his blood pressure is 130/80 mm Hg and his pulse rate is 76/minute; when he stands, his blood pressure falls to 95/40 mm Hg, his pulse rate does not change, and he experiences his usual dizziness and blurred vision. With the Valsalva maneuver—forcibly exhaling against a closed glottis—there is neither an increase nor a decrease in heart rate or blood pressure. Body warming with a heating cradle fails to produce sweating. Bladder catheterization after voiding reveals nearly 200 mL residual urine, and slow instillation of fluid into the bladder produces an urge to void but reduced reflex contraction.

Basal levels of plasma norepinephrine are normal but fail to rise on standing. Subcutaneous injection of 0.25 mg epinephrine produces a normal pressor and tachycardic response. Computerized tomographic scan of the head, electromyography, and cerebrospinal fluid are normal.

Treatment of his postural syncope includes sleeping with his head elevated, wearing an elastic garment that compresses the lower abdomen, and daily oral administration of 9α-fluorohydrocortisone. His urinary retention is treated with oral bethanechol.

Comment

Although this patient has mild symptoms of parkinsonism (see Case 35), his functional disability is the result of autonomic dysfunction (Figure 13–1). Impotence and bladder distention with a preserved sense of urinary urgency reflect efferent parasympathetic dysfunction. A fall in blood pressure greater than 30/15 mm Hg on standing and failure of the heart rate to increase when his blood pressure drops or during the Valsalva maneuver reflect sympathetic dysfunction, which theoretically could involve either the afferent or the efferent limb of the reflex arc. Failure to sweat in response to body warming indicates impairment of

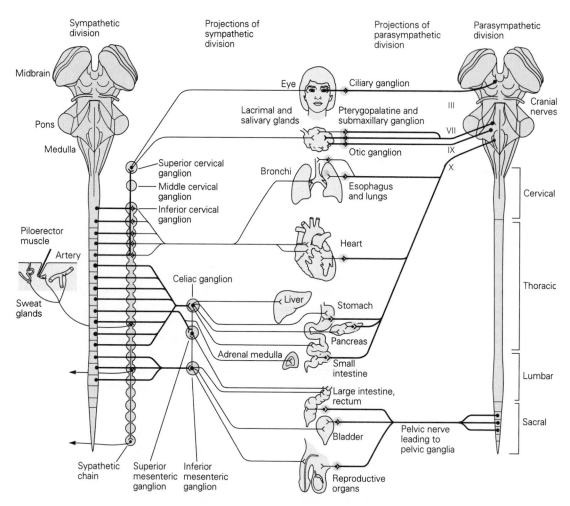

Sympathetic division

Projections of sympathetic division

Projections of parasympathetic division

Parasympathetic division

Midbrain

Pons

Medulla

Piloerector muscle

Artery

Sweat glands

Superior cervical ganglion

Middle cervical ganglion

Inferior cervical ganglion

Celiac ganglion

Adrenal medulla

Sypathetic chain

Superior mesenteric ganglion

Inferior mesenteric ganglion

Eye

Lacrimal and salivary glands

Bronchi

Liver

Stomach

Pancreas

Small intestine

Large intestine, rectum

Bladder

Reproductive organs

Ciliary ganglion

Pterygopalatine and submaxillary ganglion

Otic ganglion

Esophagus and lungs

Heart

Pelvic nerve leading to pelvic ganglia

III

VII

IX

X

Cranial nerves

Cervical

Thoracic

Lumbar

Sacral

Figure 13–1. The autonomic nervous system. The sympathetic division is shown on the left and the parasympathetic division on the right. In contrast to somatic motor innervation of skeletal muscle, in the autonomic nervous system two neurons link the central nervous system with organs of the periphery. Sympathetic *preganglionic* neurons are found in the intermediate zone of the spinal cord (T1–L3); their axons exit the spinal cord through the ventral roots and project either to paravertebral ganglia in the sympathetic trunk or to prevertebral ganglia further away from the spinal cord (notably the celiac, superior mesenteric, and inferior mesenteric ganglia). From neurons in these ganglia, *postganglionic* axons project to organ targets. Parasympathetic preganglionic neurons are found in the brainstem and sacral spinal cord (S2–S4); their axons project to peripheral ganglia, from which postganglionic axons project to organ targets. (Reproduced with permission from Kandel ER, Schwartz JH, Jessell TM. 1999. *Principles of Neural Science*, 4th ed. New York: McGraw-Hill.)

the efferent sympathetic pathway, which theoretically could be anywhere from the hypothalamus to the postganglionic peripheral sympathetic nerves.

A disorder of the postganglionic sympathetic nerves would result in reduced basal levels of plasma norepinephrine, failure of norepinephrine levels to rise when the patient stands, and, reflecting denervation supersensitivity, an excessive rise in blood pressure and heart rate in response to subcutaneous epinephrine (which stimulates both α- and β-adrenergic receptors). By contrast, although this patient's plasma norepinephrine levels do not rise when he stands, his basal plasma norepinephrine levels are normal, and he does not demonstrate a hypersensitive response to parenteral epinephrine; these findings indicate preganglionic sympathetic dysfunction (Figure 13–2).

The term *multiple system atrophy* (MSA) refers to variable combinations of symptoms and signs reflecting neuronal degeneration within the autonomic nervous system, the basal ganglia, the cerebellum, the corticobulbar/corticospinal system, and the spinal cord. When autonomic symptoms predominate, particularly postural hypotension, the eponym *Shy-Drager syndrome* is applied. Parkinsonism is often present, sometimes the result of degeneration within the substantia nigra and therefore responsive to levodopa, but more often secondary to degeneration of both the substantia nigra and the striatum (*striatonigral degeneration*) and therefore levodopa resistant. (Loss of striatal neurons means that levodopa, after its conversion to dopamine, no longer has a target on which to act.)

Cell loss in the cerebellar cortex, inferior olives, and pontine nuclei (olivopontocerebellar atrophy) causes ataxic symptoms such as tremor, dysmetria, and dysarthria, and corticobulbar and corticospinal degeneration causes weakness, clumsiness, spasticity, brisk tendon reflexes, and extensor plantar responses. Cranial motor neurons and spinal anterior horn cells are sometimes affected, producing atrophic weakness; some patients develop stridor (inspiratory vocalization), dysphagia, or sleep apnea.

Autonomic symptoms and signs are secondary to degeneration of preganglionic sympathetic efferent neurons within the intermediolateral cell columns of the thoracic spinal cord, of parasympathetic neurons within the dorsal vagal nuclei and the sacral spinal cord, and of catecholaminergic neurons in the ventrolateral medulla. Medullary catecholaminergic neurons project not only to sympathetic neurons of the intermediolateral cell columns of the spinal cord but also

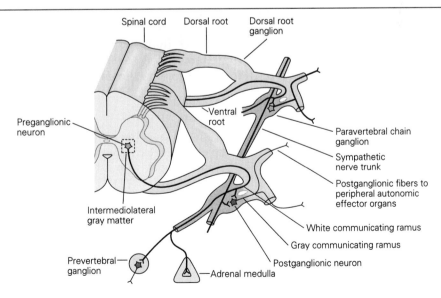

Figure 13–2. Anatomical organization of sympathetic preganglionic and postganglionic axons. [Reproduced with permission from Kandel ER, Schwartz JH, Jessell TM. 1999. *Principles of Neural Science*, 4th ed. New York: McGraw-Hill. Adapted with permission from Loewy AD, Spyer KM (eds). 1990. *Central Regulation of Autonomic Function.* New York: Oxford University Press.]

rostrally to the hypothalamus and to brain stem areas involved with sleep control (the locus coeruleus, raphe nuclei, and pontine cholinergic nuclei) and respiration (ventral respiratory neurons). Loss of projections to the hypothalamus probably accounts for a number of frequently encountered findings in patients with MSA, for example, lack of vasopressin increase following tilt-induced hypotension, impaired corticotrophin response to hypoglycemia, and impaired growth hormone response to the α_2-agonist clonidine. Loss of projections to other brain stem areas probably accounts for disturbances of cardiorespiratory control, particularly during sleep.

In some patients involvement of the parasympathetic (Edinger-Westphal) nucleus of the oculomotor nerve produces anisocoria and abnormal pupillary reactivity to light and near vision; on the other hand, the occasional presence of iris atrophy and hypersensitive pupillary responses to cholinergic drugs suggest involvement of the parasympathetic ciliary ganglion. The nuclei of the tractus solitarius (the major brain stem relay for visceral sensation) and the locus coeruleus (the source of nearly all the norepinephrine within the central nervous system) are also affected. With rare exceptions, the paravertebral and prevertebral sympathetic ganglia are normal.

The cause of this disease (or diseases) is unknown. A tantalizing clue is the presence in oligodendrocytes and neurons of filamentous cytoplasmic inclusions containing α-synuclein, a protein normally present in nerve endings. α-synuclein is also present in the Lewy bodies of Parkinson disease (see Case 35) and in intracellular inclusions of several other disorders, including diffuse Lewy body dementia, Hallervorden-Spatz disease (a rare hereditary movement disorder), and an atypical form of Alzheimer disease. Although the pathogenic role of α-synuclein in these disorders is unclear, some investigators refer to them collectively as α-synucleinopathies.

Treatment of postural hypotension includes salt-retaining corticosteroids. Bladder dysfunction is treated with cholinergic agonists. (Some patients paradoxically develop hyperactive detrusor contraction in response to bladder filling, perhaps reflecting loss of inhibitory influences from the substantia nigra and striatum. In such patients, anticholinergic medication sometimes improves urinary symptoms.) The disease is relentlessly progressive, however, and death usually occurs within several years.

SELECTED REFERENCES

Benarroch EE, Smithson IL, Low PA, et al: Depletion of catecholaminergic neurons of the rostral ventrolateral medulla in multiple systems atrophy with autonomic failure. Ann Neurol 1998;43:156.

Kaufman H: Multiple system atrophy. Curr Opin Neurol 1998;11:351.

Mathias CJ: Autonomic disorders and their recognition. N Engl J Med 1997;336:721.

McLeod JG, Tuck RR: Disorders of the autonomic nervous system: Part 1. Pathophysiology and clinical features. Ann Neurol 1987;21:419.

McLeod JG, Tuck RR: Disorders of the autonomic nervous system: Part 2. Investigation and treatment. Ann Neurol 1987;21:519.

Tu P-h, Galvin JE, Baba M, et al: Glial cytoplasmic inclusions in white matter oligodendrocytes of multiple system atrophy brains contain insoluble α-synuclein. Ann Neurol 1998;44:15.

Wenning GK, Shlomo YB, Magalhaes M, et al: Clinical features and natural history of multiple system atrophy. An analysis of 100 cases. Brain 1994;117:835.

▶ CASE 39

A 47-year-old woman, who has smoked a pack of cigarettes daily for 30 years, notices that her pupils are of unequal size. On examination in room light her left pupil is 2 mm in diameter and her right pupil is 4 mm; in the dark her right pupil enlarges to 6 mm, but her left pupil remains the same. Both pupils react directly and consensually to light and near vision. The left palpebral fissure is several millimeters smaller than the right as a result of both mild ptosis of the upper eyelid and upside-down ptosis of the lower eyelid. Warming with a heating cradle reveals decreased sweating over her entire left face. Findings on the rest of her physical and neurological examination are normal.

Following the instillation of two drops of 10% cocaine in each eye, the right pupil enlarges to 8 mm but the left remains unchanged. A day later 1% hydroxyamphetamine is instilled into each eye and, again, the right pupil enlarges but the left does not.

Radiography reveals a mass lesion in the apex of the left lung.

Comment

The first question to ask in assessing unequal pupils (*anisocoria*) is whether they signify abnormality. Twenty percent or more of normal people have pupillary inequality of up to nearly 1 mm. Such physiological anisocoria can vary from day to day. If pupillary inequality is considered pathological, the question is whether the larger or the smaller pupil is normal. When anisocoria is greater in light than in darkness, or when there is a reduced or absent light reflex in the eye with the larger pupil, parasympathetic dysfunction is causing mydriasis. When anisocoria is greater in darkness than in light, with normal light reactivity in each eye, sympathetic dysfunction is causing miosis. Sympathetic nerves supply not only the pupillodilator muscles of the iris but also smooth (Müller's) muscles in the upper and lower lids; mild ptosis therefore often accompanies miosis in patients with sympathetic lesions. When sympathetic innervation to the sweat glands and blood vessels of the face is also affected, there may be ipsilateral facial dryness and conjunctival redness. The triad of miosis, ptosis, and reduced facial sweating is called *Horner syndrome.*

A lesion anywhere along the sympathetic pathway—hypothalamus, lateral brainstem, cervical or upper thoracic spinal cord, sympathetic chain, superior cervical ganglion, internal carotid artery, or first division of the trigeminal nerve—can result in ipsilateral miosis with or without ptosis and reduced facial sweating. When the lesion is intraparencyhmal—for example, infarction of the lateral medulla (see Case 50)—other symptoms and signs will likely be present. Peripheral lesions can also cause additional symptoms, for example, pain or impaired sensation over the forehead from a meningioma compressing the first division of the trigeminal nerve.

The most common cause of acquired Horner syndrome in adults is lung cancer damaging the superior cervical ganglion, and sometimes miosis is the sole presenting sign. Such a lesion might affect cervical nerve roots or the proximal brachial plexus as well. Most of the sweat glands of the face receive their sympathetic innervation from fibers that ride along the external carotid artery; a sympathetic lesion proximal to the bifurcation of the common carotid artery will therefore cause reduced sweating over the entire ipsilateral face. When the lesion is distal to the bifurcation, reduced sweating will be restricted to the medial forehead and upper nose.

When the lesion is proximal to the superior cervical ganglion, pupillodilator muscles of the iris remain directly innervated; a lesion at or distal to the superior cervical ganglion denervates the pupillodilator muscles. Topical cocaine, which blocks reuptake of catecholamines at nerve endings, causes mydriasis by prolonging the action of norepinephrine at synapses formed by sympathetic nerve endings and iris smooth muscle. Cocaine will fail to produce pupillary dilatation when there are lesions anywhere along the sympathetic pathway; even if sympathetic nerve endings are still anatomically present on the iris, they are not firing and so there is no norepinephrine present in the synapse. By contrast, hydroxyamphetamine, which stimulates release of catecholamines from nerve endings, will continue to produce pupillary dilatation when a sympathetic lesion is proximal to the superior cervical ganglion but will produce no response (as in this patient) when the ganglion or its fibers have been destroyed.

SELECTED REFERENCES

Giles CL, Henderson JW: Horner's syndrome: An analysis of 16 cases. Am J Ophthalmol 1958;46:289.

Keane JR: Oculosympathetic paresis: Analysis of 100 hospitalized patients. Arch Neurol 1979;36:13.

Morris JGL, Lee J, Lim CL: Facial sweating in Horner's syndrome. Brain 1984;107:751.

Thompson HS, Mensher JH: Adrenergic mydriasis in Horner's syndrome. Hydroxyamphetamine test for diagnosis of postganglionic defects. Am J Ophthalmol 1971;72:472.

14

Mixed Disorders:
Somatosensory, Motor, and Autonomic

▶ CASE 40

A 54-year-old man has had 6 years of slowly progressive numbness and weakness of his distal limbs. Symptoms began as a constant painless tingling in his feet; after a few years similar sensations appeared in his fingers, and the paresthesias in his feet changed to numbness. During the next 4 years sensory symptoms spread to his knees and wrists and he had increasing unsteadiness walking and difficulty writing or manipulating objects. He attributes this difficulty to both weakness and incoordination. There are no symptoms referable to the autonomic nervous system.

On examination there is atrophy of muscles below his knees and in his hands. Strength of toe and ankle dorsiflexion and intrinsic hand muscles is graded 3/5 bilaterally; a lesser degree of weakness affects plantar flexion and forearm muscles. Vibratory sensation and proprioception are decreased in his toes, ankles, and fingers; pinprick, touch, and temperature sensation are reduced distal to his elbows and knees. Gait is broad based and unsteady, and he can neither walk tandem nor stand with his feet together and eyes closed. Tendon reflexes are absent throughout. Mentation and cranial nerves are normal.

Motor nerve conduction velocity of the median nerve in the forearm is 25 m/second, with a compound muscle action potential of 3.0 mV (both markedly reduced). Peroneal nerve stimulation fails to generate a potential from the toe extensors, and the median nerve sensory action potential is absent at the wrist. Fibrillations and positive waves are present at electromyographic study of the anterior tibial and opponens muscles. Cerebrospinal fluid (CSF) protein is elevated at 95 mg/dL. Serum protein electrophoresis reveals a γ-globulin spike. The serum immunoglobin M (IgM) level is 960 mg/dL (normal range 50–311); immunoglobin G and A levels are normal. Serum immunofixation identifies an IgM κ paraprotein, and immunoblot reveals that it binds to myelin-associated glycoprotein. A bone marrow biopsy is normal, and further studies do not identify malignant plasma cell dyscrasia or lymphoma. Sural nerve biopsy reveals IgM with κ light chains on myelin sheaths but no amyloid. Teased fiber preparations and electron microscopy reveal segmental demyelination and remyelination with lesser degrees of axonal loss and Wallerian degeneration.

He receives plasmapheresis every few days, and within a month his serum IgM levels decline and his strength and coordination improve. Attempts to increase the interval between plasmaphereses to 2 weeks result in a rise in IgM levels and a worsening of symptoms. Receiving small doses of cyclophosphamide, he is able to increase his plasmapheresis intervals to every few weeks.

Comment

Sensorimotor peripheral neuropathy has produced glove-and-stocking sensory loss, greatest for modalities conveyed by large myelinated nerves, plus distal limb weakness in this patient. The unsteady gait and incoordination of his hands are the result of both weakness and impaired proprioception. Electrodiagnostic studies confirm disease of peripheral sensory and motor nerves; the slow nerve conduction velocities are consistent with demyelination. Nerve biopsy reveals not only demyelination (and remyelination) but also the presence of IgM globulin directed against a component of myelin called myelin-associated glycoprotein (MAG). The same IgM is circulating in large amounts in the blood, but diagnostic workup fails to reveal the presence of plasma cell malignancy.

Elevated serum levels of monoclonal γ-globulins (M-proteins) are found in plasma cell malignancies (multiple myeloma and Waldenström macroglobulinemia); they also occur in the absence of evident underlying disease (monoclonal gammapathy of undetermined significance—MGUS). Particularly in the setting of MGUS, they can retain their capacity as antibodies and sometimes bind to epitopes within peripheral nerves. The result is peripheral neuropathy. A well-documented example, exemplified by this patient, is the binding of IgM to MAG resulting in segmental demyelination and probably secondary axonal degeneration. In contrast to the chronic mostly sensory neuropathy described in Case 1 and the acute mostly motor neuropathy described in Case 22, peripheral neuropathy caused by IgM autoantibodies produces variable degrees of both weakness and sensory loss, which in the absence of treatment progresses over many years. Antibodies directed against MAG (probably an adhesion molecule for interactions between axons and Schwann cells) most often cause early sensory loss with the later appearance of weakness. (By contrast, antibodies directed against GM_1 ganglioside—one of a group of glycosphingolipids present in neuronal membranes—produce a purely motor neuropathy.) Peripheral neuropathy has been produced in mice by injection of serum from patients with M-protein neuropathy, and the disorder is treated symptomatically with measures such as plasmapheresis or immunosuppression that lower the serum autoantibody levels.

As noted in Case 1, peripheral neuropathies caused by primary axonal or neuronal damage produce weakness or sensory loss that is usually greatest distally, affecting the feet before the hands; a likely explanation is impaired axonal transport, which would be expected to affect maximally that part of a nerve farthest from its cell body. Peripheral neuropathies caused by primary demyelination also often produce stocking-glove symptoms, and here an additional factor may be present. In a disorder that randomly damages myelin along the entire length of all the nerves (the elevated CSF protein in the patient probably reflects involvement of proximal nerve roots), statistical probability predicts that long nerves will be more affected than short nerves. Compensatory sprouting of fibers from short nerves, moreover, will have a better chance of reaching their distal targets than will sprouting from long nerves.

SELECTED REFERENCES

Dyck PJ, Low PA, Windebank AJ, et al: Plasma exchange in polyneuropathy associated with monoclonal gammopathy of undetermined significance. N Engl J Med 1991; 325:1482.

Latov N, Hays AP, Sherman WH: Peripheral neuropathy and anti-MAG antibodies. Crit Rev Neurobiol 1988;3:301.

Notermans NC, Wokke JHJ, Lokhorst HM, et al: Polyneuropathy associated with monoclonal gammopathy of undetermined significance. N Engl J Med 1994;117:1385.

Ropper AH, Garson KC: Neuropathies associated with paraproteinemia. N Engl J Med 1998;338:1601.

▶ CASE 41

For several months an 82-year-old man has had increasing difficulty controlling his right hand in tasks such as writing and buttoning. He also experiences a continuous pins-and-needles sensation in his fourth and fifth fingers on the right. He is otherwise healthy except for mild intermittent pain in his neck, shoulders, elbows, hips, and knees, which he attributes to arthritis.

On examination there is atrophy of intrinsic hand muscles on the right, notably the first dorsal interosseous (between the thumb and index finger). The thenar eminence is not atrophic, however. His fourth and fifth fingers are hyperextended at the metacarpophalangeal joints and flexed at the interphalangeal joints (clawhand). The following muscles are rated 3/5 strength: dorsal and ventral interossei, thumb adductor, lumbricals of the fourth and fifth fingers, deep flexors of the fourth and fifth fingers, and ulnar wrist flexor. Other muscles have normal strength, including the opponens, the short abductor and flexors of the thumb, and the lumbricals of the index and third fingers. Pinprick and touch sensation are decreased over his fifth finger, the medial (ulnar) side of his fourth finger, and the medial palm and dorsal surface of his hand; sensation over the rest of his hand and arm is preserved. Normal tendon reflexes include the biceps, triceps, pronator, and finger flexors. Findings on his neurological examination are otherwise normal.

Electrical stimulation of the right ulnar nerve reveals markedly reduced amplitude of the compound action potential of the first dorsal interosseous muscle and focal slowing of conduction velocity across the elbow. Electromyographic study of the first dorsal interosseous and the deep flexor muscles of the fourth and fifth fingers on the right reveals fibrillations and positive waves indicative of denervation; individual motor units are polyphasic and of increased duration. Nerve conduction velocities of the median and radial nerves are normal, as are electromyographic studies of muscles innervated by them.

He is referred to a neurosurgeon for consideration of decompressive elbow surgery.

Comment

Nearly everybody aged 82 has *osteoarthritis* of the neck, which can result in compression of one or more cervical nerve roots; if the C8 root is involved, weakness can affect intrinsic hand muscles, and sensory loss can involve the medial fingers and hand. In this man, however, weakness is restricted to muscles innervated by the ulnar nerve. A clawhand deformity affects only his fourth and fifth fingers because the lumbrical muscles of those fingers are innervated by the ulnar nerve, whereas the lumbricals of the second and third fingers are innervated by the median nerve. Similarly, his sensory loss, which splits the fourth finger and spares the forearm, describes an ulnar nerve territory more than a C8 root territory.

Electrodiagnostic studies confirm ulnar neuropathy and localize the damage to the elbow, probably the result of osteoarthritis and entrapment. Surgical decompression of the nerve—or actually moving it out of its groove—has a good chance of arresting the progression of symptoms. If atrophy has not progressed to the point that reinnervation is no longer possible, symptomatic improvement might occur. The presence in the first dorsal interosseous muscle of a compound action potential and of prolonged high-amplitude motor units indicative of reinnervation supports such a favorable prognosis.

SELECTED REFERENCES

Dawson DM, Hallett M, Wilbourn AW: *Entrapment Neuropathies,* 3rd edition. Lippincott-Raven, 1998.

Miller RG: Injury to peripheral nerves. Muscle Nerve 1987;10:698.

Parry GJ: Electrodiagnosis studies in the evaluation of peripheral nerve and brachial plexus injuries. Neurol Clin 1992;10:921.

▶ CASE 42

Two weeks after a flu-like illness a 37-year-old man abruptly develops pain in his left shoulder, upper arm, and base of the neck. Over the next 3 days the pain becomes increasingly severe; aching in quality and constant, it is aggravated by movement of the shoulder and upper arm but not of the neck. Four days after the onset of pain he awakens with marked weakness of the left upper arm and shoulder.

On examination there is tenderness to deep palpation at the left axilla. Complete paralysis affects left shoulder abduction (supraspinatus muscle to first 15°, deltoid beyond 15°) and external rotation (infraspinatus). Graded at 3/5 strength are internal rotation of the shoulder (upper pectoralis, subscapularis, and teres major) and elbow flexion (biceps, brachialis, and brachioradialis). Mildly weak are elbow extension (triceps), wrist extension (wrist extensors), and forearm suppination (suppinator). Other muscles have normal strength; in particular, there is no scapular winging (serratus anterior), he can symmetrically adduct his shoulder blades (rhomboids), and he can fully shrug his shoulders (trapezius). There is mild sensory impairment to touch, pinprick, and cold over his left lateral shoulder and upper arm. The left biceps and pectoralis reflexes are absent and the left triceps reflex is decreased.

Nerve conduction velocities are slowed across the left brachial plexus. Compound action potentials are absent in paralyzed muscles and reduced in amplitude in weak muscles. Evidence of denervation—fibrillations and positive waves—is not seen. Computerized tomographic (CT) scans of his neck, shoulder, and upper chest are normal, as is cerebrospinal fluid.

Over the next few days his pain gradually subsides, but weakness persists. He receives no treatment other than a protective sling and physical therapy. A month later strength begins to improve, and 6 months later his neurological examination is normal.

Comment

This man's weakness and sensory loss involve muscles and skin areas innervated by multiple cervical nerve roots and multiple peripheral nerves (see Figure 5–1 and Table 4–1). Total paralysis affects some but not all muscles supplied by the C5 and C6 roots and by the axillary and suprascapular nerves. Lesser degrees of weakness affect muscles supplied by the C5, C6, and C7 roots and the subscapular, musculocutaneous, lateral pectoral, and radial nerves. Conspicuously spared are the rhomboids (C4, C5, and dorsal scapular nerve) and the serratus anterior (C5, C6, C7, and long thoracic nerve). Impaired sensation could be attributed to involvement of the C5 and C6 roots, yet the lateral forearm and thumb, also supplied by C6, have normal sensation. Alternatively, sensory loss could be attributed to involvement of the axillary and radial nerves, but, again, if radial nerve injury were to result in sensory loss, the area affected would likely include the dorsal hand. In other words, the findings on this man's examination are inconsistent with damage at the level of either the cervical nerve roots or the peripheral nerves; they are consistent, however, with damage distal to the roots and proximal to the peripheral nerves, namely at the brachial plexus.

Spontaneous brachial plexus neuropathy (also known as brachial plexopathy, brachial neuritis, or neuralgic amyotrophy) has a course typically like this patient's: severe shoulder pain followed by weakness and a lesser degree of sensory loss, with complete or nearly complete recovery. The disorder often follows a viral illness or administration of a vaccine, suggesting autoimmunity and molecular mimickry, yet corticosteroid treatment does not seem to hasten recovery.

Damage may affect the brachial plexus proximal enough to involve its earliest branching nerves—the dorsal scapular and the long thoracic—or, as with this patient, involve the plexus more distally. When the brunt of injury involves the upper trunk of the plexus, weakness and sensory loss are greatest in the shoulder and upper arm (*Erb's palsy*). When the lower trunk is involved, weakness and sensory loss are greatest in the hand (*Klumpke's palsy*).

If a cervical root lesion is not readily excluded by neurological signs and electrodiagnosis, CT or magnetic resonance imaging of the cervical spine can identify root compression by neoplasm, osteoarthritic spur, or herniated cervical disk. Other conditions that must be considered in such patients are carcinomatous infiltration of the brachial plexus, radiation damage, peripheral nerve trauma or entrapment, and rotator cuff injury.

SELECTED REFERENCES

Editorial Committee for the Guarantors of Brain: *Aids to the Examination of the Peripheral Nervous System*. W.B. Saunders, 1986.

England JD, Sumner AJ: Neuralgic amyotrophy: An increasingly diverse entity. Muscle Nerve 1987;10:60.

Kori SH, Foley KM, Posner JB: Brachial plexus lesions in patients with cancer: 100 cases. Neurology 1981;31:45.

Subramony SH: Neuralgic amyotrophy (acute brachial neuropathy). Muscle Nerve 1988;11:39.

▶ CASE 43

Two days after sustaining a gunshot wound to his right upper arm, a 22-year-old man develops pain in his right hand, which over the next several months increases in intensity. Burning in quality and continuous, the pain initially occupies the palmar surfaces of his thumb, index and third fingers, and lateral hand, but by the time he is examined, 6 months after the injury, it has spread into his forearm and the rest of his hand. The pain is resistant to oral analgesics and exquisitely sensitive to external stimuli; even the lightest touch or a cold draft aggravates it, as does dependency of the limb or emotional upset. He has noticed that his right palm sweats continuously.

On examination he is agitated and depressed, resisting any movement or touching of his right hand, the skin of which is thin, shiny, blotchy, cool, and damp, particularly over the palmar area innervated by the median nerve. There is no decrease in the threshold for touch or pain sensation; rather, touch is interpreted as painful (allodynia) and pinprick produces overreaction and aftersensation (hyperpathia). Strength cannot be tested because of the pain, but there is full range of movement of his right wrist and fingers. Findings on his neurological examination are otherwise normal.

Radiographs of his hands reveal demineralization on the right. He refuses electrodiagnostic studies. Injection of normal saline onto the right stellate ganglion produces no change in his symptoms. Injection of 1% procaine hydrochloride to the same area is followed by prompt relief of pain.

▶ Comment

S. Wier Mitchell originally described *causalgia* (literally, burning pain) in soldiers of the American Civil War who had sustained bullet or shrapnel injuries to peripheral nerves. Pain compared to a red-hot iron occurred most often in the palm or dorsum of the foot, gradually spreading and associated with thin, red, shiny, eczematous skin. Stress, anxiety, and external stimuli (including even noise or bright light) exacerbated the pain, yet wrapping the hand in a rag soaked with cold water seemed to lessen it.

Today the term *reflex sympathetic dystrophy* (RSD) is applied to the vasomotor, sudomotor, and dystrophic abnormalites that accompany causalgic pain. Edema and hyperthermia or hypothermia of the skin progress to hyperhidrosis, cyanosis, brittle cracked nails, and loss of hair. Eventually, there is skin atrophy, bone demineralization, and ankylosis. (Similar vasomotor and sudomotor changes are encountered in other traumatic and nontraumatic peripheral nerve disorders, not just those leading to causalgia.)

Unknown to Weir Mitchell, causalgic pain, although refractory to analgesics, often responds to chemical or surgical sympathectomy. (In fact, some workers include response to sympathectomy as a criterion for calling pain causalgic.) The mechanism most often proposed to explain the clinical features of causalgia is ephaptic (nonsynaptic) short-circuiting between damaged sensory and sympathetic fibers. An alternative view is that areas of axonal demyelination or sprouting contain increased numbers of sodium and calcium channels as well as α-adrenergic receptors, resulting in ectopic pacemakers and increased sensitivity to locally released and circulating catecholamines.

Inconsistent with either of these mechanisms, RSD can occur without evident nerve injury, for example, following arthrodesis, contusion, or sprain. In such patients, an exaggerated regional inflammatory response provoked by oxygen-derived free radicals or neuropeptides has been invoked. More skeptical investigators have attributed pain relief following sympathectomy to interruption of visceral nociceptive afferent fibers rather than to efferent sympathetic block. Others have invoked a placebo effect.

Two features of causalgia—the gradual spread of pain and trophic changes outside the territory of the originally injured nerve and the tendency of sympathectomy to be less effective the longer it is delayed—suggest that over time clinically significant changes occur within the central nervous system. Experimentally, receptive fields of spinal (and cortical) sensory neurons become altered following peripheral nerve injury. Such rearrangement could change the responses of spinal cord neurons to normal inhibitory influences (centralization of pain). In animal models persistent pain induces changes in neural plasticity at the level of transcriptional control (eg, *c-fos, c-jun*) of genes that encode neuropeptides (eg, substance P, enkephalin) and neuropeptide receptors. Experimentally, selective destruction of substance P receptor-expressing neurons in lamina I of the dorsal horn abolishes allodynia and hyperpathia in response to injection of capsaicin (which stimulates release of substance P from primary afferent C fibers—see Case 1), but it does not affect responses to normal nonneuropathic pain stimuli.

Some workers invoke the gate-control theory of pain to explain certain features of causalgia (Figure 14–1). Application of a cool damp cloth to reduce pain might stimulate large-diameter afferents (Aα or Aβ fibers), facilitating spinal cord interneurons that normally inhibit (gate) projection neurons conveying nociceptive information to the brain. Consistent with such a view, transcutaneous nerve stimulation, postulated to relieve pain by generating an artificial barrage of nerve impulses to large axons, reportedly alleviates pain in some (but not all) patients with causalgia.

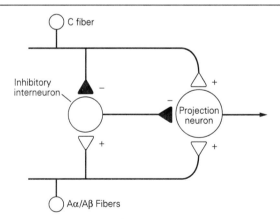

Figure 14–1. The gate control hypothesis is based on the interaction of four classes of neurons in the dorsal horn of the spinal cord: nonmyelinated nociceptive afferents (C fibers), myelinated nonnociceptive afferents (Aα and Aβ fibers), projection neurons, and inhibitory interneurons. Nociceptive and nonnociceptive neurons excite the projection neuron, the output of which determines the intensity of pain. The inhibitory interneuron is spontaneously active and normally inhibits the projection neuron, thereby reducing the intensity of pain. It is excited by the myelinated nonnociceptive afferent and inhibited by the nonmyelinated nociceptive afferent. C fiber firing thus produces pain by both direct and indirect actions on the projections neuron. (Reproduced with permission from Kandel ER, Schwartz JH, Jessell TM. 1991. *Principles of Neural Science*, 3rd ed. Norwalk, CT: Appleton & Lange.)

SELECTED REFERENCES

Iadacola MJ, Caudle RM: Good pain, bad pain. Science 1997;278:239.

Jänig W, Levine JD, Michaelis M: Interactions of sympathetic and primary afferent neurons following nerve injury and tissue trauma. Prog Brain Res 1996;113:161.

Max MB, Gilron I: Sympathetically maintained pain. Has the emperor no clothes? Neurology 1999;52:905.

Mitchell SW: *Injuries of Nerves and Their Consequences*. J.B. Lippincott, 1872. (Excerpt in Arch Neurol 1970;22:90.)

Stanton-Hicks M, Jänig W, Hassenbusch S, et al: Reflex sympathetic dystrophy: Changing concepts and taxonomy. Pain 1995;63:127.

van der Laan L, ter Laak HJ, Gabreels-Festen A, et al: Complex regional pain syndrome type I (RSD). Pathology of skeletal muscle and peripheral nerve. Neurology 1998;51:20.

▶ CASE 44

For several years a 35-year-old man has had intermittent low back pain precipitated by abrupt bending or twisting and lasting 2 or 3 days. While lifting heavy cartons, he develops more persistent lumbosacral pain that radiates down the back of his left leg to his heel when he bends forward or coughs. Lying on his side with knees and hips flexed minimizes it. Spending much of the next 2 weeks in bed brings little relief, and during this time he notes that his left lateral foot and sole feel asleep.

On examination, as he lies supine with the left hip and knee flexed, he reports little pain, but when his left knee is then extended, pain radiates from his low back down the posterior left leg to his heel. There is decreased sensation to pinprick and light touch over his left lateral foot and sole. Strength is difficult to assess because of pain, but plantar flexion of the left big toe seems slightly weaker than the right. Tendon reflexes of the left gastrocnemius and biceps femoris muscles are decreased. Findings on the neurological examination are otherwise normal.

Radiography of his lumbosacral spine is normal. Electrodiagnostic studies reveal normal nerve conduction velocities in both legs, reduced amplitude of the left sural nerve sensory action potential, and fibrillations and positive waves (indicative of denervation) in the left gastrocnemius, hamstrings, and upper sacral paraspinal muscles. Magnetic resonance imaging (MRI) of the lower spine reveals a large protrusion, anteriorly and to the left, of the intervertebral disk between L5 and S1.

Comment

For years this man has had the kind of pain often ascribed to pulled muscles but probably representing trauma to a pain-sensitive intervertebral disk. (Muscle spasm felt on examination in such patients usually signifies a compensatory splinting reaction, not the primary event.) He then traumatizes the disk sufficiently to cause herniation of its soft interior (the nucleus pulposus) posteriorly into the sac containing the lumbosacral nerve roots (the cauda equina). Compression of a lower lumbar or upper sacral nerve root produce characteristic radicular pain—shooting from the low back (or sometimes the buttock) down the back of the leg. L4 root pain typically shoots into the ankle, L5 into the big toe, and S1 into the heel. Sensory loss and weakness in this patient are consistent with a lesion of either the S1 root or the posterior tibial branch of the sciatic nerve. The decreased hamstring reflex places the lesion well above the division of the sciatic nerve into its two major branches, and electromyographic evidence of paraspinal muscle involvement places it at the root level.

The L5 root exits through the spinal foramen at L5–S1, the level of this man's protruded disk, yet it is his S1 root that is compressed. This is because at this level the L5 root, on its way through the foramen, is suffciently lateral to be missed by the protruded disk, which, instead, compresses the next root passing down. Very large disk protrusions sometimes affect more than one root.

Surgery for *herniated disks* has a discouragingly high failure rate and so is usually considered a last resort. Indications for surgery include, as in this patient, no improvement after a week or two of bed rest; intractable pain is often a consequence of the protruded fragment breaking off and lying free in the sac, in which case no amount of bed rest will restore it to where it belongs. Another indication for surgery is unacceptable neurological symptoms and signs such as severe weakness or loss of bladder control.

SELECTED REFERENCES

Borenstein D: Epidemiology, etiology, diagnostic evaluation, and treatment of low back pain. Curr Opin Rheumatol 1992;4:226.

Frymoyer JW: Back pain and sciatica. N Engl J Med 1988;318:291.

Shapiro S: Cauda equina syndrome secondary to lumbar disc herniation. Neurosurgery 1993;332:743.

▶ CASE 45

For several months a 37-year-old man has had midthoracic back pain, low-grade fevers, chills, night sweats, and weight loss. He is a former intravenous heroin abuser but has not used drugs parenterally for the past 3 years. During the past 2 weeks he has had progressive weakness of his legs, greater on the left, plus urinary frequency and urgency.

On examination, when he lies supine he can barely lift his left leg off the bed, and other left leg muscles have 3/5 strength. His right leg is only mildly weak. Both legs have increased tone, greater on the left. Pinprick and temperature sensation are markedly decreased below T10 on the right and mildly decreased below the same level on the left. Sacral dermatones are included in the pinprick and sensory loss. Proprioception is decreased in the left toes and ankle but normal on the right. Tendon reflexes are brisker in the left leg than the right with clonus at the knee and ankle, and there is a left Babinski sign. The lower abdominal and cremasteric reflexes are absent on the left.

A plain radiograph reveals destruction and collapse of the T8 and T9 vertebral bodies, including the interverterbral disk space. Magnetic resonance imaging (MRI) on cross-sectional plane reveals greater vertebral body destruction on the left, with leftward extension of the lesion into the paravertebral soft tissues and anterolateral compression of the spinal cord. The peripheral white blood count is 6000/mm^3, with 40% polymorphonuclear leukocytes and a selective decrease in CD4 T-lymphocytes. The erythrocyte sedimentation rate is 82 mm/hour, and a purified protein derivative skin test is positive.

At surgical decompression the lesion consists of granulomas with caseating necrosis and giant cells; histological stain for acid fast bacilli is positive. Following surgery his weakness and sensory loss improve. Western blot and enzyme-linked immunosorbent assay for human immunodeficiency virus (HIV) are positive. Over the next several weeks, as he receives multiple drugs for HIV and tuberculosis, his symptoms improve further.

Comment

After several months of back pain and nonspecific constitutional symptoms, this man developed *Brown-Séquard syndrome* (named after one of the most colorful figures in the history of clinical neurology, a man who, among other things, self-reported rejuvenated sexual prowess after eating extracts of monkey testis. The response was, of course, a placebo effect, but the field of endocrinology was off and running.) The patient's spinal cord compression maximally affected his left lateral corticospinal tract, spinothalamic tract, and dorsal column. The lateral corticospinal tract crosses in the lower medulla, and so its involvement within the spinal cord produces motor signs ipsilateral to the lesion (ie, spastic weakness, hyperactive tendon reflexes, an extensor plantar response, and loss of superficial abdominal and cremasteric reflexes). Similarly, information carried in the dorsal columns crosses within the medulla (after the system's first synapse at the medullary cuneate and gracile nuclei); proprioceptive and discriminative tactile sensory loss will therefore also be ipsilateral to a unilateral spinal cord lesion. By contrast, the anterolateral system, including the spinothalamic tract, consists of axons of neurons situated in the contralateral dorsal horn of the spinal cord and is crossed from its very origin; affective or nondiscriminative sensory loss (pinprick, temperature, and nondiscriminative tactile sensation) will therefore be contralateral to a unilateral spinal cord lesion.

Consistent with extrinsic compression—and in contrast to what would be expected with an intramedullary spinal cord lesion—this patient's sacral dermatomes, represented in the most superficial (outer) layers of his spinothalamic tract, were affected. Because the lesion was not strictly unilateral, he also had symptoms and signs of a spastic bladder.

The Brown-Séquard syndrome defines anatomical localization, not disease process. If a single lesion is present, a Brown-Séquard syndrome localizes that lesion to the spinal cord. Conversely, if pinprick and temperature sensation, proprioception, and strength are all decreased on the same side of the body, the lesion is either distal to the spinal cord (ie, in nerve roots or peripheral nerves) or rostral to the spinal cord (ie, above the crossing of the lateral corticospinal tracts and the dorsal column-medial lemniscus system).

SELECTED REFERENCES

DeMeyer W: Anatomy and clinical neurology of the spinal cord. In: Joynt RJ (ed): *Clinical Neurology*, Volume 3 (pp. 1–32). Lippincott Williams & Wilkins, 1992.

Smith AS, Weinstein MA, Mizushima A, et al: MR imaging characteristics of tuberculous spondylitis vs. vertebral osteomyelitis. AJNR 1989;10:619.

▶ CASE 46

A 17-year-old boy is shot through the midthoracic spine. In an emergency room he has no voluntary movement of either leg and no sensation to pinprick, touch, temperature, or vibration below T6; proprioception is absent in his ankles, knees, and hips. His legs are flaccid, tendon reflexes are absent, and plantar responses are bilaterally silent. A computerized tomographic scan confirms that the bullet passed through the spinal canal at T5, and he is treated with spinal immobilization. After removal of 400 mL urine from a distended bladder, an indwelling catheter is placed.

Over the next week there is no return of strength, sensation, or reflexes, and his legs remain flaccid. There is gastric and intestinal atony (paralytic ileus) and no voluntary defecation. Penile erection does not occur, and his abdominal, cremasteric, and bulbocavernosus reflexes are unobtainable. Sweating is absent below T6.

Three weeks after the injury, plantar stimulation produces brief dorsiflexion of the big toes, and the bulbocavernosus reflex returns. Over the next several weeks there is gradual return of tone and tendon reflexes in his legs, and plantar stimulation produces not only dorsiflexion of his toes but also flexion at his ankles, knees, and hips (*triple flexion*). Voluntary movement in his legs and sensation below T6 remain absent, yet he complains of a dull burning pain in his lower back, abdomen, and perineum. With removal of the urinary catheter, there is irregular involuntary contraction of the bladder and expulsion of urine. Reflex defecation also appears. Noxious stimuli to his legs now produce full flexion at ankle, knee, and hip, accompanied by urination and by sweating and piloerection below the level of the injury (*mass reflex*). A warm environment, however, produces sweating above T6 but not below it.

Eight months after the injury, strong noxious stimuli continue to produce flexor responses in his legs, whereas milder stimuli, such as stroking the skin or squeezing a muscle, produce leg extension. Extensor reflexes are also precipitated by abrupt shifts in posture. Both flexor and extensor reflexes are decreased by oral baclofen. A year after the injury he is performing intermittent bladder catheterization twice daily and, with physical therapy and braces, learning to walk. His pain, which had been treated with nonsteroidal antiinflammatory drugs, has largely cleared.

Comment

The clinical stages that follow spinal cord transection—flaccid areflexia (*spinal shock*) followed by spastic hyperreflexia—are not entirely understood. Spinal shock clearly results from the removal of suprasegmental descending systems that facilitate spinal motor neurons, but their identity is uncertain. Lesions selectively destroying a corticospinal tract (such as an infarct within the internal capsule—see Case 28) sometimes produce acute flaccid hemiplegia, but in such patients muscle tone usually returns within a few days. Animal studies implicate damage to the reticulospinal and vestibulospinal tracts in the production of spinal shock.

By contrast, spasticity, increased tendon reflexes, flexor and extensor responses, and abnormal autonomic reflexes point to loss of suprasegmental inhibitory influences, but their identities are also uncertain. It has been suggested that deafferentation of spinal neurons from descending projections creates a state of denervation hypersensitivity, rendering them more sensitive to various neurotransmitters.

Spinal cord transection also produces complete sensory loss below the level of the lesion—secondary to transection of the dorsal columns and the anterolateral system, including the spinothalamic tracts—and there is autonomic dysfunction, particularly loss of bowel and bladder control. Suprasacral lesions result in hyperactivity and dysynergia of the bladder detrusor muscle (supplied by parasympathetic nerves) and the striated sphincter (supplied by somatic motor nerves); with lesions above T6 there is also dysfunction of the smooth muscle sphincter (supplied by sympathetic nerves). Lesions above the origin of the sympathetic greater splanchnic nerve (T4–T9) cause postural hypotension.

The treatment of spinal cord transection is intensive and prolonged. The acute loss of normal autonomic responses—gastric atony, paralytic ileus, and hypotension—can be life threatening, and urinary tract infection, which develops in nearly everyone with an indwelling bladder catheter, can progress to sepsis. Decubitus ulcers—easier to prevent than treat—become infected and can progress to osteomyelitis. Suppositories and enemas are often required for either constipation or fecal incontinence. Nutrition must be maintained, and immobilization can cause hypercalcemia and renal stones.

Urinary or decubitus infection and a distended bladder or rectum can act as interoceptive stimuli capable of triggering muscle spasms in the legs. As noted in this patient, spasms are often accompanied by sweating and piloerection below the level of the lesion, presumably the result of disinhibited sympathetic neurons of the intermediolateral cell column. Heat stimuli, however, which do not induce autonomic responses below the level of the lesion, do produce sweating and flushing above the lesion, and sometimes there is headache, hypertension, and reflex bradycardia. This exaggerated autonomic response has been attributed to circulating norepinephrine released by disinhibited sympathetic nerve endings caudal to the lesion and to epinephrine released by the adrenal gland. (Such a response is seen in patients with catecholamine-producing tumors of the adrenal medulla—pheochromocytomas.)

In some patients flexor spasms ultimately predominate over extensor spasms, and in others the reverse is true. Flexor spasms are more likely with high spinal cord injury, and if they are allowed to occur repeatedly the patient can develop paraplegia in flexion, with muscle contractures (electrically silent fixed shortening). Patients with paraplegia in extension, on the other hand, can sometimes bear their own weight (spinal standing). Unwanted spasms that do not respond adequately to oral baclofen (a GABA-agonist believed to act at substance P–modulated synapses in the dorsal horn of the spinal cord) can be treated with intrathecal baclofen delivered by a self-administered pump.

Pain below the level of injury is also not well understood; as in this patient it usually clears spontaneously over several months. Such pain has been attributed to sensation carried by sympathetic splanchnic nerves entering the spinal cord above the level of injury, although in a contrary view it has been observed that the pain is abolished by anesthetizing the stump of the upper intact segment of the spinal cord.

SELECTED REFERENCES

Ditunno JF, Forman CS: Chronic spinal cord injury. N Engl J Med 1994;330:550.

Kneisley LW: Hyperhydrosis in paraplegia. Arch Neurol 1977;34:536.

Kuhn RA: Functional capacity of the isolated spinal cord. Brain 1950;73:1.

Meinecke FW: Sequelae and rehabilitation of spinal cord injuries. Curr Opin Neurol Neurosurg 1991;4:714.

▶ CASE 47 _____

A 31-year-old woman notes decreased sensation in her left hand after sustaining a painless burn. On examination, there is decreased pinprick and temperature sensation over her left third, fourth, and fifth fingers and her medial hand and forearm. Findings on her neurological examination are otherwise normal, including touch sensation, proprioception, and strength. Cervical spine radiographs, nerve conduction studies, and electromyography are normal.

Over the next year she develops similar sensory symptoms in her right hand, and her left hand becomes weak, causing her to drop things. Examination now reveals loss of pinprick and temperature sensation over the C5–T1 dermatomes on the left and the C6–T1 dermatomes on the right. Moderately severe weakness affects the intrinsic muscles in her left hand. Electrodiagnostic studies reveal normal conduction velocities and sensory action potentials, but there is now evidence of denervation in her left first dorsal interosseous and opponens muscles. Magnetic resonance imaging (MRI) reveals an intramedullary spinal cord lesion extending longitudinally from C5 to T2; on both T1 and T2 images the lesion produces signals identical to cerebrospinal fluid (CSF).

Over the next few years her left hand weakness worsens and the area of sensory loss extends bilaterally to dermatomes C4 through T6 on the left and C5 through T3 on the right. Following a fall she develops weakness in both legs, greater on the left, and nocturnal urinary urgency.

On examination 6 years after the onset of her illness, her left intrinsic hand muscles are markedly weak and atrophic; there is hyperextension at metacarpalphalangeal joints and flexion at interphalangeal joints (clawing) as well as dorsal rotation of the thumb (simian hand). Finger and wrist flexors and extensors, long thumb abductor, and pronator teres muscles are moderately weak, and the right intrinsic hand muscles are mildly weak. Proprioception is decreased in her left hand and leg, and pinprick and temperature sensation are mildly decreased on the right below T3. Both legs are hypertonic and weak, the left moderately and the right mildly, and her gait is stiff and unsteady. At MRI the intramedullary spinal cord lesion now extends from C3 to T7.

Comment

The Greek word *syrinx* means *tube*; *syringomyelia* refers to a pathological cavitation running longitudinally in the central part of the spinal cord. In many cases the syrinx is associated with posterior fossa anomalies, namely congenital failure of opening of the outlets of the fourth ventricle (the foramina of Magendie and Luschka) and Type I Chiari malformation (displacement of the cerebellar tonsils downward through the foramen magnum). In such patients the syrinx is attributed to obstruction of CSF flow and as a consequence diversion of CSF into the cervical spinal cord, either through a still patent central canal (hydromyelia) or along the Virchow-Robin perivascular spaces. In other cases a syrinx forms adjacent to preexisting spinal cord pathology such as an astrocytoma or traumatic myelopathy. Some cases are cryptogenic—the cavity is not connected to the central canal, and there is no associated spinal cord or posterior fossa abnormality.

Whatever the cause, syringomyelia tends to produce segmentally distributed sensory loss, weakness, and atrophy. Sensory loss is typically dissociated—there is loss of pain and temperature sensation (conveyed by the spinothalamic tracts) but preservation of proprioception, discriminative touch, and vibratory sensation (conveyed mostly or entirely by the posterior columns). Loss of pain and temperature sensation is the result of damage to second order sensory neurons in the dorsal horn of the spinal cord and their projections, which cross anterior to the central canal to form the spinothalamic tract (Figure 14–2). If a syrinx is situated asymmetrically in one dorsal horn, pain and temperature loss may be asymmetric, as in this patient, and if a syrinx enlarges longitudinally within one dorsal horn, there may be ipsilateral loss of pain and temperature sensation over a considerable number of segments. Burning or aching pain is often present at the borders of sensory loss. A more centrally located syrinx involves decussating pain and temperature fibers from both dorsal horns, producing bilateral segmental loss of pain and temperature sensation, sometimes in a cape or shawl distribution (dermatomes C4–C5) or affecting both hands (C6–C8).

Fibers conveying proprioception, discriminative touch, and vibratory sensa-

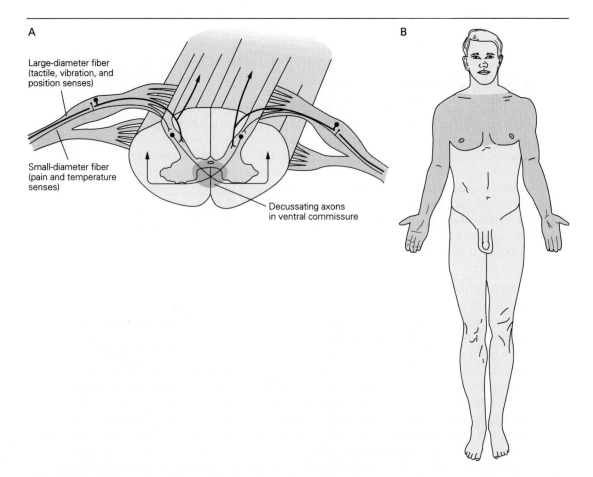

Figure 14–2. A. In syringomyelia the cavity (gray area) often initially affects crossing fibers conveying pain and temperature sensation en route to their entry into the ascending anterolateral system. **B.** The result is segmental dissociated sensory loss (gray dermatomes), with sparing of proprioception and tactile sensation. (Reproduced with permission from Martin JH. 1996. *Neuroanatomy Text and Atlas*, 2nd ed. Stamford, CT: Appleton & Lange. Adapted with permission from Kandel ER, Schwartz JH, Jessell TM. 1991. *Principles of Neural Science*, 3rd ed. Norwalk, CT: Appleton & Lange.)

tion pass into the posterior columns immediately on entering the spinal cord; they are therefore usually spared early in the course of syringomyelia. Segmental weakness, atrophy, and loss of tendon reflexes occur when the syrinx enlarges sufficiently to involve motor neurons in the anterior horns. As with sensory loss, weakness may begin asymmetrically, eventually, as in this patient, becoming bilateral. A syrinx within the thoracic spinal cord can destroy motor neurons innervating paraspinal muscles, resulting in kyphoscoliosis. If neurons within the intermediolateral cell column at spinal segments C8–T2 are affected, a Horner syndrome may result (see Case 39).

As a syrinx continues to enlarge, there is involvement of white matter tracts and the appearance of spastic weakness in one or both legs, urinary urgency, and unilateral or bilateral loss of proprioceptive, vibratory, and touch sensation. Less often, involvement of the spinothalamic tracts results in contralateral loss of pain and temperature sensation below the level of the lesion, sometimes with sacral sparing. (Fibers conveyng pain and temperature sensation from sacral dermatomes are most superficially located within the spinothalamic tract and therefore least likely to be damaged by intramedullary expanding lesions such as a syrinx; see Case 45.)

Syringobulbia occurs when a syrinx extends into (or, rarely, begins within) the brain stem. Symptoms and signs, usually unilateral and referrable to the medullary or pontine tegmentum, include loss of pain and temperature sensation over the face, dysarthria (tongue weakness), dysphagia (palatal and pharyngeal weakness), hoarseness (laryngeal weakness), nystagmus, diplopia, vertigo, and trigeminal pain. An associated Chiari malformation can produce cerebellar signs, and such patients often have hydrocephalus, which can cause gait ataxia and altered mentation.

Treatment of syringomyelia is surgical. If a Chiari malformation is present, surgical decompression of the posterior fossa and upper cervical cord often produces improvement in symptoms referrable to the Chiari malformation itself; symptoms referable to the syrinx are less often relieved by such a procedure. Syringostomy consists of placing a shunt to drain the cavity's fluid into the pleural or peritoneal space. The long-term benefit of such a procedure is controversial.

SELECTED REFERENCES

Donauer E, Rascher K: Syringomyelia: A brief review of ontogenetic, experimental and clinical aspects. Neurosurg Rev 1993;16:7.

Isu T, Susaki H, Takamura H, Kobayashi N: Foramen magnum decompression with removal of the outer layer of the dura as treatment for syringomyelia occurring with Chiari I malformation. Neurosurgery 1993;33:844.

Milhorat TH, Capocelli AL, Anzil AP, et al: Pathological basis of spinal cord cavitation in syringomyelia: Analysis of 105 autopsy cases. J Neurosurg 1995;82:802.

Oldfield EH, Muraszko K, Shawker TH, Patronas NJ: Pathophysiology of syringomyelia associated with Chiari I malformation of the cerebellar tonsils: Implications for diagnosis and treatment. J Neurosurg 1994;80:3.

► CASE 48

A 68-year-old man develops pins-and-needles sensation in both feet, and over the next year the paresthesias spread to his ankles and fingers. His feet feel increasingly numb, and he has progressive difficulty walking; to compensate for his stiff-legged wide-based gait he begins using a cane. Easily fatigued, he has difficulty concentrating and thinks his memory is not as good as it used to be. He has also lost several pounds, and his tongue has become sore.

On examination his tongue is reddened, and his nailbeds and conjunctivae are pale. He appears depressed and distractable and, although fully oriented, he recalls only two of three unrelated words after 5 minutes. There is increased tone in both legs but no evident weakness. His gait is broad based and stiff; he can barely stand unaided with his feet together and eyes open, and he falls when his eyes are closed. Proprioception is absent in his toes, ankles, and fingers; vibratory sensation is absent at his ankles, knees, and hands and reduced at his iliac crests and lumbar spine. Pinprick, temperature, and touch sensation are absent in his feet and saddle area and reduced in his hands and in his legs and trunk below a midthoracic level. Tendon reflexes are 2+ in his arms, 3+ at his knees, and 4+ (transient clonus) at his ankles. Bilateral Babinski signs are present.

Hematocrit is 28%, white blood cell count is 6000/mL, and mean red cell corpuscular volume is 120 μm^3; a peripheral blood smear reveals greater than 5% hypersegmented neutrophils. Serum vitamin B_{12} (cobalamin) level is 70 pg/mL. His blood contains antibodies to intrinsic factor. Serum methylmalonic acid concentration is more than 5000 nmol/L (normal: 110–950 nmol/L); serum homocysteine concentration is 150 μmol/L (normal: 6–29 μmol/L). Serum folic acid concentration is normal.

A Schilling test is performed; following oral administration of 2 μg radiolabeled cyanocobalamin and intramuscular administration of 1000 μg unlabeled cyanocobalamin no radioactivity is detected in the urine, indicating that the orally administered vitamin B_{12} has not been absorbed. When the same procedure is repeated, this time with intrinsic factor given together with the oral radiolabeled cyanocobalamin, radioactivity is detected in the urine, indicating that the orally administered vitamin B_{12} has now been absorbed.

Following the Schilling test he is treated with intramuscular cyanocobalamin 100 μg daily for 4 weeks and monthly thereafter. Within 24 hours of receiving cyanocobalamin, he reports an increased sense of well-being. Over the next week his tongue and mouth become less sore, his concentration and memory improve, and his reticulocytes increase to 30%. There is then gradual hematological and neurological improvement.

On examination a year later his only residual neurological symptoms are paresthesias in his feet and mildly unsteady gait; vibratory, pinprick, and touch sensation are mildly decreased at his feet and ankles and proprioception is reduced in his toes. He cannot walk tandem, and he is unsteady when standing with his feet together and eyes closed. Mental status, strength, muscle tone, and reflexes are normal as are his hematocrit, mean red cell corpuscular volume, peripheral blood smear, and serum concentrations of cobalamin, methylmalonic acid, and homocysteine.

Comment

Paresthesias and sensory loss in the distal extremities suggest peripheral sensory neuropathy; sensory loss below a particular spinal segment (a sensory level) suggests myelopathy. Increased muscle tone, hyperactive tendon reflexes, and extensor plantar responses indicate central rather than peripheral nervous system disease, and altered mentation signifies cerebral dysfunction. This man has a disorder that affects both peripheral and central nervous system myelin, namely pernicious anemia, an absence of gastric intrinsic factor that results in malabsorption of cobalamin (vitamin B_{12}).

The term *subacute combined degeneration* (or *combined systems disease*) refers to the myelopathy, which is the most prominent neurological lesion in most patients with cobalamin deficiency of any cause (including gastrectomy and strict vegetarianism). Swelling and vacuolization of myelin sheaths begin in the posterior columns of the upper thoracic or lower cervical spinal cord, spreading caudally and rostrally and soon including the corticospinal tracts. Paresthesias in the legs progressing to a spastic-ataxic gait are therefore the most common early neurological symptoms, and vibration and position sense are usually impaired before touch, pain, or temperature sensation. In some patients damage to peripheral nerve myelin produces paresthesias and impaired sensation distally in all four limbs and may produce loss of tendon reflexes at the same time that Babinski signs indicate upper motor neuron disease.

Cobalamin deficiency causes fatigue secondary to anemia; it also damages the brain, producing a spectrum of mental symptoms that includes difficulty concentrating, irritability, memory loss, somnolence, depression, paranoia, and psychosis (*megaloblastic madness*). Involvement of optic nerve myelin causes impaired vision and optic atrophy.

Intracellular vitamin B_{12} has two active forms. Methylcobalamin is a coenzyme with methionine synthetase in the conversion of homocysteine to methionine. In this reaction cobalamin receives a methyl group from methyltetrahydrofolate and then donates it to homocysteine; demethylated tetrahydrofolate, the active form of folic acid, is essential for purine and pyrimidine synthesis, and when it is unavailable, the result is megaloblastic anemia. The second active form of vitamin B_{12}, deoxyadenosylcobalamin, is a coenzyme with methylmalonyl-coenzyme A (CoA) mutase in the conversion of methylmalonyl-CoA to succinyl-CoA.

In contrast to the anemia, the mechanisms responsible for myelin damage in cobalamin deficiency are uncertain. It has been suggested that failure of the methylmalonyl-CoA mutase reaction results in accumulation of methylmalonyl-CoA and its precurser propionyl-CoA, resulting in disordered membrane lipid formation and myelin synthesis. Methionine synthetase deficiency has also been implicated in the neurological lesions. In a hereditary disease in which methionine synthetase activity is deficient but methylmalonyl-CoA mutase activity is normal, myeloneuropathy occurs. Moreover, the anesthetic nitrous oxide inactivates methylcobalamin and the methionine synthetase reaction; chronic exposure to nitrous oxide (most often from recreational sniffing or huffing) results in myeloneuropathy indistinguishable from subacute combined degeneration.

That the anemia of cobalamin deficiency is actually the result of activated folate deficiency explains why giving folic acid to such patients can prevent or improve the anemia without affecting the neurological lesions. In fact, over one-fourth of patients with neuropsychiatric abnormalities due to cobalamin deficiency have neither anemia nor macrocytosis. Another important diagnostic point is that serum cobalamin levels do not reflect body stores and may remain normal for years after gastrectomy, falling only as liver stores of cobalamin are finally depleted. (The situation is very different from thiamine deficiency, which can produce neurological disease in only a few weeks; see Case 74.) Low serum cobalamin levels, moreover, are often encountered in elderly people with no evidence of hematological or neurological disease. A more sensitive indicator of clinically significant cobalamin deficiency than the serum cobalamin concentration is an elevation of serum methylmalonic acid and homocysteine levels, which rapidly fall with treatment.

SELECTED REFERENCES

Green R, Kinsella LJ: Current concepts in the diagnosis of cobalamin deficiency. Neurology 1995;45:1435.

Healton EB, Savage DG, Brust JCM, et al: Neurologic aspects of cobalamin deficiency. Medicine 1991;70:228.

Lindenbaum J, Healton EB, Savage DG, et al: Neuropsychiatric disorders caused by cobalamin deficiency in the absence of anemia or macrocytosis. N Engl J Med 1988;318:1720.

Shevell MI, Rosenblatt DS: The neurology of cobalamin. Can J Neurol Sci 1992;19:472.

▶ CASE 49

A 62-year-old man with a 3-year history of retrosternal pain on exertion is found to have an aortic aneurysm next to the eighth and ninth thoracic vertebrae. At surgery it is necessary to divide four consecutive pairs of intercostal arteries; the aorta is cross-clamped and a graft is inserted during an occlusion period of 14 minutes. Awakening from anesthesia, he is paraplegic except for incomplete dorsiflexion of his left ankle. His legs are flaccid with absent tendon and plantar reflexes. Pinprick and temperature sensation are absent below the umbilicus, but light touch, vibratory sensation, and proprioception are intact. His lower superficial abdominal reflexes are absent, and there is urinary retention. Magnetic resonance imaging is consistent with spinal cord infarction.

Over the next several months, receiving physical therapy, he gradually improves. On examination 4 months after his surgery he is able to walk using two canes. He has nocturnal urinary frequency but normal sphincter control; his legs are only mildly weak and spastic, with brisk tendon reflexes and Babinski signs. Pinprick and temperature sensation are mildly decreased below the first lumbar dermatome.

Comment

Like the patient in Case 46 this man has an obvious spinal cord lesion affecting his corticospinal tracts (paraplegia, with early flaccidity and areflexia and later spasticity and hyperreflexia) and spinothalamic tracts (loss of pain and temperature sensation below the level of the lesion). Unlike that patient, however, he has no impairment of tactile, vibratory, or proprioceptive sensation, conveyed (mostly) in the posterior columns. This dissociation is explained by the vascular anatomy of the spinal cord (Figure 14–3).

Blood supply to the spinal cord is derived rostrally from branches of the vertebral and subclavian arteries and caudally from branches of the aorta. At the cervicomedullary junction paired branches of the vertebral arteries join to form the anterior spinal artery, which runs longitudinally the length of the cord in the anterior sulcus and is supplied along its course by a series of unpaired radicular arteries that arise from the aorta and its branches. In most people the anterior spinal artery is discontinuous, particularly at thoracic levels, and in some people

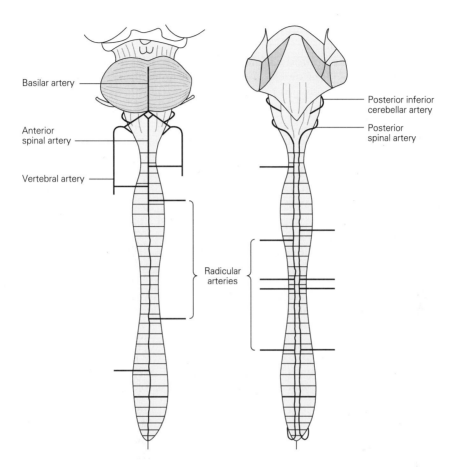

Figure 14–3. Schematic ventral (**left**) and dorsal (**right**) views of the arterial supply to the spinal cord. (Reproduced with permission from Martin JH. 1996. *Neuroanatomy Text and Atlas*, 2nd ed. Stamford, CT: Appleton & Lange. Adapted with permission from Carpenter MB, Sutin J. 1983. *Human Neuroanatomy.* Baltimore: Williams & Wilkins.)

the entire caudal two-thirds of the spinal cord is supplied by a single segmental artery (the great radicular artery of Adamkiewicz), which anastomoses with the anterior spinal artery at a low thoracic or upper lumbar level.

The anterior (ventral) two-thirds of the spinal cord is supplied by penetrating branches of the anterior spinal artery. The posterior (dorsal) third of the spinal cord is supplied by penetrating branches of paired posterior cerebral arteries, which are supplied not only by the same radicular arteries that supply the anterior spinal artery but also, to varying degrees, by smaller radicular arteries of their own. The posterior third of the spinal cord thus has a richer and more dependable blood supply than does the anterior two-thirds. As a consequence, even though *spinal cord infarction* is rarely the result of disease within the anterior spinal artery itself but rather follows sustained hypotension, aortic dissection, aortic surgery, or atherosclerosis within the aorta or its large radicular branches, the infarcted area usually involves the area of the cord supplied by the anterior spinal artery and spares the area supplied by the posterior spinal arteries. The result is the anterior spinal artery syndrome—below the lesion there is paralysis and loss of pain and temperature sensation but preserved proprioceptive, tactile, and vibratory sensation.

Low cervical lesions produce paralysis of intercostal muscles, and breathing is then entirely dependent on the diaphragm; lesions above C3–C5, the level of origin of the phrenic nerve, produce diaphragmatic paralysis as well. Autonomic symptoms are also common, particularly bladder dysfunction, and, with lesions above the midthoracic level, postural hypotension.

As with occlusive stroke of the brain, the prognosis following spinal cord infarction is uncertain; improvement of the degree experienced by this patient is not unusual, particularly when there is some preserved strength in the legs from the outset. Animal research, moreover, reveals that the mammalian spinal cord, when disconnected from suprasegmental controls, possesses sufficient plasticity in its neuronal connections to produce, autonomously, patterns of firing essential for locomotion. Such central pattern generators mean that a spinal cord can re-learn to walk. The implications for physical therapy are obvious.

Magnetic resonance imaging may or may not identify spinal cord infarction but it can usefully exclude other lesions such as neoplasm or infection.

SELECTED REFERENCES

Cheshire WP, Santos CC, Massey EW, Howard JF: Spinal cord infarction: Etiology and outcome. Neurology 1996;47:321.

Davidoff RA: The dorsal columns. Neurology 1989;39:1377.

Sandson TA, Friedman JH: Spinal cord infarction: Report of 8 cases and review of the literature. Medicine 1989;68:282.

Wickelgren I: Teaching the spinal cord to walk. Science 1998;279:319.

▶ CASE 50

A 65-year-old hypertensive man suddenly experiences occipital headache, vertigo, nausea, vomiting, and burning pain in his left face and forehead. In the emergency room he falls to the left on attempting to stand or walk, and his left arm and leg display dysmetria on finger-to-nose and heel-to-shin testing and adiadochokinesis on rapid successive and alternating movements. His voice is hoarse, and he has persistent hiccuping. Bilateral nystagmus, both horizontal and rotatory and present in all directions of gaze, is most marked when he looks to the right. His pupils react to light, but the left is 2 mm smaller than the right; there is mild ptosis on the left, with inverted ptosis of the left lower lid. Pinprick and temperature sensation are markedly decreased over his left face, with the borders of loss corresponding to the territory of the trigeminal nerve, including his left tongue, gums, and inner cheek. His left corneal reflex is absent. Touch sensation on his face is normal. His palate deviates to the right, and his gag reflex is absent on the left even though he feels the stimulus equally well on both sides of his pharynx. Pain and temperature sensation are decreased over his right posterior scalp, neck, arm, trunk, and leg. Touch and vibratory sensation and proprioception are normal bilaterally. Mental status, strength, and tendon and plantar reflexes are normal.

Head computerized tomographic scan is normal. Magnetic resonance imaging (MRI), however, reveals probable infarction of the left dorsolateral medulla and inferior cerebellar peduncle. Magnetic resonance angiography shows occlusion of the left vertebral artery and nonfilling of the left posterior inferior cerebellar artery.

Over the next several months, receiving physical therapy, antihypertensive medication, and daily aspirin, he slowly improves. Examined 5 months after his stroke, he walks unaided but tends to veer or fall to the left on turning or walking tandem. There is mild residual ataxia of his left limbs. He can now tell sharp from dull and warm from cold over his left face. Sensation on his right side is normal over the face, scalp, neck, shoulder, and arm; below the nipple there is moderate-to-severe loss of pinprick and temperature sensation, and in the areas of greatest impairment, pinprick and cold elicit perverted sensations of tingling or warmth.

Comment

When single lesions are presumed, location within the posterior fossa is suggested by (1) bilateral long tract (motor or sensory) signs, (2) crossed (eg, left face and right limb) motor or sensory signs, (3) cerebellar signs, (4) stupor or coma (from involvement of the ascending reticular formation), (5) disconjugate eye movements or nystagmus, and (6) involvement of cranial nerves not usually affected by single cerebral hemispheric lesions (eg, unilateral deafness or pharyngeal weakness). This patient has four such findings.

Taken alone, each of his multiple symptoms and signs could be caused by a lesion in any of several different locations. Vertigo, nausea, vomiting, and rotatory nystagmus implicate the vestibular system but do not by themselves define the lesion as peripheral (the vestibular labyrinth within the inner ear or the eighth cranial nerve—see Case 12) or central (the vestibular nuclei or their connections, including the flocculonodular lobe of the cerebellum—see Case 14). Gait ataxia could be a consequence of vertigo or could signify a lesion of the cerebellum, its inflow or outflow projections, or its more distant connections. Unilateral dysmetria and adiadochokinesis are cerebellar signs but, again, the lesion could be affecting either the cerebellum itself or its afferent or efferent projections.

Pain and numbness on one side of the face could be due to a peripheral lesion involving the trigeminal nerve or a central lesion involving sensory pathways, including the contralateral parietal lobe. The fact that pain and temperature sensation are completely lost whereas touch is spared makes a lesion of either the trigeminal nerve or the parietal lobe unlikely, and the sharply demarcated boun-daries of the facial sensory loss, corresponding precisely to the territory of the trigeminal nerve, would be highly unlikely with a lesion involving the sensory cortex. The facial sensory loss is readily explained, however, by a lesion affecting either the spinal trigeminal tract and nucleus or its crossed ascending projections, which carry pain and temperature sensation. Because the lesion spares the primary (main) trigeminal sensory nucleus and its crossed and uncrossed central connections, touch sensation on the face is spared. Similarly, loss of pain and temperature sensation over the right arm, trunk, and leg, with sparing of touch sensation and proprioception, implicates the spinothalamic tract within either the upper cervical spinal cord or the lower brain stem.

Pupillary miosis and ptosis of both upper and lower lid (Horner syndrome—see Case 39) could be due to a lesion anywhere along the sympathetic pathway including the lateral brain stem, the cervical or upper thoracic spinal cord, the sympathetic chain, the superior cervical ganglion, the internal carotid artery, and the first division of the trigeminal nerve. Dry skin on the same side of the face, reflecting reduced sweating, places the sympathetic lesion proximal to the bifurcation of the common carotid artery into the internal and external carotid arteries. Finally, hoarseness, asymmetry of palatal movement, and loss of the efferent arc of the gag reflex could be the result of damage to muscles of the palate, pharynx, or larynx, to the peripheral nerves that supply them (the special visceral efferent components of the vagus and, to a lesser degree, the glossopharyngeal), or to the nucleus ambiguus. (Because the nucleus ambiguus receives bilateral projections from the primary motor cortices of the frontal lobes, a unilateral supranuclear lesion would be unlikely to produce these signs.)

If each symptom or sign in this patient carries a number of plausible localizations, their combination can be explained by one localization only, namely the dorsolateral medulla, affecting the vestibular nuclei, the inferior cerebellar peduncle, the spinal trigeminal tract and nucleus, the spinothalamic tract, the descending sympathetic pathway, and the nucleus ambiguus (Figure 14–4). MRI reveals an infarct in the territory of the posterior inferior cerebellar artery (PICA) and the lateral medullary branches of the vertebral artery. The constellation of symptoms and signs resulting from such a lesion is known as *Wallenberg syndrome.* (Adolf Wallenberg, describing a single patient in 1895, correctly localized the lesion without the aid of either MRI or autopsy.)

Headache is common in occlusive stroke and might be due to vascular distention produced by the occlusion. Hiccups, often a feature of lateral medullary infarction, could be secondary to involvement of medullary respiratory centers or of vagus nerve fibers. Some patients have more serious autonomic signs, including episodic hypotension and hypertension, tachycardia, and loss of automatic respiration (Ondine's curse). Difficulty swallowing can be a feature of Wallenberg syndrome, but it tends to clear even when unilateral pharyngeal weakness persists.

Some patients with lateral medullary infarction have loss of pain and temperature sensation on the contralateral face, presumably from involvement of the

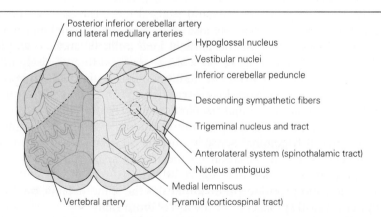

Figure 14–4. Medulla and its arterial supply, showing structures affected by damage within the territory of the posterior inferior cerebellar artery and lateral medullary arteries. (Reproduced with permission from Martin JH. 1996. *Neuroanatomy Text and Atlas*, 2nd ed. Stamford, CT: Appleton & Lange.)

crossed projections from the contralateral spinal trigeminal nucleus now ascending near the spinothalamic tract. Recovery of this patient's sensory loss over the arm and upper trunk, also not unusual, is explained by the somatotopy of the spinothalamic tract; medial fibers representing the neck, arm, and upper trunk are sometimes less damaged than lateral fibers representing the leg and lower trunk.

In addition to the dorsolateral medulla, the PICA supplies the posterior inferior cerebellum, and cerebellar infarction is often additionally present. In such cases damage to both the inferior cerebellar peduncle and the cerebellum itself contributes to the gait and limb ataxia. In some patients cerebellar signs include abnormal eye movements, for example, hypometric or hypermetric saccades.

Conspicuously absent in Wallenberg syndrome are tongue weakness, pyramidal signs, and contralateral loss of proprioception and discriminative touch, for the medial location of structures subserving these functions—the hypoglossal nucleus, the pyramidal tract, and the medial lemniscus—is outside the territory of the PICA and lateral medullary arteries. In this patient, pharyngeal sensation is preserved because the lesion is not medial enough to affect the solitary tract and nucleus.

SELECTED REFERENCES

Caplan LR: Vertebrobasilar occlusive disease. In: Barnett HJM, Mohr JP, Stein BM, Yatsu FM (eds): *Stroke: Pathophysiology, Diagnosis, and Management,* 3rd edition. Saunders, 1998.

Kim JS, Lee JH, Lee MC: Patterns of sensory dysfunction in lateral medullary infarction. Clinical-MRI correlation. Neurology 1997;49:1557.

Soffin G, Feldman M, Bender MB: Alterations of sensory levels in vascular lesions of the lateral medulla. Arch Neurol 1968;18:178.

Wallenberg A: Acute bulbar disturbance (embolus of the left posterior inferior cerebellar artery). Arch Psychíat Nervenkrankheit 1895;27:504.

▶ CASE 51

Two weeks after being treated for a myocardial infarction a 48-year-old man suddenly develops left hemiparesis, left lateral deviation of gaze, double vision, and right facial weakness. On examination there is moderately severe weakness of his right face, including the forehead, and of his left arm and leg. Tendon reflexes are hyperactive on the left, and there is a left Babinski sign. A complete right conjugate gaze palsy is present for both saccadic and pursuit eye movements, and there is complete paralysis of right eye adduction for all movements except convergence, during which adduction is observed. When abducted, his left eye displays left-beating nystagmus. Vertical eye movements are full. Proprioception and two-point discrimination are mildly impaired in his left arm and leg, and stereognosis is reduced in his left hand, but pain and temperature sensation are normal.

Magnetic resonance imaging (MRI) reveals probable infarction in the right paramedian pons involving tegmentum and base. Cardiac echo identifies an akinetic segment of the left ventricular wall, and on the presumption of cardioembolism he receives heparin anticoagulation. Two days later he becomes lethargic, and on examination, in addition to the above signs, there are now bilateral Babinski signs, complete left-sided facial sensory impairment to pain, temperature, and touch, mild cerebellar ataxia of his right arm, right pupillary miosis, right-sided deafness, and right-sided palatal myoclonus. MRI reveals blood within the area of infarction and extending laterally in the tegmentum. Heparin is stopped, and for the next month he remains neurologically unchanged.

Comment

Right facial weakness could be due to a lesion affecting the seventh cranial nerve peripherally, the facial nucleus in the pons, or, suprasegmentally, the motor cortex of the contralateral frontal lobe or its corticobulbar projections; involvement of the frontalis (forehead) muscle suggests but does not prove that the lesion is of lower-motor-neuron type.

Left hemiparesis, hyperactive tendon reflexes, and a Babinski sign signify corticospinal system damage, but if there were no additional signs, the lesion could be in the left cervical spinal cord or, above the pyramidal decussation, anywhere along the right corticospinal tract from medulla to frontal lobe. Taken together, however, right facial weakness and left hemiparesis are explained by a lesion of the right pons, where the facial nucleus and the intraparenchymal facial nerve are adjacent to the corticospinal tract (Figure 14–5). Such a lesion also explains the abnormal eye movements.

With its right medial location, the patient's infarct has destroyed three structures that participate in horizontal eye movements, namely the abducens nucleus, the median longitudinal fasciculus, and the pontine paramedian reticular formation (PPRF, also known as the pontine horizontal gaze center) (see Figure 3–7). His right horizontal gaze palsy could be the result of damge to either the PPRF or the right abducens nucleus. The abducens nucleus contains not only

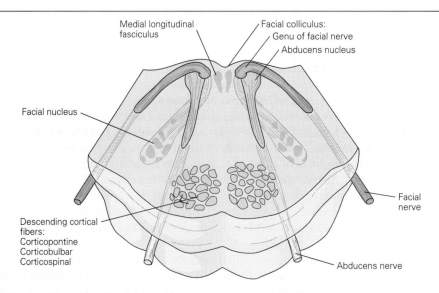

Figure 14–5. Pons, showing anatomical relationship of the corticospinal/corticobulbar tract, the facial nerve, and the abducens nerve. (Reproduced with permission from Martin JH. 1996. *Neuroanatomy Text and Atlas*, 2nd ed. Stamford, CT: Appleton & Lange. Adapted with permission from Williams PL, Warwick R. 1975. *Functional Neuroanatomy of Man.* Philadelphia: W.B. Saunders.)

neurons that innervate the lateral rectus muscle via the abducens (sixth cranial) nerve, but also interneurons that, via the contralateral median longitudinal fasciculus, stimulate neurons within the oculomotor nucleus of the mesencephalon that innervate the medial rectus muscle; the resulting simultaneous firing of lateral and medial rectus muscles produces conjugate gaze. His inability to adduct the right eye except during convergence is the result of damage to the right median longitudinal fasciculus; preservation of convergence confirms that neurons innervating the medial rectus muscle are themselves intact (hence the term *internuclear ophthalmoplegia*). The undamaged oculomotor nuclei also allow vertical eye movements, both downward and upward. Nystagmus of the abducting eye contralateral to a median longitudinal fasciculus lesion is a common feature; a possible mechanism is that attempted adduction of the ipsilateral eye produces abduction overshoot of the contralateral eye, followed by periodic inward drifting and saccadic overcorrection.

This patient's eye movement disturbance is known as *one-and-a-half syndrome*. If normal conjugate gaze to one side is rated a 1, full conjugate gaze would rate a 2; loss of conjugate gaze in one direction and adduction in the other therefore represents loss of $1\frac{1}{2}$ movements out of 2.

The patient's initial left-sided sensory loss involves proprioception and discriminative modalities, a consequence of damage to the appropriately named medial lemniscus. The more laterally placed spinothalamic tract, conveying pain and temperature sensation, and the trigeminal systems, conveying facial sensation, are initially spared but become damaged when the infarct becomes hemorrhagic. Other signs also appear as the lesion enlarges. An ipsilateral Babinski sign is likely the result of pressure on the contralateral corticospinal tract. Ataxia of the right arm could indicate damage to crossing fibers of either the right superior cerebellar peduncle or the right middle cerebellar peduncle. Light-reactive miosis is the result of damage to descending sympathetic fibers. Deafness likely indicates damage to the cochlear nuclei; more rostral projections—the lateral lemnisci and above—carry information from both ears, and so unilateral deafness does not follow unilateral damage to supranuclear auditory pathways.

Right-sided palatal myoclonus—rhythmic involuntary movements of the palate and pharyngopalatine arch at 40 to 200 per minute—is less readily explained. It is seen most often with acute lesions affecting the Mollaret triangle—comprising the dentate nucleus of the cerebellum, the crossing projections of the dentate nucleus to the contralateral red nucleus, the red nucleus itself, and projections from the red nucleus through the central tegmental tract to the ipsilateral inferior olive (which is somatotopically related to the contralateral dentate nucleus). The lesion responsible for this patient's palatal myoclonus most likely affects the right central tegmental tract.

SELECTED REFERENCES

Fisher CM: Some neuro-ophthalmological observations. J Neurol Neurosurg Psychiatry 1967;30:383.

Kataoka S, Hari A, Shirakawa T, Hirose G: Paramedian pontine infarction. Neurological/topographical correlation. Stroke 1997;28:809.

Lapresle J, Ben Hamida M: The dentato-olivary pathway. Arch Neurol 1970;22:135.

Pierrot-Deseilligny C, Chain F, Serdaru M, et al: The one-and-a-half syndrome. Brain 1981;104:665.

Smith JL, Cogan D: Internuclear ophthalmoplegia. Arch Ophthalmol 1959;61:687.

▶ CASE 52

A 46-year-old man experiences horizontal diplopia when he reads. Over the next few weeks the double vision becomes present on looking at far as well as near objects, and his eyelids become droopy. He begins having difficulty controlling movements of his right arm. On examination there is impaired adduction of his left eye on attempted saccades, pursuit, and convergence. Upward and downward eye movements are also limited on the left; on attempted downgaze, his left eye intorts. Incomplete ptosis is present bilaterally, and there is limited upward movement of his right eye. The left pupil is 2 mm larger than the right pupil and is less reactive to light, both directly and consensually. His right limb movements are clumsy; tremor and dysmetria are present on finger-to-nose and heel-to-knee testing, and rapid successive and alternating movements produce adiadochokinesis. His right arm and leg also appear choreic—in addition to tremor and clumsiness the limbs seem to generate irregular involuntary movements, even at rest. The nasolabial fold is mildly flattened on the right, and he seems to talk out of the left side of his mouth. Strength is difficult to test on the right because of incoordination, but his arm and leg seem mildly weak. Tendon reflexes are brisker on the right than on the left, and the right plantar response is less prominently downward. Pain, temperature, and touch sensation are mildly reduced on the entire right side, including his face. Proprioception is reduced in his right fingers and toes.

Magnetic resonance imaging reveals a gadolinium-enhancing mass in the left midbrain tegmentum, most likely a glioma.

Comment

Most of this man's signs can be easily explained. The right-sided weakness and sensory loss include the face; therefore, damage to the corticobulbar/corticospinal tract is rostral to the facial nucleus in the pons, and damage to the spinothalamic tract, medial lemniscus, and trigeminothalamic sensory pathways is rostral to the principal and spinal trigeminal nuclei of the pons and medulla. Combined with a left oculomotor nerve palsy, these signs place the lesion in the left midbrain (Figure 14–6).

The patient's *oculomotor palsy* has features that would not be encountered with peripheral nerve damage but are quite consistent with an intraparenchymal lesion. Of the subnuclei within the oculomotor complex that innervate individual extraocular muscles, fibers innervating the medial rectus, inferior rectus, and inferior oblique muscles are uncrossed, fibers innervating the superior rectus muscle are crossed, and fibers innervating the levator palpebrae are both crossed and uncrossed. A lesion involving the left oculomotor complex and its intraparenchymal outflow tract will therefore not only affect all these muscles ipsilaterally but also produce ptosis and limited upward gaze contralaterally. (Vertical gaze palsy with intact horizontal eye movements is associated with midbrain lesions that involve the rostral interstitial nucleus of the median longitudinal fasciculus, a vertical gaze center comparable to the horizontal gaze center in the paramedian pontine reticular formation.)

Left eye intorsion on attempted downgaze signifies preservation of the fourth (trochlear) cranial nerve, which, innervating the superior oblique muscle, contributes to downward gaze when the eye is adducted and intorts it when the eye is in primary gaze or abducted. The larger less reactive pupil is

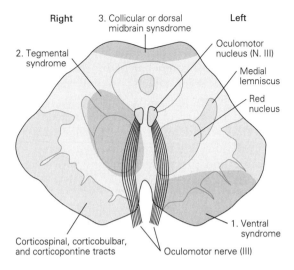

Figure 14–6. Midbrain, showing relationship of the oculomotor nuclei and outflow tracts, the corticospinal tracts, the medial lemniscus, and the red nucleus. Not shown are crossing fibers of the superior cerebellar peduncle, projecting to the thalamus. In the ventral syndrome, ipsilateral oculomotor palsy is combined with contralateral weakness of the face and limbs. In the tegmental syndrome, ipsilateral oculomotor palsy is combined with contralateral ataxia. In the dorsal syndrome (Parinaud syndrome) there is paralysis of upward gaze sometimes combined with impaired pupillary reactivity to light. Larger lesions produce combinations of these signs. (Reproduced with permission from Kandel ER, Schwartz JH, Jessell TM. 1991. *Principles of Neural Science*, 3rd ed. Norwalk, CT: Appleton & Lange. Adapted with permission from Gatz AJ. 1996. *Manter's Essentials of Clinical Neuroanatomy and Neurophysiology*, 3rd ed. Philadelphia: Davis.)

the result of damage to the parasympathetic Edinger-Westphal nucleus or its outflow tract.

Less easily attributable are the clumsiness and abnormal movements of the right arm and leg. The superior cerebellar peduncle, arising from the dentate and interposed deep nuclei of the cerebellum, cross at the midbrain and either synapse in the red nucleus or continue on to the ventral thalamus; a lesion interrupting crossed cerebellar outflow projections causes contralateral intention tremor, dysmetria, and adiadochokinesis. (The crossed cerebellar projections onto the red nucleus and thalamus will ultimately be countered by the crossing of the corticospinal tract in the medulla and the rubrospinal tract in the midbrain; therefore, this patient's cerebellar signs are on the right, contralateral to the lesion; see Case 34.)

In some patients with midbrain lesions, movements are reduced in rate and amplitude to a degree that suggests parkinsonism, and sometimes tremor persists at rest or involuntary movements appear that resemble chorea or athetosis. Corticospinal tract lesions often impair the rate and amplitude of movements, particularly distally, out of proportion to weakness (see Case 28), but a midbrain tegmental lesion, by damaging projections from the substantia nigra to the striatum, can produce true parkinsonian signs (see Case 35). Proprioceptive loss not only aggravates limb ataxia but if severe can produce continuous involuntary movements of the fingers or hands (pseudoathetosis). Also possibly contributing to the movement disturbance in this patient is damage to the red nucleus.

Participating in a number of pathways, the red nucleus receives projections from the deep nuclei of the cerebellar hemispheres and from the cerebrum (principally the motor cortex). It sends projections through the crossed rubrospinal tract to brain stem and spinal cord motor neurons, through the superior cerebellar peduncle back to the cerebellar deep nuclei, and, via the central tegmental tract, inferior olive, and inferior cerebellar peduncle, to the cerebellar cortex. Interruption of the rubrospinal tract, which is mainly facilitory to flexor muscles, probably contributes to extensor posturing (decerebrate rigidity), but because the red nucleus is traversed by efferent projections of deep cerebellar nuclei, the symptoms and signs that would result from damage to the red nucleus alone have never been defined. So-called rubral tremor—a coarse, rhythmic movement resembling wing-beating and precipitated by any movement of the limb—follows lesions of the superior cerebellar peduncle whether or not the red nucleus is additionally damaged.

A number of eponyms are applied to brain stem syndromes, for example, Weber syndrome (oculomotor palsy with contralateral hemiparesis), Claude syndrome (oculomotor palsy with contralateral tremor and ataxia), and, as would describe this patient, Benedikt syndrome (oculomotor palsy with contralateral cerebellar and corticospinal signs). In each case a brain stem lesion is indicated by the combination of cranial nerve signs on one side and long-tract motor or sensory signs on the other. Rather than memorizing eponyms, a clinician should understand the anatomy that explains the symptoms and signs.

SELECTED REFERENCES

Bucy PC, Keplinger JE: Tumors of the brain stem with special reference to ocular manifestations. Arch Ophthalmol 1959;62:541.

Büttner-Ennever J, Büttner U, Cohen B: Vertical gaze paralysis and the rostral interstitial nucleus of the median longitudinal fasciculus. Brain 1982;105:125.

Silverman JE, Liv GT, Volpe NJ, Galetta SL: The crossed paralyses. Arch Neurol 1995; 52:635.

▶ CASE 53

A 34-year-old woman awakens with continuous dull pain behind her left ear and the following day notices that her left face is droopy. Over the next 24 hours left facial weakness becomes pronounced; she dribbles saliva from the left side of her mouth, and food collects between her lips and teeth on the left. She also finds that loud noises produce discomfort in her left ear.

On examination 4 days later the left nasolabial fold is flattened. Marked weakess affects her left facial muscles, including the frontalis and the platysma. She cannot close her left eye, and when she attempts to do so, the eyeball diverts upward (Bell phenomenon). Left-sided lower facial weakness is evident both on voluntary tasks—pressing her lips together or showing her teeth—and on spontaneous smiling.

Tested with sugar, taste sensation over the anterior tongue on the left is decreased. With the stethoscope in her ears, she reports that the examiner's voice sounds louder on the left. Although she describes an overflow of tears in the left eye, comparisons of the two sides using filter paper reveal decreased tear production on the left. The external auditory canals and tympanic membranes are normal bilaterally, as are other findings on her neurological examination.

She begins a 10 day course of prednisone and is given a patch to wear over her left eye during sleep. Ten days later there is a slight return of left facial movement and electromyographic evidence of denervation (fibrillations and positive waves) in the left facial muscles. Six months later strength has further improved but remains incomplete. When she blinks, the left side of her mouth twitches synchronously, and when she bares her teeth, her left palpebral fissure narrows. She describes increased lacrimation in her left eye when she eats.

Comment

Unilateral facial weakness, taken alone, could be the result of a lesion involving either the central or the peripheral nervous system. Centrally, such weakness could follow damage to the contralateral frontal lobe (eg, from a small infarct involving that part of the motor cortex responsible for facial movement). Peripherally, facial weakness could follow damage to the facial nerve distal to its exit through the stylomastoid foramen (eg, from carcinoma of the parotid gland). Facial weakness could also follow damage to pathways between these sites, including, contralaterally, descending corticobulbar projections from the motor cortex to the pons and, ipsilaterally, the pontine facial nucleus, the intraparenchymal seventh nerve outflow tract, and the proximal portion of the facial nerve itself, either at the cerebellopontine angle, within the internal auditory canal, or along its passage through the petrous portion of the temporal bone.

In this patient, paralysis of all the facial muscles, including the frontalis, suggests (but does not prove) a lower-motor-neuron lesion involving the nucleus, the outflow tract, or the peripheral nerve. So does the involvement of emotional as well as volitional facial movement. (Upper-motor-neuron facial weakness tends to spare the frontalis muscle as well as emotional—mimetic—facial movements; see Case 28.) It is involvement of other facial nerve functions, however, that localizes this woman's lesion to the peripheral seventh nerve proximal to the geniculate ganglion within the temporal bone (see Figure 3–10).

Emerging from the pons, the seventh nerve enters the internal auditory canal in close apposition to the auditory nerve. It then passes through a canal of its own, in which is situated the geniculate ganglion, containing sensory neurons subserving general sensation within the external auditory canal and taste over the anterior two-thirds of the tongue. Just distal to the geniculate ganglion, parasympathetic secretomotor fibers branch off to supply, via the greater superficial petrosal nerve and the pterygopalatine ganglion, the lacrimal gland and mucus-secreting glands of the nose and palate. Further distal to the ganglion two branches successively arise, namely the nerve to the stapedius muscle (which dampens the effect of loud noise on the ossicles of the middle ear) and the chorda tympani (which carries afferent fibers subserving taste and efferent parasympathetic fibers to the sublingual and submandibular salivary glands).

Loss of taste on this woman's anterior tongue places the lesion proximal to the takeoff of the chorda tympani. Intolerance to loud noise places it proximal to the branch to the stapedius. Decreased tear production places it proximal to the parasympathetic branch to the lacrimal gland. It would be unlikely that each of these functions would be affected by a lesion at the internal auditory meatus or the cerebellopontine angle, for the closely apposed eighth nerve is not affected. It would be nearly impossible for each of these functions to be affected by an intraparenchymal pontine lesion in the absence of other brain stem signs.

During recovery the patient develops synkinesis; when she blinks there is simultaneous involuntary movement of the ipsilateral muscles of her mouth, and when she voluntarily contracts the muscles of her mouth there is simultaneous involuntary narrowing of her ipsilateral palpebral fissure. Synkinesis has been attributed both to misdirection of regenerated fibers and to ephaptic conduction (nonsynaptic spread of impulses between fibers of the nerve at the site of injury). Unilateral lacrimation during eating (crocodile tears) signifies synkinesis between the sublingual/submandibular salivary glands and the lacrimal gland.

In diabetic patients, spontaneous unilateral facial weakness with subsequent gradual recovery is often secondary to microinfarction affecting the peripheral facial nerve. In nondiabetics, spontaneous facial weakness—*Bell palsy*—most often occurs without evident cause. In the mid-1990s investigators using polymerase chain reaction identified herpes simplex genome in the geniculate ganglion and seventh nerves of patients with Bell palsy, and subsequent studies suggested benefit from the antiviral drug acyclovir.

Acute facial paralysis is also associated with herpes zoster; in such cases vesicles are observed within the external auditory canal, implicating involvement of the seventh nerve's somatic sensory branch.

SELECTED REFERENCES

Hauser WA, Karnes WE, Annis J, Kurland LT: Incidence and prognosis of Bell's palsy in the population of Rochester, Minnesota. Mayo Clin Proc 1971;46:258.

Miller H: Facial paralysis. Br Med Bull 1967;3:815.

Murakami S, Mutsuhiko M, Nakashiro Y, et al: Bell's palsy and herpes simplex virus: Identification of viral DNA in endoneurial fluid and muscle. Ann Intern Med 1996;124:27.

▶ CASE 54

A 56-year-old woman has had 6 weeks of left facial numbness and intermittent left-sided headaches. The numbness has gradually increased, ultimately involving both her face and her tongue on the left. She also notices horizontal diplopia, more pronounced when she looks at distant than at near objects.

On examination there is decreased sensation to pinprick, temperature, and touch over her left face and anterior scalp as far back as the vertex; the sensory loss spares the pinna of her ear, the angle of her jaw, her posterior scalp, and her neck but includes her nasal mucous membranes, inner cheek, anterior tongue, and gums. The afferent limb of the corneal reflex is absent on the left; neither eye blinks when her left cornea is touched, but both eyes blink when her right cornea is touched. As she opens her mouth, her jaw deviates to the left, and when she bites down forcibly, the masseter and temporalis muscles are less firmly contracted on the left. There is limited abduction of her left eye. Eye movements are otherwise full, and her pupils are equal and reactive. Findings on her neurological examination, including other cranial nerves, are otherwise normal.

A magnetic resonance image reveals a 1-cm-diameter lesion, enhancing with gadolinium, in the floor of the left middle fossa involving Meckel's cave (the site of the trigeminal ganglion) and the apex of the petrous bone. Subsequent workup discloses an occult carcinoma of the lung.

Comment

Taken alone, impaired sensation on the left side of the face could be due to a lesion on the left involving the trigeminal nerve (including its ganglion or root), or the left lower brain stem (including the primary or spinal sensory nuclei or their root entry zones) or to a lesion on the right involving ascending sensory pathways (including the ventroposterior nucleus of the thalamus and the parietal lobe). The following factors indicate a peripheral lesion:

1. The sensory loss is sharply restricted to the territories of the ophthalmic, maxillary, and mandibular divisions of the trigeminal nerve, including the oral and nasal cavities.
2. There is weakness of masticatory muscles on the left, including leftward jaw deviation as a result of left pterygoid muscle weakness.
3. Although weakness of the lateral rectus muscle follows lesions involving either the abducens nerve within the pons, the abducens nerve along its peripheral course, or the muscle itself, lateral rectus weakness in this patient is most readily explained by a lesion at the apex of the petrous bone, where the trigeminal and abducens nerves travel in close proximity.
4. There are no other symptoms and signs referable to the brain stem or the cerebrum.

Tumors presenting as *trigeminal neuropathy* include meningiomas, schwannomas, and metastases. In the preantibiotic era it was not unusual for middle ear infection to spread to the apex of the petrous bone, affecting both the trigeminal and abducens nerves (Gradenigo syndrome).

SELECTED REFERENCES

Foley JM: The cranial mononeuropathies. N Engl J Med 1969;281:905.
Gass H: Unilateral numbness of the face and the nasal cisternogram. Neurology 1969; 19:66.
Lecky BRF, Hughes RAC, Murray NMF: Trigeminal sensory neuropathy. A study of 22 cases. Brain 1987;110:1463.
Rush JA, Younge BR: Paralysis of cranial nerves III, IV, and VI. Cause and prognosis in 1000 cases. Arch Ophthalmol 1981;99:76.

▶ CASE 55

A 27-year-old typist develops persistent horizontal diplopia. A few days later, her gait is unsteady, and she experiences numbness of all her fingertips, greater on the left. On examination there is mild left abducens paresis, horizontal nystagmus on either right or left lateral gaze, up-beating nystagmus on upward gaze, mild left facial weakness, mild gait unsteadiness, decreased pinprick sensation in all fingertips, and decreased vibratory sensation in her toes.

Somatosensory evoked response testing shows delay of the P-1 potential for the left sural nerve. Visual evoked response testing shows delay of the P-1 potential bilaterally. T2-weighted magnetic resonance imaging (MRI) shows areas of increased signal bilaterally in the frontal periventricular areas and in the left midbrain and pons.

Her gait unsteadiness worsens, her left arm becomes clumsy, and abnormal eye movements now include up-beating nystagmus on primary gaze, down-beating nystagmus on downward gaze, and bilateral limited adduction with preserved convergence (ie, internuclear ophthalmoplegia). Her mood is inappropriately euphoric. She receives a course of corticosteroids, with much improvement in all her symptoms and signs.

A few months later her neurological examination is normal except for a childish demeanor with unexpected outbursts of laughter. Over the next 3 years her only symptom is intermittent visual blurring of her left eye, and her visual acuity and fundi remain normal bilaterally. She then develops ataxia of gait and of both arms and diffusely hyperactive tendon reflexes. Improvement follows another course of corticosteroids, but gait and limb ataxia persist, and her mood becomes increasingly labile. Her gait ataxia then worsens, and she develops urinary urgency, frequency, nocturia, and occasional incontinence.

On examination there are now jerky interruptions of pursuit eye movements, up-beating nystagmus on upward gaze, and bilateral arm dysmetria, intention tremor, and adiadochokinesis. Her gait is broad based with titubation, tendon reflexes are hyperactive with ankle clonus, and there is decreased vibratory sensation in both feet. She is facetious and flirtatious with bursts of loud laughter, but attentiveness, memory, language, and cognition are otherwise normal.

At this time, 8 years after the onset of her illness, she begins weekly injections of interferon-beta-1a but over the next year her gait and limb ataxia worsen; severe intention tremor of her legs and trunk prevent standing. Recent memory becomes impaired, and bilateral optic atrophy is noted, worse on the left, with reduced visual acuity and an afferent pupillary defect on that side.

Comment

The clinical diagnosis of *multiple sclerosis* is based on multiple lesions in space and time. This woman's initial symptom—horizontal diplopia—could theoretically have resulted from a primary disturbance of the extraocular muscles (eg, myasthenia gravis), the third or fourth cranial nerves (eg, diabetic cranial neuropathy), or intraparenchymal brain stem structures. Impaired sensation could similarly have been either extra- or intraparenchymal in origin. In the presence of normal proprioception, her gait ataxia suggested a lesion of the cerebellum or its connections. The only possible *single* lesion to explain each of her initial symptoms would be in the brain stem. (Her sensory loss would then be attributed to bilateral damage to the medial lemnisci and the spinothalamic tracts.) Although possible, it is unlikely that a single lesion would produce such findings, and so diagnostic studies were undertaken to identify multiple lesions. Somatosensory evoked response testing showed that her sensory symptoms were more plausibly attributable to impaired conduction in sensory pathways at the level of the spinal cord. Visual evoked response testing showed that although she had normal visual acuity, there were subclinical conduction abnormalities of her visual pathways. T2-weighted MRI demonstrated not only the brain stem lesion that would appropriately explain her abnormal eye movements and ataxia, but also additional periventricular lesions in the white matter of both cerebral hemispheres. A diagnosis of multiple sclerosis was made, and concomitant with a course of corticosteroid treatment, her symptoms and signs remitted. Over the next decade, however, she experienced repeated attacks that increasingly left lasting neurological dysfunction in their wake. By the time immunosuppressive therapy with interferon-beta became available, she was functionally incapacitated by spasticity and ataxia and displayed emotional and cognitive disturbance.

Multiple sclerosis is characterized pathologically by multiple areas of inflammation, demyelination, and glial scarring in white matter of the central nervous system. In acute lesions there is perivenous infiltration of lymphocytes and plasma cells, followed by the appearance of microglial phagocytes—macrophages—and breakdown of myelin sheaths, layers of which are peeled off by processes of macrophages (Figure 14–7). Oligodendrocyte cell loss and astrocytosis occur, but early lesions tend to spare axons. Remyelination then occurs but tends to be incomplete. There may then be recurrent attacks or, as commonly occurs by middle age, the pattern of illness changes from relapsing-remitting to chronic progressive. Axonal damage then occurs, resulting in permanent functional disability.

What initiates the immune attack in multiple sclerosis is unknown. Epidemiological studies are suggestive of both genetic susceptibility and exposure during childhood to an infectious agent. Appropriate host defenses to a virus might be associated with molecular mimicry between nervous system antigens and viral antigens or with epitope spreading, in which tissue inflammation leads to nonspecific up-regulation of major histocompatibility complex class I and class II molecules on cell surfaces and activation of normally quiescent T cells. The result would be autoimmune attack on innocent bystander myelin. Neither a virus nor an autoantigen has been convincingly identified, however. Pathological studies describe different types of demyelination—based on the loss or preservation of oligodendrocytes—that do not depend on the stage of the lesion but rather are specific for a given patient. Perhaps, as with some other autoimmune disorders such as systemic lupus erythematosis, multiple sclerosis represents a diathesis or susceptibility to a multiplicity of causes.

Inflammation and demyelination result in impaired saltatory conduction from one note of Ranvier (where sodium channels are concentrated) to the next.

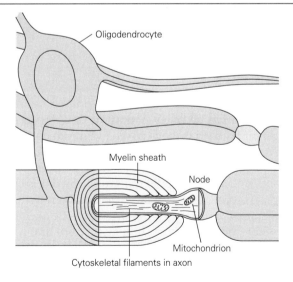

Figure 14–7. Oligodendrocyte processes forming a myelin sheath around an axon in the central nervous system. In multiple sclerosis myelin is destroyed by the body's own immune system. (Reproduced with permission from Kandel ER, Schwartz JH, Jessell TM. 1999. *Principles of Neural Science*, 4th ed. New York: McGraw-Hill. Adapted with permission from Bunge RP. 1968. Glial cells and the central myelin sheath. Physiol Rev 48:197.)

When symptoms resolve within a few days of onset—too soon for remyelination to occur—axonal conduction was probably blocked physiologically rather than pathologically, presumably by inflammation and edema; such lesions are detected by contrast-enhanced T1-weighted MRI, which reflects breakdown of the blood–brain barrier. When symptoms resolve over weeks, demyelination has been followed by remyelination; such lesions are detected by T2-weighted MRI, which reflects myelin loss or incomplete remyelination. When symptoms become permanent, axonal loss has occurred; such lesions are detected with MRI spectroscopy for N-acetylaspartate, a marker for neurons and neuronal processes.

Some patients with multiple sclerosis experience precipitation of symptoms by metabolic or environmental stimuli, particularly temperature (Uhthoff phenomenon). Partially remyelinated fibers are vulnerable to temperature elevations as small as 0.5 °C; vigorous exercise in such patients can trigger visual blurring, paresthesias, or weakness. 4-Aminopyridine blocks fast potassium channels, prolongs the duration of nerve action potentials, and restores conduction in demyelinated nerve fibers; this drug has been beneficial in some multiple sclerosis patients with temperature-sensitive symptoms.

SELECTED REFERENCES

Compston A (ed): *McAlpines Multiple Sclerosis,* 3rd edition. Chruchill-Livingstone, 1998.

Liblau RS, Fontaine B: Recent advances in immunology in multiple sclerosis. Curr Opin Neurol 1998;11:293.

Lucchinetti CF, Brück W, Rodriguez M, Lassman H: Distinct patterns of multiple sclerosis pathology indicates heterogeneity on pathogenesis. Brain Pathol 1996;6:259.

Miller DH, Grossman RI, Reingold SC, McFarland HF: The role of MR techniques in understanding and managing multiple sclerosis. Brain 1998;121:3.

Simon JH, Jacobs LD, Campion M, et al and the Multiple Sclerosis Collaborative Research Group: Magnetic resonance studies of intramuscular interferon beta-1a for relapsing multiple sclerosis. Ann Neurol 1998;43:79.

Trapp BD, Peterson J, Ransohoff, et al: Axonal transection in the lesions of multiple sclerosis. N Engl J Med 1998;338:278.

▶ CASE 56

A 31-year-old woman slips and falls at home, landing on her sacrum. Except for pain in the sacral area she has no other symptoms until the following day, when she complains to her husband that she is weak and numb on the right side.

On examination her mental status is normal, and she appears neither anxious nor depressed. Right-sided weakness of wrist extension, hip flexion, and ankle dorsiflexion is difficult to quantitate; the muscles seem to give way abruptly to any counterforce. All other muscles are of normal strength, including finger extensors, hip adductors, knee extensors, and toe dorsiflexors. There is decreased sensation over the entire right side including face, scalp, limbs, and trunk. Vibratory sensation is felt to the immediate left but not the immediate right of midline over the forehead, chin, and sternum. Proprioception is absent at all joints of the right arm and leg, yet she is able accurately to perform finger-to-nose testing bilaterally with her eyes closed. Her gait is not ataxic, but she walks holding her right leg stiffly with the knee fixed in extension and the ankle fixed in dorsiflexion. She reports that sounds are fainter in her right ear, and she sees colors less brightly with her right eye. When a 512-Hz tuning fork is held over her mid-forehead, the sound does not lateralize to either side, and her fundi and pupils are normal. Muscle tone and tendon and plantar reflexes are normal. She is admitted for observation, and over the next 48 hours, with no specific treatment except encouragement, her symptoms and signs gradually clear.

Comment

This woman's symptoms and signs do not plausibly reflect a lesion of either the central or the peripheral nervous system. If the right-sided weakness were secondary to corticospinal tract, nerve root, or peripheral nerve damage, it would not be restricted to the particular muscles affected. In particular, wrist extensor and ankle dorsiflexor weakness, if corticospinal tract in origin, would likely be accompanied by widespread weakness, particularly distally, and if secondary to root or peripheral nerve injury, would be accompanied by weakness in muscles innervated by the same root or nerve. Moreover, when she walks, she awkwardly stiffens her entire right leg and forcibly contracts her allegedly weak right ankle dorsiflexors. Her sensory findings are equally implausible; she splits vibratory sensation across bony midlines, and she flawlessly performs finger-to-nose testing in the absence of proprioception. There is no asymmetry of reflexes or tone, and her visual and auditory findings, if real, would require separate lesions involving one eye or its optic nerve and one ear or its auditory nerve.

A problem with patients such as this is that although most of the symptoms and signs are obviously spurious, it is possible that one or more of them do actually signify neurological pathology; the others represent psychiatric overlay—that is, suggestibility. Multiple sclerosis is always a consideration in a young person with unexplained neurological symptoms, and sometimes hospitalization is justifiable even when the likelier diagnosis is conversion or malingering. Admission also allows a nonconfrontational face-saving interval, during which secondary gain, monetary or otherwise, can sometimes be identified and symptoms can gradually (or, in some cases, abruptly) clear. When symptoms persist, psychiatric consultation is appropriate.

SELECTED REFERENCES

Couprie W, Wijdicks EFM, Rooijmans HGM, van Gijn J: Outcome in conversion disorder: A follow-up study. J Neurol Neurosurg Psychiatry 1995;58:750.

Lazare A: Current concepts in psychiatry: Conversion symptoms. N Engl J Med 1981; 305:745.

Marsden CD: Hysteria: A neurologist's view. Psychol Med 1986;16:277.

15

Disorders of Consciousness

► CASE 57

A 56-year-old hypertensive man collapses on the sidewalk. Rushed to an emergency room, he is unresponsive to verbal stimuli, including commands to look up or down. Blood pressure is 190/100 mm Hg, pulse is 92/minute and regular, and temperature is 100.4 °F. Respirations are 12/minute, shallow, and regular. Pupils are pinpoint with a barely discernible reaction to light. Spontaneous horizontal eye movements are absent, but several times per minute his eyes move conjugately and briskly downward, returning immediately to the primary position. There is no response to the oculocephalic maneuver or to ice water caloric testing. His limbs are flaccid with tendon reflexes of normal amplitude; plantar stimulation produces a bilateral flexor response of his legs (including dorsiflexion of his toes). There is no facial grimace or upper limb movement to any painful stimulus.

Computerized tomography reveals a hemorrhage of his pons involving both the tegmentum and the base bilaterally. He is admitted to an intensive care unit and undergoes endotracheal intubation.

The following day there is no spontaneous eye movement, and caloric testing again produces no response. His pupils are now 3 mm and no longer react to light. Corneal reflexes are absent, the limbs are still flaccid, and tendon reflexes are still present, but there is no longer any response to plantar stimulation or other noxious stimuli. He is not triggering the respirator, and he remains apneic after being disconnected from the respirator for a period sufficient to raise his arterial pCO_2 to 65 mm Hg. Blood pressure is 130/80 mm Hg, and temperature is 101 °F. Urine assay for drugs and toxins, including sedatives, is negative. An electroencephalogram is flat-line—that is, there is no evidence of cerebral electrical activity.

Six hours later his examination is unchanged. Criteria for brain death having been met, ventilatory support is terminated.

Comment

This man's initial examination revealed the three signs most characteristic of *pontine hemorrhage,* namely, coma, pinpoint reactive pupils, and absent horizontal eye movements. Coma was secondary to destruction of the reticular activating system, the most caudal extent of which is within the pons. Miosis was secondary to transection of descending sympathetic projections and to disinhibition of the parasympathetic Edinger-Westphal nucleus. Because sympathetic lesions do not interrupt the parasympathetically mediated light reflex, pupillary reactivity was still present (see Figure 7–3). As with miosis secondary to morphine or heroin overdose, the degree of pupillary constriction was so marked that light reactivity was difficult to detect without a magnifying glass.

Loss of horizontal eye movement was the result of damage to the pontine paramedian reticular formation (PPRF, the pontine horizontal gaze center), the sixth nerve nuclei (which mediate horizontal gaze as well as ipsilateral abduction), and their various projections (see Figure 7–4). Less well understood is ocular bobbing, consisting of conjugate downward movements of the eyes several times per minute at irregular intervals. Ocular bobbing signifies damage to the pontine tegmentum and is therefore nearly always accompanied by absence of spontaneous or reflex horizontal eye movements. The downward movement thus might represent roving eye movements, which are horizontal during normal non–rapid eye movement (non-REM) sleep or in stuporous patients with functioning brain stems, but which become vertical in patients lacking the circuitry required for horizontal eye movement.

Respiratory patterns are often abnormal following pontine hemorrhage, but unpredictably so (see Figure 7–2). Most ominous, short of apnea, is ataxic (irregularly irregular) breathing. Cheyne-Stokes respiration occurs but must be differentiated from cluster breathing, which carries a worse prognosis. Apneustic breathing, with prolonged inspiratory pauses, more often follows pontine infarction than pontine hemorrhage, perhaps reflecting a lesser degree of damage.

On initial examination plantar stimulation produced flexion of the legs (including dorsiflexion of the toes—a Babinski response—which, physiologically, is flexion), but there was neither facial grimace nor upper limb movement to painful stimulation. Total lack of motor response to stimuli could reflect deep coma, complete paralysis, or both. The presence of only reflexic leg movements in this patient suggests that they were mediated, like his preserved tendon reflexes, through the spinal cord. He never demonstrated extensor responses of either his arms or his legs, perhaps because the hemorrhage destroyed the descending vestibulospinal and reticulospinal projections that must be intact for such posturing to occur.

The following day there were no eye movements of any kind, and the pupils were larger and unreactive to light; probably the lesion extended rostrally to involve the oculomotor nucleus. He was apneic even with a degree of arterial hypercarbia that would normally produce hyperventilation; probably the lesion extended caudally to involve areas within the pontomedullary reticular formation that control respiration. He met criteria for brain death, meaning that the only parts of his central nervous system still viable were his spinal cord and perhaps the vasomotor control centers of his medullary reticular formation (see Table 7–2). Although there have been dramatic exceptions in children, brain death in adults is short lived; cardiac asystole nearly always occurs within a few days or weeks. When organ donation is being considered, therefore, brain death is documented as soon as possible.

Whether or not the subject is a potential organ donor, however, brain death in most countries means legal death, with criteria that can be unambiguously tested. It is both economically absurd and morally repellant to provide protracted ventilatory support to a dead person.

SELECTED REFERENCES

Guidelines for the determination of death: Report of the medical consultants on the diagnosis of death to the President's Commission for the Study of Ethical Problems in Medicine and Biomedical and Behavioral Research. Neurology 1982;32:395.

Nakajima K: Clinicopathological study of pontine hemorrhage. Stroke 1983;14:485.

Plum F, Posner JB: *The Diagnosis of Stupor and Coma,* 3rd edition. F.A. Davis, 1980.

Shewmon DA: Chronic "brain death." Meta-analysis and conceptual consequences. Neurology 1998;51:1538.

Susac JO, Hoyt WF, Daroff RB, Lawrence W: Clinical spectrum of ocular bobbing. J Neurol Neurosurg Psychiatry 1970;33:771.

► CASE 58

While rollerblading, an 18-year-old boy is rendered briefly unconscious after falling. In an emergency room his examination is normal, and he is discharged. Several hours later he is observed to be confused and sleepy. Brought back to the emergency room, he now gives monosyllabic replies to loud verbal stimuli and is too inattentive to cooperate with the examiner. Blood pressure is 110/70 mm Hg, pulse is 80/minute and regular, and respirations are 15/minute and regular. The right pupil is 6 mm and the left pupil is 4 mm in diameter; both react to light. When he is undisturbed, his eyes rove smoothly and conjugately past the midline in both directions. When he is stimulated, the eye movements become saccadic. His limbs move symmetrically and purposefully to noxious stimuli and offer resistance to passive movement. Tendon reflexes are brisker on the left, and the left plantar response is extensor. At funduscopic examination the retinal veins appear abnormally widened compared to the arteries, but there are no hemorrhages or papilledema.

Computerized tomography (CT) reveals a large right-sided epidural hematoma, with a 6 mm right-to-left shift of midline structures at the level of the pineal gland. There is partial obliteration of the quadrigeminal and ambiens cisterns by the inferomedial right temporal lobe. A small fracture is present in the right calverium.

Following CT he responds only to painful stimuli with left-sided extensor posturing. Respirations are 30/minute and regular, pulse is 58/minute and regular, and blood pressure is 160/100 mm Hg. The right pupil is 8 mm in diameter and unreactive to light; the left pupil is 6 mm in diameter and reacts sluggishly. The eyes no longer rove, and because neck radiographs have not been obtained, oculocephalic testing is not performed. Plantar responses are bilaterally extensor.

Emergency endotracheal intubation is carried out, and he receives hyperventilation and mannitol in a rapid intravenous infusion. At surgery the hematoma is evacuated, and a bleeding middle meningeal artery is cauterized. Immediately after the operation his pupils are equal and reactive. At discharge a week later he is neurologically normal.

Comment

Briefly impaired consciousness following head injury, with spontaneous recovery over minutes or a few hours and no evident residua except (sometimes) transient posttraumatic amnesia, is termed *concussion.* This boy exemplifies why a CT scan is necessary after such an injury; without it his skull fracture and epidural hematoma would not have been identified before he deteriorated clinically. Neurosurgical intervention, when it finally occurred, was just in time.

The patient's signs typified transtentorial herniation of a lateral (uncal) type. Progressive loss of consciousness resulted from compromise to the ascending reticular activating system, probably initially at the level of the thalamus, which was distorted by right-to-left shift, and later at the level of the midbrain, which was distorted by the lateral shift and compressed by a herniated temporal lobe within the incisura.

Pupillary changes are explained by stretching or compression of the oculomotor nerves passing through the incisura over the tentorial edge (see Figure 7–3). In such a situation, pupillary dilatation and loss of light reactivity usually precede oculomotor paralysis, attributable to the presence of parasympathetic pupilloconstrictor fibers on the surface of the oculomotor nerve, rendering them particularly vulnerable to extrinsic compression. Had the patient's deterioration gone unchecked, both pupils might have become smaller and unreactive as midbrain damage affected both parasympathetic and sympathetic pathways.

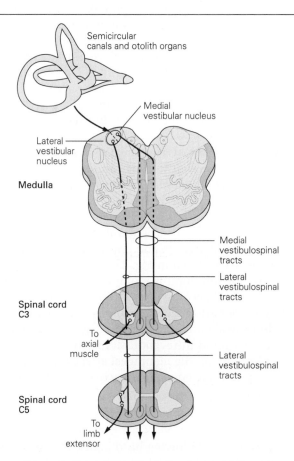

Figure 15–1. Vestibulospinal projections to axial and limb motor neurons. Disinhibition of this system can result in extensor posturing. (Reproduced with permission from Kandel ER, Schwartz JH, Jessell TM. 1991. *Principles of Neural Science*, 3rd ed. Norwalk, CT: Appleton & Lange.)

The patient's hyperventilation was probably the result of brain stem dysfunction rather than an appropriate response to hypoxia or acidosis (see Figure 7–2). Had rostrocaudal deterioration continued, breathing would likely have become increasingly irregular, finally progressing to apnea.

Extensor posturing in response to noxious stimuli implies upper brain stem dysfunction with preservation of vestibulospinal and reticulospinal projections arising from the lower pons and medulla (Figure 15–1). Although flexor and extensor posturing are common features of transtentorial herniation—sometimes sequentially, with flexor (decorticate) postures evolving into extensor (decerebrate) postures as rostrocaudal damage progresses—they are also associated with metabolic derangements such as hepatic encephalopathy and barbiturate intoxication (see Figure 7–1).

Bradycardia and hypertension during transtentorial herniation (or primary brain stem damage) is called the Cushing response after the American neurosurgeon who described it. The pathophysiological mechanism is uncertain, and the response is unpredictably present. It is most often encountered in children.

Hyperventilation reduces intracranial pressure by producing hypocarbia, which in turn causes cerebral vasoconstriction and reduced cerebral blood volume. Mannitol, an osmotic diuretic, draws water out of both normal and swollen brain, producing rapid and dramatic shrinkage. Patients tend to become refractory to both hyperventilation and mannitol, but their administration can buy precious time when emergency surgery is being arranged.

SELECTED REFERENCES

Cordobés F, Lobato RD, Rivas JJ, et al: Observations on 82 patients with extradural hematoma. Comparison of results before and after the advent of computerized tomography. J Neurosurg 1981;54:179.

Fisher CM: The neurological examination of the comatose patient. Acta Neurol Scand 1969;45(Suppl 36):1.

Ropper AH: Lateral displacement of the brain and level of consciousness in patients with an acute hemispheral mass. N Engl J Med 1986;314:953.

Simon RP: Respiratory manifestations of neurological disease. In: Goetz CG, Tanner CM, Aminoff MJ (eds): Handbook of Clinical Neurology, Volume 19 (63): Systemic Diseases, Part 1 (pp. 477–501). Elsevier Science Publishers BV, 1993.

White RJ, Likavec MJ: The diagnosis and management of head injury. N Engl J Med 1992;327:1507.

▶ CASE 59

Hospitalized for bronchopneumonia, a 55-year-old unemployed accountant becomes anxious and tremulous. Two days after admission his tremor has increased, and he is flushed, sweaty, and nauseated. The next day he is unaware of his surroundings, asserting that he is at a friend's apartment. Marked inattentiveness and agitation then supervene, and he no longer answers questions, gazing wildly about and shouting at what seem to be hallucinated people or objects. He is coarsely tremulous, with tachycardia, tachypnea, systolic hypertension, temperature of 103 °F, and profuse sweating.

A history is obtained of longstanding alcoholism, and he is treated with large parenteral doses of a benzodiazepine sedative. Studies to exclude other possible causes of acutely altered mental status, including computerized tomography (intracranial hemorrhage), cerebrospinal fluid (meningitis), liver function tests (hepatic encephalopathy), arterial blood gases (hypoxia, acid-base disturbance), blood glucose (hypoglycemia), and blood cultures (sepsis), are negative. After 5 days of intensive care, including heavy sedation, cardiac, respiratory, and blood pressure monitoring, cooling, attention to fluid and electrolyte balance, and administration of thiamine and other vitamins, treatment is gradually withdrawn. A few days later his mental status is normal except for mild impairment of recent memory.

Comment

Some drugs, for example, cocaine and other psychostimulants, cause delirium as an acute toxic effect. By contrast, sedatives such as ethanol and barbiturates cause delirium as a withdrawal phenomenon after protracted heavy use. Unlike other recreationally abused drugs such as opioids, cocaine, and Δ^9-tetrahydrocannabinol (the psychoactive ingredient in marijuana), which bind to specific receptors in the brain, *ethanol* appears to act nonspecifically by disrupting the phospholipid bilayer of cell membranes; the result is increased membrane fluidization and secondary alteration of proteins and ion channels. A number of neurotransmitter systems are indirectly affected by these conformational changes. In addition, however, ethanol may have more specific and selective actions at certain receptor-gated ion channels. Ethanol inhibits neurotransmission at excitatory glutamate receptors of the N-methyl-D-aspartate (NMDA) type, perhaps acting at the glycine coagonist site (see Figure 12–20). Ethanol augments neurotransmission at γ-aminobutyric acid (GABA) receptors (Figure 15–2).

The clinical effects of ethanol are the result of a net inhibitory action on particular regions of the brain. With moderate dosage there is sedation (reticular activating system) and impaired hand–eye coordination (parietal association cor-

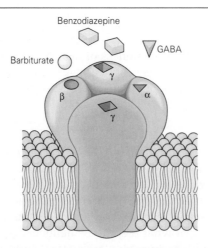

Figure 15–2. The γ-aminobutyric acid (GABA) receptor complex. There are three subunit types, which together form the chloride channel. GABA binds to the α-subunit. Barbiturates bind to the β-subunit. Benzodiazepines bind to the γ-subunit. (Reproduced with permission from Kandel ER, Schwartz JH, Jessell TM. 1999. *Principles of Neural Science*, 4th ed. New York: McGraw-Hill.)

tex). Heavy dosage produces coma and respiratory depression. (Hyperactivity and jocularity signify disinhibition, not stimulatory action of ethanol—the superego is soluble in ethanol.) Chronic use produces down-regulation of GABA neurotransmission and up-regulation of glutamate neurotransmission, resulting in tolerance—the need for increasing doses to achieve the desired effect—and, on abrupt abstinence, withdrawal hyperexcitability, variably manifested as seizures, hallucinations, or, as in this patient, delirium tremens.

SELECTED REFERENCES

Brust JCM: Ethanol. In: *Neurological Aspects of Substance Abuse.* Butterworth-Heinemann, 1993.
Isbell H, Fraser HF, Wikler A, et al: An experimental study of the etiology of "rum fits" and delirium tremens. Q J Stud Alcohol 1955;16:1.
Lustig HS, Chan J, Greenberg DA: Ethanol inhibits excitotoxicity in cerebral cortical cultures. Neurosci Lett 1992;135:259.
Pohorecky LA, Brick J: Pharmacology of ethanol. Pharmacol Ther 1988;36:335.
Tabakoff B, Hoffman PL: Alcohol addiction: An enigma among us. Neuron 1996;16:909.
Tsai G, Gastfriend DR, Coyle JT: The glutamatergic basis of human alcoholism. Am J Psychiatry 1995;152:3.

▶ CASE 60

A 21-year-old woman is found apneic and pulseless following ingestion of sedatives combined with ethanol. She receives cardiopulmonary resuscitation. In an emergency room, pulse and blood pressure are now obtainable, but she is still apneic, her pupils are dilated and unreactive to light, there are no spontaneous or reflexic eye movements, and she neither grimaces nor moves her limbs to painful stimuli. An hour later respirations have returned, and 12 hours later her pupils are smaller and react to light. During the next week there is stimulus-induced flexion of the arms, fist clenching, inversion of the feet, plantar flexion, head turning to the right, yawning, and grunting. Painful stimuli produce, variably, flexion of the limbs or opisthotonus and upward deviation of the eyes.

Over the next several months she has sleep–wake cycles but never shows evidence of cognitive function or awareness of her environment. Because of a tendency to become apneic during sleep, she receives continued ventilatory support. Her eyes rove fully in both horizontal directions, mostly conjugate but with occasional disconjugate interruptions. She does not follow moving objects with her eyes, look toward a loud verbal stimulus, move her eyes in any direction to command, or blink to threat. The oculocephalic maneuver produces conjugate horizontal deviation of the eyes opposite in direction to the head turning, and cold water introduced into each ear produces conjugate deviation of the eyes toward the stimulus without nystagmus. Limb movements are stereotypically stimulus dependent and never purposeful in appearance.

Carotid and vertebral angiography are normal. An electroencephalogram during her wakeful state shows mostly low-voltage beta activity (faster than 12 Hz); during apparent sleep there is mostly slower activity in the theta (5–7 Hz) and delta (1–4 Hz) range.

Despite severe weight loss and the development of limb contractures and decubitus ulcers, she remains neurologically unchanged until her death from infection 9 years later. Computerized tomography 5 years after her cardiac arrest shows widespread cerebral and cerebellar atrophy.

Comment

Persistent vegetative state refers to patients who are awake but not aware (see Table 7–1). In contrast to patients who are brain dead, vegetative patients have brain stem reflexes (pupillary, oculovestibular, corneal, gag), their limbs move to stimuli and sometimes move spontaneously, and they demonstrate sleep–wake cycles behaviorally and electroencephalographically. There is no evidence, however, of inner or outer awareness or a functioning mind.

Coma, defined clinically as lack of response to stimuli, is never persistent; over hours, days, or weeks there is either death or some degree of recovery, including survival in the vegetative state. Rarely have vegetative patients improved further after more than a few weeks; with aggressive nursing care, however, they can he kept alive for decades.

The anatomic basis of the vegetative state is a nonfunctioning cerebral cortex, although the lesion itself might be either cortical or subcortical, including the cerebral white matter and the thalamus. Brain stem structures are largely preserved. When vegetative state follows cardiac arrest, autopsy often reflects the vulnerability of certain types of neurons to anoxia and of certain brain regions to hypoperfusion (ischemia). Neuronal loss is particularly severe in the third and fourth layers of the cerebral cortex (laminar necrosis), the Ammon's horn (*cornu Ammonis,* CA) region of the hippocampus, and the Purkinje cell layer of the cerebellum. The vulnerability of these cells to anoxia might be related to glutamate excitotoxicity. Anatomically, damage tends to be maximal in cortical border zones (watersheds) between major surface arteries and end zones of deeper penetrating arteries. Such regional infarction frequently affects the parasaggital cortex of the frontal and parietal lobes (the border zone of the middle and anterior cerebral arteries) and the globus pallidus (the end zone of the anterior choroidal artery). Regional damage of this type is a consequence of hypotension and decreased cerebral perfusion; brain areas most distally perfused are rendered most ischemic.

The patient described above is Karen Ann Quinlan, whose plight in 1975 launched a legal and ethical debate that led to the development of medicolegal guidelines for the care of persistently vegetative patients. Neuropathological study of her brain, reported in 1994, revealed parasaggital border-zone infarcts as well as occipital lobe infarction (likely a consequence of transtentorial herniation and compression of the posterior cerebral artery as it passed through the incisura). These lesions, however, were considered insufficient to account for her vegetative state. The major brain damage was bilateral in the thalamus. Such localization, which has been described in other vegetative patients, raises the possibility that the thalamus is involved with cognition and awareness as well as arousal.

As discussed in Cases 57 and 58, arousal and wakefulness are traditionally viewed as dependent on the reticular activating system, which consists of projections from the brainstem reticular formation to thalamic reticular, midline, and intralaminar nuclei and their projections to the cerebral cortex. Independent of the thalamus, however, the cerebral cortex can be activated by noradrenergic, cholinergic, and serotonergic systems that originate in the brain stem, hypothalamus, and basal forebrain. Arousal might therefore continue to occur after extensive thalamic damage, but attentiveness and cognition, dependent on thalamic binding of separate computational circuits (parallel distributed processing), would no longer be possible. The brain of a comatose patient lacks consciousness because it cannot be aroused. The brain of a vegetative patient lacks consciousness because, although arousable, it lacks mental content.

SELECTED REFERENCES

Andrews K: Prediction of recovery from post-traumatic vegetative state. Lancet 1998; 351:1751.

Dougherty JH, Rawlinson DG, Levy DE, Plum F: Hypoxic-ischemic brain injury and the vegetative state: Clinical and neuropathologic correlation. Neurology 1981;31:991.

Jennett B, Plum F: Persistent vegetative state after brain damage. Lancet 1972;1:734.

Kinney HC, Korein J, Panigrahy A, et al: Neuropathological findings in the brain of Karen Ann Quinlan—the role of the thalamus in the persistent vegetative state. N Engl J Med 1994;330:1469.

Multi-Society Task Force on PVS: Medical aspects of the persistent vegetative state. N Engl J Med 1994;330:1499, 1572.

▶ CASE 61

A 50-year-old woman begins having attacks of daytime sleepiness. Most often when sitting quietly or engaging in boring activity, but sometimes when conversing or eating, she is overcome by a desire to sleep. Awakening after 5 to 15 minutes, she feels refreshed. Over the next several months the attacks increase in frequency to several per day. A year after the onset of these symptoms she notices that emotional experiences, particularly laughter, trigger weakness; her jaw drops, her head falls forward, and her knees buckle. Weakness is also sometimes present on awakening in the morning, and she often has brief formed visual hallucinations when she is drowsy.

Findings on physical and neurological examination are normal. A multiple sleep latency test is performed; over the course of the day she is asked to fall asleep every 2 hours, and electroencephalography reveals sleep latency of less than 5 minutes and rapid eye movement activity at the onset of sleep.

Treatment with methylphenidate is followed by reduction in the frequency and severity of her sleep attacks, but her episodic weakness continues, on one occasion resulting in a serious fall. When clomipramine is included in her therapy, she no longer experiences such weakness.

Comment

The classic tetrad of *narcolepsy* consists of (1) repeated attacks of irresistable sleepiness, (2) emotionally triggered weakness (*cataplexy*), (3) inability to move during the onset of sleep or on awakening (*sleep paralysis*), and (4) hallucinatory experiences during drowsiness or on awakening (*hypnagogic hallucinations*). Daytime sleepiness is temporarily relieved by 5 to 15 minutes of sleep, but soon returns. Cateplexy and sleep paralysis usually last no more than a few minutes. Patients are fully aware of the hallucinatory nature of their visual experiences, describing them as dream-like.

Each of these four symptoms is a feature of the rapid eye movement (REM) stage of sleep, during which dreaming is accompanied by a loss of muscle tone, bursts of rapid eye movement are superimposed on the slower eye movements of other sleep stages, and electroencephalographically there is low-voltage, desynchronized, fast activity. During REM sleep, which occupies about 25% of sleep time in young adults, there is an increased threshold for arousal by environmental stimuli, yet the subject is more likely than in other sleep stages to awaken spontaneously.

In most normal adults REM sleep occurs several times during the night but does not appear until the subject, over a period of 60 to 90 minutes, has passed through and then retraced the other four stages of sleep (Figure 15–3). In narcolepsy (and in some other disorders, eg, depression) sleep onset is more abrupt than usual, and REM sleep appears within a few minutes (Figure 15–4). Narcolepsy can be viewed as a disorder in which the temporal boundaries of wakefulness, non-REM sleep, and REM sleep are blurred and features of REM sleep intrude into wakefulness. Some narcoleptic patients have amnestic periods during which their behavior appears automatic, superficially resembling nocturnal sleepwalking, partial complex seizures, or psychogenic fugue states. Such episodes are accompanied electroencephalographically by drowsy and sleep patterns intermixed with wakefulness. During nocturnal sleep, narcoleptics display frequent awakenings and body movements, reduced time spent in stages 3 and 4, and decreased total sleep.

Neither psychogenic nor epileptic in origin, narcolepsy is of unknown cause. A nearly 100% association with the HLA-DQB1 allele of the major histocompatibility complex (MHC) suggests genetic influence involving chromosome 6, but the gene has not been more precisely located or characterized. (An intriguing aspect of this association is that sleep deprivation impairs immune responses and that infections—as well as certain cytokines—cause sleepiness). There is no evidence for immunological attack in the brain in narcolepsy, however, and in

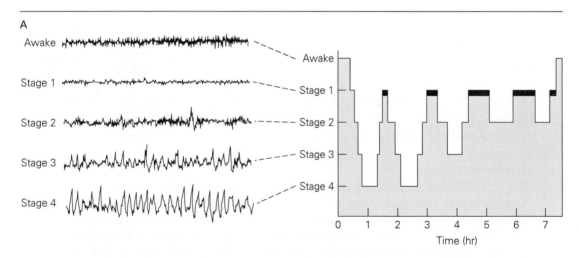

Figure 15–3. Stages of sleep. **A.** Electroencephalographic (EEG) recordings during different stages of wakefulness and sleep. Each record spans 30 seconds. Low-voltage activity at 9–11 Hz α and 18–30 Hz β characterizes an awake brain. As a person falls asleep, the EEG progresses through stages of increasingly slow wave activity. Stage 2 is characterized by brief bursts of waxing and waning waves (sleep spindles). Stages 3 and 4 are referred to as slow wave or delta sleep. Rapid eye movement (REM) is electroencephalographically similar to stage 1 sleep but differs from it by the presence of rapid eye movements and diffuse loss of muscle tone.

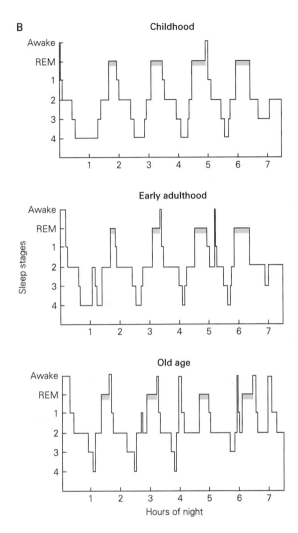

Figure 15–3. *(continued)* **B.** Pattern of normal sleep in childhood, early adulthood, and old age. Stage 4 sleep is reached after approximately 45 minutes; the sleep stages then recur in reverse order over a similar time span, with REM sleep appearing approximately 1.5 hours after sleep onset. As the cycle repeats itself during the night the time spent in slow wave sleep decreases and the time spent in REM sleep increases. Dreaming is more likely to be reported if one is awakened during REM sleep than if one is awakened during slow wave sleep. (Reproduced with permission from Kandel ER, Schwartz JH, Jessell TM. 1991. *Principles of Neural Science,* 3rd ed. Norwalk, CT: Appleton & Lange.)

breeds of narcoleptic/cataplectic dogs, the canine gene is not located within the MHC complex.

Autopsies of narcoleptic patients do not show obvious brain abnormalities. Studies of humans and narcoleptic/cataplectic dogs reveal decreased concentration of dopamine and its metabolite homovanillic acid in cerebrospinal fluid and increased dopamine D_2 receptor density in the basal ganglia, consistent with impaired dopamine release and secondary receptor up-regulation. Narcoleptic dogs also have increased concentrations of cholinergic M_2 receptors in the pontine reticular formation. Canine cataplexy is inhibited by drugs that increase synaptic norepinephrine and serotonin and exacerbated by α_1-adrenergic antagonists; the

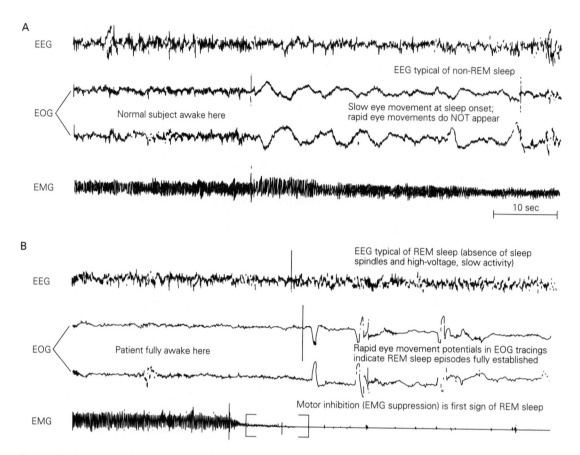

Figure 15–4. Narcoleptic sleep onset compared to normal sleep onset **A.** With normal sleep onset the electroencephalogram (EEG) gradually changes from a waking pattern to lower frequencies coupled with rolling eye movements on the oculogram (EOG) and continued muscle activity on the electromyogram (EMG). **B.** In narcolepsy sleep onset is preceded by several seconds of markedly reduced muscle activity (bracketed in the EMG tracing); there then appear conjugate rapid eye movements, and the EEG resembles stage 1 sleep. Sleep spindles are not present, and there is no high-voltage slow activity. [Reproduced with permission from Kandel ER, Schwartz JH, Jessell TM. 1991. *Principles of Neural Science*, 3rd ed. Norwalk, CT: Appleton & Lange. Adapted with permission from Dement W, Guilleminault C, Zarcone V. 1975. The pathologies of sleep: A case series approach. In: Tower DB (ed): *The Nervous System*, Volume 2 *The Clinical Neurosciences.* Raven Press (pp. 501–518).]

exacerbation is blocked by the cholinergic antagonist atropine, whereas cholinergic agonists (which induce REM sleep) exacerbate cataplexy.

These observations are consistent with studies of normal sleep. REM and non-REM sleep are probably regulated by interaction between serotonergic neurons of the dorsal raphe nuclei, noradrenergic neurons of the locus coeruleus, and cholinoreceptive neurons of the gigantocellular nucleus. Acetylcholine appears to activate REM; serotonin and norepinephrine, by inhibiting REM-selective cholinergic neurons, appear to suppress it, but the specific interactions of these systems are otherwise uncertain, as is the nature of their disruption in narcolepsy.

In human narcoleptics dextroamphetamine and methylphenidate, which stimulate release of norepinephrine at synaptic nerve endings, prevent sleep attacks but have no effect on cataplexy. By contrast, tricyclic antidepressants, which block synaptic reuptake of norepinephrine and serotonin, prevent cataplexy, hypnagogic hallucinations, and sleep paralysis but have no effect on sleep attacks. A recently developed drug, modafinil, appears to promote wakefulness without acting through dopamine, norepinephrine, or serotonin systems (or, like caffeine, inhibiting the neuromodulator adenosine); it may modulate the activity of the hypothalamic suprachiasmatic nucleus, the major component of the brain's circadian clock (see Case 62).

SELECTED REFERENCES

Aldrich MS: The clinical spectrum of narcolepsy and idiopathic hypersomnia. Neurology 1996;46:393.

Beardsley T: Waking up. Sci Am, July 1996: page 14.

Fry JM: Treatment modalities for narcolepsy. Neurology 1998;50(Suppl 1):S43.

Mahowald MW: Synchrony, sleep, dreams, and consciousness. Clues from K-complexes. Neurology 1997;49:909.

McCarley RW: Neurophysiology of sleep; basic mechanisms underlying control of wakefulness and sleep. In Chokroverty S (ed): *Sleep Disorders Medicine,* 2nd edition. Butterworth-Heinemann, 1998.

Mignot E: Genetic and familial aspects of narcolepsy. Neurology 1998;50(Suppl 1):S16.

▶ CASE 62

A 52-year-old man begins having nocturnal insomnia, impotence, and loss of libido. Two months later he is sleeping only 1 hour per night and is disturbed by vivid dreams, during which he gets out of bed and engages in seemingly purposeful activity. He also develops episodic rhinorrhea, salivation, lacrimation, sweating, and increased body temperature. Three months after the onset of symptoms he has no normal sleep and his dreaming episodes are increasingly frequent. His breathing becomes irregular with episodes of apnea, and there is tachycardia and hypertension. His gait is clumsy and his speech is slurred.

On examination his pupils are small and hyporeactive. Left alone, he lapses into a stupor-like state with complex purposeful gesturing and irregular breathing; he is easily awakened from this state.

Over the next few months he develops intention tremor and tactile-evoked myoclonus. Neuropsychological studies 7 months after the onset of symptoms reveal fluctuations of attentiveness but normal thought processes and short-term memory. His speech gradually becomes unintelligible, and he has episodes of agitation with screaming and dystonic posturing. Hyperactive tendon reflexes and Babinski signs are present. More intense stimuli are required to arouse him from his stupor-like state, and 9 months after the onset of symptoms he dies of uncontrollable pneumonia.

Electroencephalography (EEG) soon after the onset of symptoms reveals normal posterior alpha activity (see Figure 11–2). At serial tracings recorded over the course of his illness the alpha rhythm gradually loses its normal reactivity to stimuli, spreads anteriorly over his entire cortex, and eventually becomes replaced by slower (theta) activity. Twenty-four-hour polygraphic recordings show quiet wakefulness alternating with periods of desynchronization, during which there are rapid eye movements (REMs), reduced muscle tone, muscular jerks, and reports of dreaming. There is no demonstrable circadian rhythm and no evidence of physiological non-REM sleep.

Blood measurements of growth hormone, prolactin, and follicle-stimulating hormone reveal complete absence of circadian oscillations. Autonomic studies, including the Valsalva maneuver, infusion of phenylephrine, and pupillary tests with homatropine and cocaine, reveal generalized autonomic failure.

Over several generations multiple relatives have been affected.

At autopsy there is marked neuronal loss and gliosis in the anterior and dorsomedial nuclei of the thalamus, with preservation of neurites passing through these areas. Neuronal loss is also present in the olivary nuclei of the medulla, other thalamic nuclei, and the cerebral and cerebellar cortices. The hypothalamus is spared.

Comment

This bizarre disorder, known as *fatal familial insomnia* (FFI), in most patients begins with insomnia, enacted dreams, and autonomic disturbances, progressing over months or years to dysarthria, ataxia, pyramidal signs, myoclonus, coma, and death. The disease is hereditary, with autosomal dominant transmission, and in the Italian family in which FFI was first described—of which the present patient is the proband—age of onset ranged from 20 to 56 years (mean, 44 years) and duration of disease ranged from 6 to 42 months (mean, 15 years).

Insomnia has many causes, including anxiety, depression, altered circadian rhythms (jet lag), nocturnal myoclonus, sleep apnea, and sedative or alcohol abuse. The neurophysiological basis of this patient's disordered sleep and autonomic function is likely the result of his thalamic lesions. Sleep became increasingly restricted to the REM stage, which occurred without the normal paralysis that accompanies dreaming (see Figure 15–3). The patient's dreams were therefore acted out.

Electroencephalographically, his alpha rhythm—a 9- to 13-Hz sinusoidal rhythm normally generated by the thalamus and observed over the parietal and occipital lobes during relaxed wakefulness—became increasingly unreactive to even painful stimuli and spread over his entire cerebral cortex. Terminally there were only theta and delta rhythms, which reflected coma, not sleep. During his dreaming episodes there was electroencephalographic desynchronization, as would be expected during the REM stage of sleep, but normal patterns of non-REM sleep—bursts of waxing and waning waves known as sleep spindles, and considered thalamic in origin—were never seen, and during sleep, as opposed to his eventual coma, there was no delta activity. Continuous 24-hour monitoring revealed no circadian rhythm to neuroendocrine and autonomic function.

In humans the suprachiasmatic nucleus (SCN) of the anterior hypothalamus is the principal generator of circadian rhythmicity, which modulates sleep–wake cycles, autonomic activity (eg, body temperature, blood pressure, and heart rate), and endocrine function (eg, secretion of growth hormone, adrenocorticotropin, and melatonin) (Figure 15–5). Circadian rhythmicity is an autonomous feature of neurons in the SCN, not an emergent property of their circuitry. Cultured SCN neurons show circadian rhythms of electrical firing, and in animals whose SCNs have been ablated, central nervous system grafting of neonatal SCN tissue restores circadian patterning. The mechanism of this oscillatory activity appears to be autoregulatory feedback; over an approximately 24-hour period certain pro-

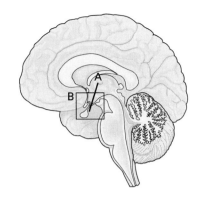

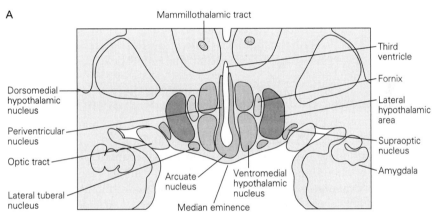

A

Mammillothalamic tract

Third ventricle

Fornix

Dorsomedial hypothalamic nucleus

Lateral hypothalamic area

Periventricular nucleus

Supraoptic nucleus

Optic tract

Amygdala

Arcuate nucleus

Ventromedial hypothalamic nucleus

Lateral tuberal nucleus

Median eminence

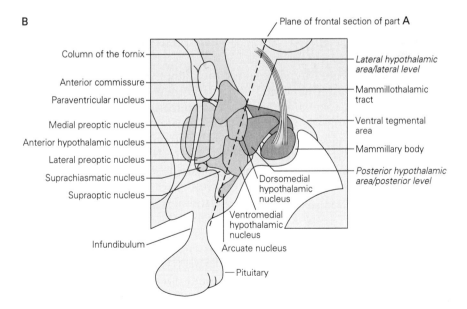

B

Plane of frontal section of part **A**

Column of the fornix

Lateral hypothalamic area/lateral level

Anterior commissure

Mammillothalamic tract

Paraventricular nucleus

Medial preoptic nucleus

Ventral tegmental area

Anterior hypothalamic nucleus

Mammillary body

Lateral preoptic nucleus

Suprachiasmatic nucleus

Posterior hypothalamic area/posterior level

Supraoptic nucleus

Dorsomedial hypothalamic nucleus

Ventromedial hypothalamic nucleus

Infundibulum

Arcuate nucleus

Pituitary

Figure 15–5. Coronal (**A**) and sagittal (**B**) views of the hypothalamus. (**B**) shows the suprachiasmatic nucleus and its relationship to other hypothalamic nuclei. (Reproduced with permission from Kandel ER, Schwartz JH, Jessell TM. 1999. *Principles of Neural Science,* 4th ed. New York: McGraw-Hill.)

teins are synthesized, interact with each other, and then suppress their own genes. Eventually released from inhibition, the genes become active again, and a new cycle begins.

The circadian clock can be environmentally modulated, particularly by light. The SCN receives a direct projection from the retina, the retinohypothalamic tract. There are also direct projections from the retina to areas of the thalamus that probably integrate photic and nonphotic information and then, projecting back to the SCN, modulate its activity. Major projections of the SCN are to other hypothalamic nuclei (with further projections to the pituitary, brain stem reticular formation, and pineal gland), and to the thalamus and basal nuclei (with further projections to neocortex, limbic structures, and basal ganglia). Disrupted circadian regulation follows discrete damage to the anterior hypothalamus. Autopsies of patients with FFI, however, fail to show hypothalamic damage; the dependence of SCN function on its thalamic connections make it reasonable, therefore, to ascribe loss of circadian rhythmicity in FFI to thalamic damage. In animals bilateral lesions of the dorsomedial thalamic nuclei result in electrical and behavioral insomnia.

A prion disease, FFI is caused by an abnormal isoform of a protein normally present in the brain and known as cellular prion protein or PrP. Altered isoforms of the protein, which are resistant to proteases, cause a number of fatal central nervous system diseases in animals and humans, including scrapie in sheep and bovine encephalopathy (mad cow disease) in cattle. Human prion diseases include kuru (a nonhereditary disorder described in natives of the New Guinea highlands), Gerstmann-Straussler-Scheinker disease (a dominantly inherited disorder), Creutzfeldt-Jacob disease (which is hereditary in 10% of cases and sporadic in 90%), and FFI. Transmission of altered prion protein produces disease in the recipient despite the absence of DNA or RNA. Thus, some of these diseases are both infectious and genetic. The neoligism *prion* is based on its two features—protein and infectious. Altered and infectious prions are collectively referred to as PrP^{sc} (for scrapie).

The currently favored hypothesis for the pathogenesis of prion diseases is that they are the result of abnormal folding. Normal PrP consists largely of α-helices. PrP^{sc}, however, contains β-strands, in which the molecule's backbone is stretched out, rendering the protein resistant to protease. PrP^{sc} is infective because when it comes into contact with normal PrP molecules, it causes them to unfold and adopt the conformation of PrP^{sc}. Like a seed crystal the original PrP^{sc} sets up a cascade, and over time insoluble protease-resistant PrP^{sc} accumulates in affected neurons, eventually destroying them. (Consistent with this hypothesis is the observation that knockout mice lacking the normal PrP gene and therefore devoid of PrP are resistant to scrapie disease when infected with PrP^{sc}.)

Sporadic prion diseases are the result of posttranslational spontaneous conformational alteration of PrP. Human genetic prion diseases are the result of mutations of the PrP^{sc} gene on chromosome 20. At least 18 mutations have been identified in families with inherited prion diseases. In FFI the mutation is at codon 178. Clinical differences between the different prion diseases are presumably the result of different conformations adopted by different isoforms of PrP^{sc}. Still unknown is how the different folding patterns produce the particular neuroanatomical patterns of each disorder—cerebral cortex and basal ganglia in Creutzfeldt-Jacob disease, resulting in dementia, spastic weakness, and extrapyramidal signs; cerebellar cortex in Gerstmann-Straussler-Scheinker disease, resulting in ataxia; and thalamus in FFI, resulting in insomnia, enacted dreams, and dysautonomia.

SELECTED REFERENCES

Czeisler CA, Duffy JF, Shanahan TL, et al: Stability precision, and near-24-hour period of the human circadian pacemaker. Science 1999;284:2177.

Hastings M: The brain, circadian rhythms, and clock genes. Br Med J 1998;317:1704.

Johnson RT, Gibbs CJ: Creutzfeldt-Jacob disease and related spongiform encephalopathies. N Engl J Med 1998;339:1994.

Manetto V, Medori R, Cortelli P, et al: Fatal familial insomnia. Clinical and pathologic study of five new cases. Neurology 1992;42:312.

Mastriami JA, Nixon R, Layzer R, et al: Prion protient conformation in a patient with sporadic fatal insomnia. N Engl J Med 1999;340:1630.

Moore RY: Circadian rhythms: Basic neurobiology and clinical applications. Annu Rev Med 1997;48:253.

Prusiner SB: Prion diseases and the BSE crisis. Science 1997;278:254.

Schwartz WJ: Understanding circadian clocks: From c-Fos to fly balls. Ann Neurol 1997; 41:289.

16

Disorders of Language, Praxis, Gnosis, and Thought

▶ CASE 63

A 55-year-old right-handed man suddenly develops difficulty speaking and weakness of his right side. Admitted to a hospital a few hours later, he is described as having right hemiparesis, with speech limited to inarticulate grunts but intact speech comprehension as evidenced by ability to follow simple commands.

Three days later he has regained some speech, and a more comprehensive neurological examination is performed. He is alert, attentive, cooperative, and appropriately anxious. His speech is nonfluent, with delayed effortful initiation and an output of less than a dozen words per minute. One- or two-word phrases are often perseveratively repeated. His speech lacks melody and rhythm and is poorly articulated. His words consist largely of nouns and verbs, often incorrectly constructed (eg, a noun lacking a plural ending or a verb with a wrong tense); strikingly absent are function words (conjunctions, prepositions, articles, pronouns, and relational adjectives), giving his speech a telegrammatic style.

Speech comprehension is normal when tested with simple commands and yes–no questions, but he makes errors when asked to point to several objects in sequence or when a command depends on grammatical structure. Shown a variety of objects, body parts, and colors, he names most of them correctly but laboriously. With some objects he offers the wrong word (eg, *clock* for *watch*), and with others he perseveratively repeats the name of the previous object. He is able to repeat single words but not phrases of two or more words.

Using his nonparalyzed left hand, he is able to write single letters to dictation, but they are poorly formed to a degree not explained by the use of his nondominant hand, and he cannot write whole words. Reading aloud is effortful but largely correct; he has greater difficulty reading individual letters and grammatical words aloud than imageable nouns. Reading comprehension is mildly impaired, particularly with grammatically complex phrases.

Right-sided facial weakness spares the forehead. His right arm is paralyzed and flaccid; his right leg is moderately weak proximally and mildly weak distally. Pinprick, temperature, and touch sensation are mildly impaired over his right face and arm, and proprioception is reduced in his right hand. Visual fields are normal to gross bedside testing. Tendon reflexes are increased in his right arm, and a right plantar response is absent.

Computerized tomography reveals abnormal lucency in the territory of the superior division of the left middle cerebral artery, including pre- and post-rolandic motor and sensory cortices and frontal and parietal opercular areas. An electrocardiogram reveals atrial fibrillation.

Comment

Aphasia is an acquired disorder of previously intact language function. It is not explained by impaired speech (dysarthria or dysphonia) or impaired thinking (dementia or psychosis), although, as this patient demonstrates, some aphasics also have abnormal articulation. Aphasia, however, refers to a disturbance of one or more of the coding processes that underlie the several components of language, including speaking, oral comprehension, writing, and reading. Aphasic deaf mutes develop defects in producing or comprehending sign language.

This patient has *Broca aphasia,* also called motor or expressive aphasia. In 1861 Paul Broca, a Parisian neurosurgeon, described a patient whose speech output was limited to the phrase "tan-tan," but who could still comprehend the speech of others. Although autopsy showed a large left cerebral lesion that included the insula and both the frontal and the parietal operculum, Broca, perhaps influenced by the phrenologist Franz Gall, attributed the patient's aphasia to involvement of the left frontal operculum, specifically the pars opercularis, known ever since as *Broca's area* (Figure 16–1). In fact, lesions restricted to Broca's area do not produce aphasia, and every case of Broca aphasia with autopsy documentation has shown more extensive damage. Nevertheless, Broca observations, in contrast to Gall's speculations, provided scientific support of the concept of cerebral localization, and within a few years, as he accumulated additional cases of aphasia, Broca was able to assert that language processing is a left hemispheric function.

No two people use language identically, and no two aphasics have identical syndromes. The defining features of Broca aphasia are nonfluent, aprosodic speech with articulatory struggle, agraphia, and relatively preserved speech comprehension and reading. Syntax (grammar) is often impaired to a greater degree than semantics (word meaning), and this dissociation may be evident in both the production and the interpretation of speech and written material. Agrammatism, or telegrammatic speech, as encountered in this patient, is unusual, however. Some patients, reminiscent of Broca first case, have recurrent utterance—their speech is limited to a single phrase, word, or phoneme.

Lesions restricted to the pars opercularis produce transient reductions in speech initiation and output. Lesions of the lower motor cortex cause severely disordered and effortful articulation (*aphemia*) without agraphia or other language abnormalities. Which cortical or subcortical structures are responsible for the additional features that define Broca aphasia is conjectural and controversial.

Aphasia is most often the result of head trauma or cerebrovascular disease, and the stroke most frequently responsible for Broca aphasia is infarction in the territory of the upper division of the middle cerebral artery. This vascular territory includes the motor cortex on the frontal convexity; therefore, most patients with Broca aphasia have hemiparesis affecting the face and arm more than the leg. By contrast, visual fields are usually normal; in most people the optic radiations are supplied by the inferior division of the middle cerebral artery and by the posterior cerebral artery.

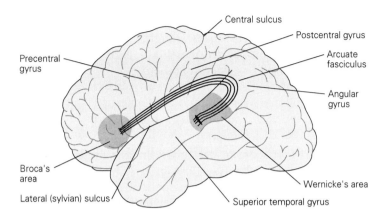

Figure 16–1. Primary language areas of the brain. The role of Broca's area (pars opercularis) in language processing is uncertain; selective damage to this region produces only transient dysarticulation, not full-blown Broca aphasia. Wernicke's area (planum temporale) is necessary, although not sufficient, for speech comprehension; selective damage to this region produces defects in auditory comprehension but not full-blown Wernicke aphasia. Whether lesions affecting the arcuate fasciculus, by disconnecting Wernicke's area from Broca's area, cause aphasia is controversial. (Reproduced with permission from Kandel ER, Schwartz JH, Jessell TM. 1991. *Principles of Neural Science*, 3rd ed. Norwalk, CT: Appleton & Lange.)

SELECTED REFERENCES

Alexander MP, Naeser MA, Palumbo C: Broca's area aphasias: Aphasias after lesions including the frontal operculum. Neurology 1990;40:353.

Broca P: Remarques sur le siege de la faculté du langage articule, suivies d'une observation d'aphemie. Bull Soc Anat (Paris) 1861;2ᵉ serie tV1:330.

Mohr JP, Pessin MS, Finkelstein S, et al: Broca asphasia: Pathologic and clinical aspects. Neurology 1978;28:311.

Tranel D: Neurology of language. Curr Opin Neurol Neurosurg 1992;5:77.

Wise RJS, Greene J, Buchel C, Scott SK: Brain regions involved in articulation. Lancet 1999;353:1057.

► CASE 64

A 53-year-old woman abruptly begins "talking out of her head." At examination a few hours later her speech is fluent to the point of logorrhea and has normal articulation and prosody. Grammatical words are present, but there is a paucity of meaningful, substantive words; rather her speech is heavily contaminated by paraphasias, both verbal (a wrong word substituted for the correct word) and literal (syllabic substitutions within a word, resulting in a nonword or neologism). Most of her speech is therefore incomprehensible to the examiner. She, in turn, has little or no comprehension of the examiner's speech, as tested by spoken commands, yes–no questions, and requests to point to objects in the room. Attempts to name objects or to repeat the examiner's words result in verbal and literal paraphasias. Writing with her right hand (which is neither weak nor clumsy), she produces well-formed legible letters strung together to make incomprehensible words. Reading aloud results in mostly paraphasias, and although she comprehends some individual written words, correctly matching them to pictures, she cannot comprehend written sentences.

Particularly striking is her evident lack of insight into her difficulty. She delivers an appropriately inflected but meaningless sentence, then pauses for the examiner's turn, seemingly unaware that her speech is incomprehensible and that she cannot comprehend the speech of others.

Findings on the neurological examination are othewise normal, including visual fields, eye movements, sensation and movement of the face and limbs, and tendon and plantar reflexes. Computerized tomography reveals an infarct involving the posterior part of the superior and middle temporal gyri as well as the supramarginal and angular gyri of the inferior parietal lobule.

Comment

The defining characteristics of *Wernicke aphasia*—also known as sensory or receptive aphasia—are fluent speech with normal intonation and articulation but a paucity of meaningful content, plus impairment of both oral comprehension and repetition; writing is always abnormal, and reading—aloud or for comprehension—is usually so. In contrast to Broca aphasia, in which grammatical words are sometimes omitted and speech consists largely of nouns or verbs, in Wernicke aphasia grammatical phrases occur but there is a dearth of semantic content. The speech may simply sound empty with occasional verbal paraphasias, or there may be nearly total replacement of meaningful words by verbal and literal paraphasias—so called neologistic jargon or jargon aphasia. With its preserved fluency and prosody, the speech may sound like a foreign language, and, indeed, Wernicke aphasia in a patient who never learned English might pass unrecognized by someone familiar only with English. Less severe forms of Wernicke aphasia can be mistaken for schizophrenic speech. A striking feature of severe Wernicke aphasia is anosognosia—inability to recognize the existence of the neurological abnormality.

In Wernicke aphasia there is disruption of the decoding operations necessary for the comprehension of spoken and (usually) written language. Auditory stimuli are no longer recognized as meaningful linguistic symbols; speech and writing, in turn, are devoid of semantic content and contaminated with word errors—paraphasias. As with Broca aphasia, the particular anatomical damage responsible for this type of aphasia has been controversial since Carl Wernicke's original description in 1874. Affected in nearly all cases is the planum temporale (Wernicke's area)—the posterior region of the superior temporal gyrus, considered, in the language–dominant hemisphere, an associative cortex crucial for language processing (and appropriately located adjacent to Heschl's gyrus, the primary auditory cortex) (see Figure 16–1). However, just as Broca's original cases involved destruction of more than Broca's area, Wernicke's cases involved destruction of more than the planum temporale, and nearly all subsequent cases of full-blown Wernicke aphasia have had additional damage in the temporal, temporo-occipital, and parietal lobes. Lesions restricted to Wernicke's area appear to produce a syndrome resembling pure word deafness—there is impaired auditory comprehension, and speech may contain paraphasic errors, but reading comprehension is relatively preserved.

In functional imaging studies—positron emission tomography or functional magnetic resonance imaging—the planum temporale is activated by both linguistic and nonlinguistic auditory stimuli; linguistic stimuli more selectively activate temporal lobe cortex ventral to the planum temporale—in the superior temporal sulcus, the middle temporal gyrus, and the inferior temporal gyrus.

SELECTED REFERENCES

Binder JR, Frost JA, Hammeke TA, et al: Function of the left planum temporale in auditory and linguistic processing. Brain 1996;119:1239.

Caplan D, Gow D, Makris N: Analysis of lesions by MR1 in stroke patients with acoustic-phonetic processing deficits. Neurology 1995;45:293.

Geschwind N, Levitsky W: Human brain: Left-right asymmetries in temporal speech region. Science 1968;161:186.

Price CJ, Wise RJS, Warburton EA, et al: Hearing and saying. The functional neuroanatomy of auditory word processing. Brain 1996;119:911.

▶ CASE 65

Awakening in the morning, a college-educated 62-year-old right-handed man discovers that he cannot see in the right half of his visual field and that written words make no sense to him. Examined several hours later, he has a dense right homonymous hemianopia; visual acuity, other cranial nerves, strength, coordination, gait, sensation, and reflexes are normal. He is alert and attentive with normal spontaneous speech, speech comprehension, and ability to name objects and body parts and to repeat unfamiliar phrases. Shown 10 color samples, he correctly names only 2, and he has difficulty pointing to colors when given their names, yet he correctly matches similar hues and declares that colors appear normal to him. Spontaneous and dictated writing are normal.

Attempting to read standard printed material aloud, he is hesitant, effortful, and incorrect, and he cannot read his own written productions aloud a few minutes later. Reading comprehension is equally impaired. He is able to read individual letters and digits aloud, hesitatingly, and with effort he correctly reads monosyllabic words after repeating their letters sequentially to himself. This strategy does not work for polysyllabic words. He can, however, identify even polysyllabic words when they are spelled aloud to him, and he can spell such words aloud himself.

Computerized tomography reveals left-sided cerebral infarction involving the medial occipital lobe, the inferomedial occipitotemporal junction, and the splenium of the corpus callosum.

Comment

Destruction of this man's left visual (calcarine) cortex has caused right homonymous hemianopia (see Figure 3–2). As a consequence, he sees only with his intact right visual cortex. The lower levels of visual analysis are unimpaired. Also intact are speech, speech comprehension, and, as evidenced by his ability to write, the processing of orthographic word forms. In the language-dominant hemisphere the angular gyrus (a region of cortex at the posterior end of the first temporal sulcus) integrates visual, auditory, and tactile information so as to allow writing; destruction of the language-dominant angular gyrus results in both alexia and agraphia. When the angular gyrus is intact but disconnected from what is seen—and in this patient it is the right visual cortex that is doing all the seeing—the result is *pure alexia*, also referred to as alexia without agraphia. Similar reading impairment occurs in the absence of homonymous hemianopia if a lesion immediately subcortical to the angular gyrus interrupts input from bilaterally intact visual cortices. This concept of alexia without agraphia as a callosal disconnection syndrome was formulated by Dejerine in his original 1892 case report.

Also reflecting intact language-processing areas is the patient's ability to spell words and to identify words spelled aloud. The relatively preserved ability to read single letters aloud probably means that letter (and digit) naming, like object and body part naming, is less dependent on visual-angular gyrus connections and the need for orthographic symbol processing than is the identification of written words. Patients with this kind of alexia, in contrast to those with angular gyrus lesions, can identify short words by reading the individual letters aloud serially. Sometimes reading individual letters is facilitated when the patient traces the letter with a finger; presumably the added tactile information compensates for the loss of visual information.

Studies of individuals with normal reading and language function offer an alternative explanation for pure alexia. Field potential recording from the inferior temporal lobe reveals a region of the anterior fusiform gyrus (also supplied by the posterior cerebral artery) that responds selectively to real words but not nonwords or other complex visual stimuli. Damage to this area has reportedly caused alexia without agraphia or other language disturbances.

Color anomia, frequently encountered, also has more than one possible explanation. Some patients cannot name colors but correctly point to colors that are named; others, like this patient, have bidirectional impairment of matching a color with its name. Some investigators have attempted to explain color anomia in terms of callosal disconnection. Others, noting the frequency with which either alexia or color anomia can occur alone, have correlated color anomia with damage to the inferomedial occipitotemporal lobe. Some pure alexics have either true color agnosia (inability not only to name colors but also to recognize or match them) or achromatopsia (see Case 10).

This man's cerebral infarct followed occlusion of his left posterior cerebral artery distal to penetrating branches that supply the midbrain and thalamus. Strength and sensation are therefore intact. Sometimes encountered in such patients are impaired verbal memory (from damage to left hippocampal and parahippocampal structures) and optic ataxia (clumsiness or difficulty pointing to targets when using the right hand in the intact left visual field, presumably the result of visual information being disconnected from the intact left motor cortex).

SELECTED REFERENCES

Benito-Leon J, Sanchez-Suarez C, Diaz-Guzman J, et al: Pure alexia could not be a disconnection syndrome. Neurology 1997;49:305.

Damasio AR, Damasio H: The anatomic basis of pure alexia. Neurology 1983;33:1573.

Dejerine J: Sur un cas de cecité verbale avec agraphie, suivi d'autopsie. Memoires Soc Biol 1891;3:197.

Geschwind N: Disconnection syndromes in animals and man. Brain 1965;88:237, 585.

Nobre AC, Allison T, McCarthy G: Word recognition in the human inferior temporal lobe. Nature 1994;372:260.

▶ CASE 66

A 59-year-old right-handed man suddenly develops right leg weakness. On examination there is flaccid paralysis of his right ankle and toes and 3/5 strength of more proximal leg muscles. His proximal right arm is mildly weak, but muscles of his right forearm, hand, and face are normal; in particular, he bares his teeth and protrudes his tongue on command. Proprioception is decreased in his right toes, and pain, temperature, and touch sensation are mildly decreased in his right foot. Tendon reflexes at the knee and ankle are less on the right than the left, and the right plantar response is silent.

Praxis is normal in his right arm and hand; on verbal command he correctly demonstrates saluting, hitchhiking, and how he would hammer a nail, strike a match, flip a coin, or use a comb. When told to perform the same acts with his left arm and hand, however, he produces incomplete and inaccurate movements despite normal strength and sensation. Performance improves somewhat when he tries to imitate the examiner's actions. When he is given an actual object (match, coin, comb), he performs the actions correctly.

Language function is normal, including writing with his right hand and naming objects held in his right hand. Attempts to write with his left hand, however, produce dysgraphic abnormalities not explained by clumsiness, and with his eyes closed he cannot name objects held in his left hand. Computerized tomography reveals infarction in the territory of the left anterior cerebral artery involving the medial frontal and parietal lobes and the anterior corpus callosum.

Comment

This man's infarction, involving the motor and sensory cortices of the medial left cerebral hemisphere, predictably resulted in weakness and sensory loss in his right leg with preserved strength, coordination, and praxis in his right hand. Praxis was impaired, however, on his good left side.

Apraxia is an inability to perform a learned motor act in response to a stimulus that normally would evoke it; the difficulty is not explained by impaired strength, sensation, comprehension, or attention. The term has been applied to a variety of motor and perceptual disturbances; the type exemplified by this patient is termed *ideomotor apraxia,* and since its original description by Hugo Liepmann nearly a century ago it has been attributed to disconnection of motor and premotor cortex either from language areas, from areas containing motor engrams (ie, movement programs), or from both.

Lesions involving the language-dominant retrorolandic parietal lobe or the arcuate fasciculus, which connects Wernicke's area to Broca's area and other frontal opercular areas, might produce such a disconnection. The result would be bilateral ideomotor apraxia—inability to perform learned acts involving the mouth and tongue (eg, blowing out a match) or the limbs (such as the tasks described above) on command. If motor engrams are intact and not disconnected from motor cortices, performance will improve with imitation or when an actual object is used. These motor engrams, representing a time-space-form representation of the movement, are believed by some investigators to be situated in the posterior superior parietal lobe, an associative area with visual, tactile, and motor connections.

This patient's ideomotor apraxia, affecting his left side only, is the result of damage to his anterior corpus callosum, which disconnects his left hemispheric language areas from his right motor and premotor cortex. The same disconnection explains his left-handed agraphia and tactile anomia. Some patients with such apraxia (termed sympathetic apraxia) perform motor acts more accurately when imitating the examiner or when holding the appropriate object in the left hand; others do not. A plausible explanation for the difference is that in over 95% of right-handed people language is processed by the left hemisphere, whereas motor programming has less predictable cerebral dominance, being largely left hemispheric in some people and bihemispheric in others. The above patient's improvement with object use suggests that his right hemisphere participated in motor programming.

SELECTED REFERENCES

Gazzaniga MS, Bogen JE, Sperry RW: Dyspraxia following division of the cerebral commissures. Arch Neurol 1967;16:606.

Geschwind N: The apraxias: Neural mechanisms of disorders of learned movement. Am Sci 1975;63:188.

Volpe BT, Sidtis JJ, Holtzman JD, et al: Cortical mechanisms involved in praxis: Observation following partial and complete section of the corpus collosum in man. Neurology 1982;32:645.

Watson RT, Heilman KM: Callosal apraxia. Brain 1983;106:391.

▶ CASE 67

A 58-year-old right-handed man suddenly develops left hemiparesis and complains that both words and music sound like noise to him. On examination speech, naming, writing, and reading are normal, but speech comprehension and repetition are impossible. Mild left hemiparesis and hemisensory loss are most evident in his arm and hand. Computerized tomography (CT) reveals bilateral lesions affecting the posterior superior temporal lobes with extension into the temporal isthmus; the right-sided lesion extends into prerolandic, postrolandic, and inferior parietal areas and, unlike the left-sided lesion, enhances with contrast material.

The diagnosis is bilateral cerebral infarction, old on the left and new on the right. Doppler and angiographic studies reveal marked stenosis of the right internal carotid artery, and he undergoes uneventful right carotid endarterectomy. Receiving speech therapy, he learns to lip-read. His speech comprehension is better when he also hears what is being said, yet speech alone continues to sound "like a foreign language." Although he had played the violin, music is incomprehensible to him, and environmental noise is bothersome.

Examined a year later, he has fluent, prosodic, grammatically correct speech with rare paraphasic errors. He cannot comprehend speech except when also lip-reading, and, although bilingual in English and French, he cannot tell which language is being spoken. He has great difficulty identifying single consonants but is nearly normal with vowels. Naming, reading, and writing are normal. He cannot recognize or sing familiar melodies, and on tests of sound recognition he makes frequent errors. He identifies a cat's meow as "a girl singing," coughing as "a man speaking a foreign language," a machine gun as "somebody climbing steps," and an airplane as "seashore waves."

Pure tone audiometry is nearly normal, with mild bilateral sensorineural hearing loss up to 2000 Hz and moderate loss above that. Evoked response testing reveals normal auditory processing at the level of the brain stem but abnormal processing in both temporal lobes, worse on the right. Other tests reveal abnormal temporal resolution of auditory stimuli; he has difficutly either detecting two successive clicks separated by short intervals or counting clicks separated at high frequency. His auditory comprehension improves when speech is presented at a slower rate.

Comment

Agnosia is a failure of recognition that cannot be explained by elementary sensory loss, intellectual impairment, aphasia, inattention, or unfamiliarity. The neuropsychologist Hans-Lukas Teuber described agnosia as "a normal percept that has somehow been stripped of its meaning." Different kinds of agnosias involve tactile, visual, and auditory recognition, and different models have been proposed to explain them.

Over a century ago Heinrich Lissauer defined two stages of recognition. During apperceptive recognition the separate sensory features of what is perceived are combined into a whole. During associative recognition what is perceived is matched to a previous experience, thereby giving it meaning. Whether the different agnosias encountered clinically are either apperceptive or associative has been controversial ever since.

This patient has lost the ability to recognize sounds despite adequate hearing as measured by audiometry. He cannot recognize spoken words even though his language function is otherwise intact (*pure word deafness*); he also has difficulty recognizing nonspeech sounds (*auditory sound agnosia*). Particularly impaired, despite previous training, is his ability to recognize (and to produce) music.

CT and evoked response testing reveal bilateral temporal lobe damage affecting areas involved in auditory processing. The larger right-sided lesion has largely destroyed the primary auditory cortex (Heschl's gyrus), adjacent auditory associative areas, and auditory radiations projecting to these cortical areas from the thalamic medial geniculate nucleus. The smaller left-sided lesion has spared the primary auditory cortex, and one might attribute the word deafness to disconnection of Heschl's gyrus from auditory associative areas of the language hemisphere, particularly the planum temporale (Wernicke's area) (see Case 64).

Disconnection models less readily explain the patient's agnosia for nonspeech sounds. Word deafness and agnosia for nonverbal sounds often occur together, as in the present case, but either can occur alone, indicating separate processing mechanisms for linguistic and nonlinguistic sounds. Both mechanisms would require intact auditory temporal acuity, which in this patient, as evidenced by the click discrimination tests, was impaired, indicating an apperceptive component to his agnosia. Whether that loss is sufficient to explain all of his abnormalities—including receptive and expressive amusia—is speculative, as is the locus of damage responsible. Auditory agnosia encompasses a number of clinical syndromes, and although they predict superior temporal lobe damage, lesions causing either word deafness, agnosia for nonverbal sounds, or receptive amusia have been unilateral as well as bilateral and subcortical as well as cortical.

SELECTED REFERENCES

Auerbach SH, Allard T, Naeser M, et al: Pure word deafness. Analysis of a case with bilateral lesions and a defect at the prephonemic level. Brain 1982;105:271.

Bauer RM: Agnosia. In: Heilman KM, Valenstein E (eds): *Clinical Neuropsychology,* 3rd edition (pp. 215–278). Oxford University Press, 1993.

Motomura N, Yamadori A, Mori E, Tamaru F: Auditory agnosia: Analysis of a case with bilateral subcortical lesions. Brain 1986;109:379.

Oppenheimer DR, Newcombe F: Clinical and anatomic findings in a case of auditory agnosia. Arch Neurol 1978;35:712.

▶ CASE 68

A 57-year-old woman is brought to the hospital after being found at home unable to move her left arm. Expressing annoyance, the patient denies that anything is wrong with her other than high blood pressure. On examination there is obvious weakness of her left face, with sparing of her forehead, and there is no spontaneous movement of her left arm or leg. She readily makes eye contact and answers questions when the examiner is to her right; when addressed from the left, however, she either ignores the question or gives answers without making eye contact. Although her eyes occasionally move to the left, they are directed to the right of midline most of the time. Asked to raise her right arm, she does so; asked to raise her left arm, she raises her right, and when asked why she did not raise her left arm, she replies that she did raise it. When each of her hands is placed within her right visual field, she identifies the right as her own and the left as the examiner's. Asked to bisect a horizontally drawn line, she places her mark well to the right of midline, and when asked to copy simple diagrams, she omits details on the left. Shown a circle and asked to put in numbers to make a clock face, she places the numbers, 1 through 12, entirely on the right side. She is, however, alert, attentive, and cooperative, and language function, orientation, and memory are intact. She does not blink to threat from the left side or report seeing objects in her left visual field, and she does not report any stimuli, including pinprick, delivered to her left face, arm, trunk, or leg. Her left limbs are flaccid and do not move in response to painful stimuli. Tendon reflexes are slightly brisker on the left, and her left plantar response is silent.

Computerized tomography shows hypodensity with mass effect, consistent with acute infarction, in the territory of the right middle cerebral artery, including the inferior parietal and posterior temporal lobes.

Over the next few weeks voluntary movement returns to her left leg, but her left face and arm remain severely weak, and her arm becomes hypertonic. She now acknowledges that her left arm is her own and that it is paralyzed. Notable, however, is an apparent lack of concern over her disability and a tendency to refer to her left arm and leg as if they were objects. Sensation remains impaired on the left, and she frequently reports tactile or painful stimuli to her left arm as felt on her right arm. A year later sensation is nearly normal on the left, and visual fields are grossly intact, but when visual or tactile stimuli are presented simultaneously and bilaterally, only the right-sided stimuli are recognized.

Comment

Acutely this woman's stroke caused not only left hemiplegia but also *hemineglect,* defined as a failure to report or respond to meaningful stimuli presented contralateral to a brain lesion and not attributable to either weakness or sensory loss. As with aphasia, neglect exists in the absence of general cognitive impairment. It can involve the contralateral half of one's own body with inability to recognize obvious hemiplegia (*anosognosia*) or the identity of one's own limbs (*hemiasomatognosia*). Some patients fail to dress or groom their abnormal sides. They may express alarm that someone else is sharing their beds.

Neglect also involves extracorporeal space (*spatial neglect*). When mild, there is a tendency to ignore stimuli contralateral to the lesion or a failure to recognize them when they are delivered simultaneously with ipsilateral stimuli. Such extinction includes auditory and visual stimuli, and since unilateral cerebral lesions do not cause contralateral deafness, auditory neglect is evidence that hemineglect is a higher order polymodal disorder, not simply a defect of sensory input. Similarly, visual extinction can be present in the absence of homonymous hemianopia, and abnormal line bisection and picture copying occur even when the tasks are performed in hemispace ipsilateral to the lesion. When severe, as in this case, hemispatial neglect produces complete psychic obliteration of contralateral space, making it impossible to assess contralateral vision or sensation. Patients have even demonstrated defective representational memory for the left side of scenes they were trying to recall; for example, a patient asked to describe a room might omit objects that would be on his left, whichever direction he was facing. Such observations suggest the existence of cerebral representational maps, with the left hemispace represented in the right hemisphere.

Right hemineglect also exists but is less frequent than left hemineglect, even when coexisting aphasia is taken into account. A proposed explanation is that hemineglect reflects hemiinattention (as against a disturbance of sensory input) and that in most people the right hemisphere participates in attention to both left and right hemispace, whereas the left hemisphere contributes to attentiveness in only right hemispace. Left hemispheric damage is unlikely to produce hemineglect because the intact right hemisphere is still attending to both left and right hemispace; by contrast, right hemispheric damage produces left hemineglect because the intact left hemisphere is attending only to right hemispace. Physiological studies in humans and animals support such a hypothesis.

The precise anatomical basis of sensory hemineglect is uncertain. Lesions usually involve the parietooccipital or temporo-occipital lobes, and the severity of the syndrome seems to depend as much on the size of the lesion as on involvement of particular cortical areas. In animals hemineglect follows lesions of either the mesencephalic reticular formation, the thalamus, or the posterior temporal and parietal lobes, and studies in monkeys have defined neurons in the posterior inferior parietal lobule that fire in response only to stimuli of importance to the animal. The inferior parietal lobule is considered a supramodal area, in which polymodal sensory information (tactile, visual, and auditory) is integrated and conveyed to frontal and limbic structures. Attention can be considered as having several components: arousal (reticular activating system), sensory/spatial (parietal), motor/intent (frontal), and emotional/motivational (limbic). Different kinds of hemineglect follow damage to each component (see Case 32).

As demonstrated by this patient, the more florrid features of hemineglect tend to clear over days or weeks. Although she became aware of her weakness and the proper ownership of her left extremities, she demonstrated an inappropriate lack of concern over her impairment (*anosodiaphoria*) and viewed her left limbs in an impersonal way. For a time, stimuli presented to her left were localized to her right (*allesthesia*). Eventually, her left-sided visual and sensory impairment consisted simply of residual extinction.

SELECTED REFERENCES

Binder JR, Marshall R, Lazar RM, et al: Distinct syndromes of hemineglect. Arch Neurol 1992;49:1187.

Bisiach E, Luzzatti C, Pernai D: Unilateral neglect, representational schema and consciousness. Brain 1979;102:609.

Heilman KM, Watson RT, Valenstein E: Neglect and related disorders. In: Heilman KM, Valenstein E (eds): *Clinical Neuropsychology,* 3rd edition (pp. 279–336). Oxford University Press, 1993.

Small M, Ellis S: Denial of hemiplegia: An investigation into the theories of causation. Eur Neurol 1996;36:353.

► CASE 69

A 55-year-old woman suddenly develops impaired vision, and computerized tomographic (CT) scan reveals bilateral temporo-occipital infarcts. Thereafter she is unable to recognize any face learned before her illness or to learn any new faces. She identifies friends and relatives by recognizing their voices.

On examination several years later, intellect and language function are intact. She is unable to identify the faces of any famous people, yet she has no difficulty recognizing faces as such, and she can distinguish facial gender, estimate facial age, and recognize the meaning of different facial expressions (sadness, anger, fear, surprise). There is a right superior homonymous quadrantanopia and a left superior homonymous quadrantanopic paracentral scotoma extending 10° out from fixation. Color perception is impaired in the entire left visual field. Stereopsis and perception of movement are normal. Computerized tomography and magnetic resonance imaging confirm bilateral temporo-occipital infarcts involving the fusiform and lingual gyri. The left lesion is larger, and the right lesion extends more posteriorly, but neither lesion involves the calcarine region of the occipital lobe.

Comment

Prosopagnosia refers to agnosia for faces; familiar persons can no longer be recognized on the basis of visual perception of their faces. Severely affected patients may be unable to recognize their own faces. It is not a global amnestic disorder; memory for specific events can be otherwise intact, and the person whose face is not recognized is readily identified by voice or other attributes such as hair style, clothes, or gait. Neither is it a selective inability to name. Depending on the anatomical extent of the lesion, some prosopagnosic patients also have alexia (see Case 65), but language function is otherwise preserved. Prosopagnosic patients often have central achromatopsia (see Case 10) or, as a consequence of damage to the visual radiations or the calcarine cortex, visual field abnormalities. Some have visual agnosia for more than faces, but prosopagnosia exists with otherwise normal or near normal visual perception.

In apperceptive prosopagnosia impaired facial recognition reflects a less specific perceptual disorder; mental manipulation of visual images is disturbed at a processing level proximal to higher association areas necessary for recognition. Such patients misjudge line orientations and simple geometric shapes, and in contrast to associative prosopagnosics, they cannot match unfamiliar faces.

Autopsies on prosopagnosic patients have revealed bilateral temporo-occipital lesions. CT reports have described unilateral lesions, and prosopagnosia has followed right hemispherectomy; such cases do not exclude the possibility of a preexisiting contralateral hemispheric abnormality. Temporo-occipital lesions involving the fusiform and lingual gyri would disconnect primary visual processing areas of the occipital lobe from higher associative areas of the temporal lobes involved in visual memory.

The particular vulnerability of facial recognition appears to be the consequence of each face's uniqueness. The normal ability to recognize thousands of faces is unlike any other nonverbal visual task, for in no other area of perception does a superordinate category—in this instance face—encompass such a large number of significant but subtly different subordinate examples—the faces of particular individuals. Some prosopagnosic patients demonstrate superordinate/subordinate dissociation in other categories, for example, the ability to identify a dog or a cat as such but not *which* dog or cat. Some have difficulty identifying their own cars, sorting their own clothes, or telling different foods from one another. Such observations suggest that prosopagnosia is the most disabling manifestation of an inability to identify the specific historic context of a particular visual stimulus when the stimulus belongs to a visually ambiguous category—that is, when a large number of its different members are visually similar.

Facial recognition appears to involve holistic processing, in contrast to recognition of most objects, which is primarily analytic. Evidence for such a dichotomy is a report of a man who, following head injury, had visual object agnosia—objects looked like blobs to him—yet he could still recognize faces. When faces were inverted, however, he could no longer recognize them, presumably because their recognition now required analytic processing.

In primates, individual neurons of the inferior temporo-occipital cortex have remarkably large and complex receptive fields, which invariably include the foveal region and, unlike the receptive fields of most neurons in the occipital cortex, include large areas of both visual hemifields. Some of these neurons respond preferentially to faces, and those that respond to frontal views of faces are aligned in separate columns adjacent to those that respond to profiles (Figure 16–2). By impairing pattern recognition at this level, temporo-occipital lesions prevent visual images from triggering specific memories; the most prominent manifestation of this disconnection is prosopagnosia.

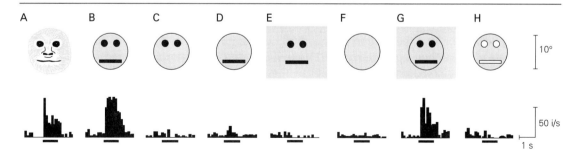

Figure 16–2. Response of a neuron in the inferior temporal cortex of a monkey to complex stimuli. The cell responded strongly to the face of a toy monkey (**A**) and to images containing two black spots and one horizontal black bar arranged on a gray disk with a circular outline (**B, G**), but not to images missing one or more of these features (**C, D, E, F, H**). (Reproduced with permission from Kandel ER, Schwartz JH, Jessell TM. 1999. *Principles of Neural Science*, 4th ed. New York: McGraw-Hill. Adapted with permission from Kobatake E, Tanaka K. 1994. Neural selectivities to complex object features in the ventral visual pathway of the macaque cerebral cortex. J Neurophys 71:856.)

SELECTED REFERENCES

Damasio A, Tranel D, Damasio H: Face agnosia and the neural substrates of memory. Neuroscience 1990;13:89.

Gorno Tempini ML, Price CJ, Josephs O, et al: The neural systems sustaining face and proper name processing. Brain 1998;121:2103.

McCarthy G, Puce A, Gore JC, Allison T: Face-specific processing in the human fusiform gyrus. J Cog Neurosci 1997;9:605.

Moscovitch M, Winocur G, Behrmann M: What is special about face recognition? Nineteen experiments on a person with visual object agnosia and dyslexia but normal face recognition. J Cog Neurosci 1997;9:555.

Tanaka K: Inferotemporal cortex and object vision. Annu Rev Neurosci 1996;19:109.

▶ CASE 70

A 58-year-old woman is brought to the hospital by her husband, who reports that several hours earlier she began acting strangely. On examination it is evident that she is blind. She cannot detect hand movements or a bright light directed to either eye, yet she denies her blindness and confabulates responses when asked to identify objects held in front of her. Disoriented to time and place, she gives the wrong year and claims she is at home in her apartment. Her pupils are equal in size and normally reactive to light. Findings on her neurological examination, including optic fundi and eye movements, are otherwise normal.

Computerized tomography reveals lucency and mild swelling in both occipital lobes, consistent with acute infarction. Over the next few weeks she continues to insist that she can see despite obvious evidence to the contrary. Her disorientation also persists, with variable misidentifications of where she is. She also describes hallucinations and delusions; for example, she reports being visited by a long-deceased relative.

Comment

Anosognosia for blindness—Anton syndrome—has been recognized for nearly a century, but its neurophysiological basis remains a mystery. Sometimes associated with lesions of the retina, optic nerves, or optic chiasm, it is most often encountered in patients with occipital lobe damage, particularly, as in this patient, infarction in the territory of both posterior cerebral arteries. Mentation is seldom otherwise intact; most patients misplace themselves in time and space, for example, admitting that they are in the hospital but maintaining that the hospital occupies a wing of their apartment building (*reduplicative paramnesia*). Formed hallucinations are also common, and belief in their reality can result in delusions, but neither disorientation nor hallucinations account for the patients' steadfast insistence that they can see.

Occipital injury alone does not readily explain Anton syndrome either, for most patients with bilateral infarction of the calcarine cortex do not deny their blindness. In addition to the occipital lobes, the posterior cerebral arteries also supply parts of the midbrain, most of the thalamus, and the inferior temporal lobes, but damage to those structures, although plausibly contributing to altered mentation in patients with posterior cerebral artery occlusion, would not explain anosognosia in patients with anterior (peripheral) lesions.

Possibly relevant to denial of blindness is *blindsight*. In the original clinical report, a man whose right calcarine cortex was removed during surgery for a vascular malformation was left with a dense left homonymous hemianopia. He declared that he could see nothing in his hemianopic visual field, yet when told to guess, he correctly identified the location and shape of objects placed there, expressing surprise that he had been able to do so. Such residual visual capacity has also been demonstrated experimentally in monkeys.

Blindsight is consistent with the existence of parallel pathways processing visual information, not all of which reach conscious experience. The major visual pathway mediating conscious visual experience is from the retina to the lateral geniculate nucleus of the thalamus and then to the primary (striate) visual cortex in the occipital lobe, but there are also direct retinal projections to other areas, for example, the pulvinar of the thalamus and the superior colliculus in the midbrain. Patients rendered blind from damage to the primary visual cortex but in whom such parallel pathways are preserved might experience a kind of visual imagery that gives them the impression they can see. In patients with peripheral blindness, in whom all visual pathways are presumably interrupted, visual imagery acquired before injury and persisting in memory might be sufficient to create a similar anosognosia.

SELECTED REFERENCES

Redlich FC, Dorsey JF: Denial of blindness by patients with cerebral disease. Arch Neurol Psychiatry 1945;53:407.
Stoerig P, Cowey A: Blindsight in man and monkey. Brain 1997;120:535.
Symonds C, Mackenzie I: Bilateral loss of vision from cerebral infarction. Brain 1957; 80:415.
Weiskranz L: Blindsight revisited. Curr Opin Neurobiol 1996;6:215.

▶ CASE 71

For 11 years, a 21-year-old woman has had attacks of incapacitating fearfulness. At age 3, she experienced two major motor (grand mal) convulsions, with loss of consciousness and tonic-clonic movements. One of the seizures was associated with fever, and the other was not. At age 10 she began having episodes of fear lasting 2 minutes to 12 hours. Remaining alert, she becomes frightened, perspires, and does not want to be left alone. These spells are not accompanied by hallucinations or stereotyped movements (automatisms). However, she also has frequent nocturnal episodes during which she crawls around the bed, moans, chews, salivates, and looks fearful. Some spells progress to major motor convulsions.

At age 21 her neurological examination and computerized tomographic scan are normal. Interictal electroencephalograms reveal multiple bilateral independent spikes that predominate in the right anterior temporal region (see Figure 11–2). During attacks of fear, rhythmic 2- to 3-Hz waves appear in the right midtemporal region, and the anterior temporal spiking increases. Nocturnal seizures with automatisms begin with either right anterior temporal or bitemporal bisynchronous rhythmic waves.

Because the seizures are refractory to anticonvulsant drugs, she undergoes right temporal lobectomy. An intraoperative electrocorticogram reveals intermittent spikes arising from a focus 2 cm behind the tip of the right temporal lobe.

The resected anterior 4 cm of the temporal lobe includes the amygdala but not the hippocampus. Pathologically there is cortical gliosis, clumping and thinning of neurons, and ectopic neurons in the subcortical white matter. Following surgery her seizures, including attacks of fear, are well controlled with anticonvulsant medication.

Comment

Epileptic seizures are caused by abnormal hypersynchronous electrical discharges of neurons in the cerebral cortex. Generalized seizures, which include *grand mal* convulsions and *petit mal* absence, involve the cerebral hemispheres diffusely from the outset (see Figure 12–19). Partial (or focal) seizures begin in one part of a cerebral hemisphere, and so clinical manifestations—whether motor, sensory, or subjective—will depend on the location of the epileptic discharge (see Cases 4, 16, and 30). *Auras* are subjective epileptic (*ictal*) symptoms that are not associated with objective signs such as altered consciousness or motor activity. Auras may consist of illusions, hallucinations, altered self-awareness (depersonalization), a sense of strangeness regarding one's surroundings (derealization), an emotional intrusion, or simply an indescribable feeling. In many patients, spread of the epileptic discharge causes further epileptic phenomena, including progression to a grand mal convulsion, and such patients may consider their aura as warning of an impending attack. An aura, however, signifies focal ictal discharge (see Case 4).

One of the most common auras is fear, which can be intense yet is undirected; it is not fear of anyone or anything, nor is it simply an appropriate emotional response to a signal that a seizure has begun. As Hughlings Jackson put it a century ago, it is "fear which comes by itself—the symptom of fear." *Ictal fear* has nearly always been associated with lesions of the inferomedial temporal lobe, either right or left sided. Electrical stimulation studies in animals and humans implicate the amygdala as the source of ictal fear. When the hippocampus is stimulated, fear occurs only when afterdischarges spread to the amygdala, but stimulation of the amygdala alone produces immediate fear.

Each of the three divisons of the amygdala is involved with an organism's response to stimuli (Figure 16–3). The basolateral nucleus receives projections from higher order sensory and association cortical areas and sends projections to other limbic areas, including the cingulate gyrus, the medial orbitofrontal cortex, the hippocampus, the dorsomedial nucleus of the thalamus (a relay nucleus that projects to association areas of the frontal lobe), and the basal nucleus of Meynert (the source of widespread cholinergic projections to the cerebral cortex). Critical for attaching conscious emotional significance to a stimulus and for imprinting the emotional response in memory, the basolateral nucleus also projects to the amygdala's central nucleus, which receives afferent imput from brain stem viscerosensory structures and projects to brain stem autonomic nuclei and the hypothalamus. The central nucleus thus modulates autonomic nervous system responses to emotionally significant stimuli. Finally, the amygdala's corticomedial nuclei receive olfactory stimuli from the olfactory bulb and project to the ventromedial nuclei of the hypothalamus; the corticomedial nuclei thus mediate the effects of olfactory stimuli on behaviors such as eating and sexual activity.

In monkeys bilateral removal of the anterior and inferomedial temporal lobes, including the amygdala, the hippocampus, and the nonlimbic temporal cortex, produces the Klüver-Bucy syndrome—placidity, lack of fear, orality (putting any object in the mouth, whether food or not), increased sexual behavior, compulsive reactivity to any visual stimulus, and apparent inability to recognize familiar objects. Loss of temporal lobe visual association areas probably accounts for the visual agnosia (see Case 69), and loss of the hippocampi probably accounts for the impaired memory. Removal of the amygdala most likely explains the absence of fear and the oral and sexual dysfunction. Symptoms reminiscent of the Klüver-Bucy syndrome have occurred in humans followng bilateral temporal lobe injury, and surgical amygdalectomy has been performed on emotionally disturbed subjects with uncontrollable fear or anger.

In addition to her subjective aura, this patient's seizures consisted of *automatisms,* complex motor activity that is inappropriate and undirected. In contrast to the stereotypic tonic or clonic motor activity produced by stimulation of the frontal lobe motor cortex (see Case 30), automatisms range from primitive movements such as chewing, licking, or swallowing to more complex actions such as perserveration of an ongoing motor task, fumbling with clothes, handling whatever object is near, wandering as if in a daze, muttering, mumbling, or humming. There is usually, but not always, amnesia for the episode. Complex and organized behavior can resemble a fugue state and, when prolonged, more often indicates postictal confusion than a continuing seizure discharge. Electroencephalographic and video monitoring are often necessary to identify precisely the transition from an ictal to a postictal state or to distinguish epileptic

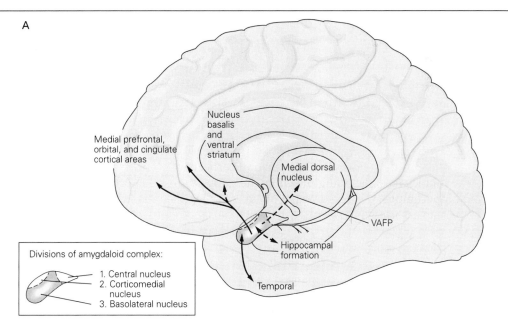

Figure 16–3. Principal connections of the amygdaloid complex, the three divisions of which are depicted in the inset. Shown here and on the next page are connections of the basolateral complex (**A**), the central nuclei (**B**), and the corticomedial nuclei (**C**). Anatomical contiguity of the amygdala, the hippocampal formation, and temporal lobe visual association areas accounts for the clustering of signs—Klüver-Bucy syndrome—following bilateral removal of the anterior and inferomedial temporal lobes. VAFP, ventral amygdalofugal pathway. (Reproduced with permission from Martin JH. 1996. *Neuroanatomy Text and Atlas,* 2nd ed. Stamford, CT: Appleton & Lange.)

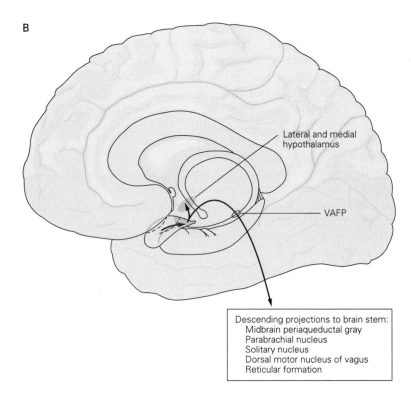

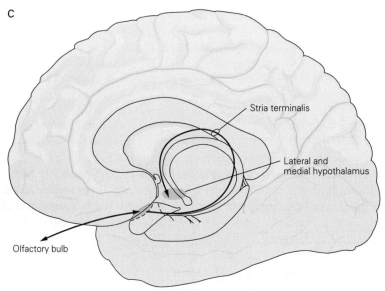

Figure 16–3. *(continued)*

automatisms from psychiatric illness. The great majority of patients with seizures of this type have lesions of the temporal lobe, but, not surprisingly, the circuitry responsible for producing such complex phenomena is uncertain. Some investigators consider automatisms a negative phenomenon—that is, ictal paralysis of temporal lobe function produces confusion, semipurposeful movements, and amnesia physiologically no different from the similar phenomena observed postictally.

SELECTED REFERENCES

Gloor P: Experiential phenomena of temporal lobe epilepsy. Facts and hypotheses. Brain 1990;113:1673.

Hermann BP, Chhabria S: Interictal psychopathology in patients with ictal fear. Examples of sensory-limbic hyperconnection? Arch Neurol 1980;37:667.

McLachlan RS, Blume WT: Isolated fear in complex partial status epilepticus. Ann Neurol 1980;8:639.

Strauss E, Risser A, Jones MW: Fear responses in patients with epilepsy. Arch Neurol 1982;39:626.

Swanson LW, Petrovich GD: What is the amygdala? Trends Neurosci 1998;21:323.

► CASE 72

A 14-year-old boy has had episodes of altered behavior since sustaining a head injury with loss of consciousness at the age of 3. During attacks he sees a room that is different from the room he is in; he seems to be in the room but does not see himself there. The room then appears to move into the distance as if he were looking at it through the wrong end of binoculars. Some spells progress to major motor seizures, during which his head and eyes turn to the right. Treatment with antiepileptic drugs is ineffective.

Electroencephalography shows high-voltage spikes over the left temporal region (see Figure 11–2). Imaging studies reveal enlargement of the temporal horn of the left lateral ventricle. At surgery there is scarring of the anterior tip of the left temporal lobe, particularly inferiorly. The anterior 5 cm of the left temporal lobe is therefore resected, but before that is done, cortical stimulation studies are performed under local anesthesia with the patient awake.

When the superior temporal gyrus is stimulated, the patient reports hearing a song, although he is unable to say if it is being sung or played by an orchestra. When stimulation of this region is repeated, he again hears a song and this time sees two boys playing, but he cannot tell what they are doing. When a more posterior superior temporal region is stimulated, he sees and hears two men sitting in armchairs singing a different song. When the middle temporal gyrus is stimulated, he sees a man and a dog walking; asked if they are in town or the country, he describes seeing only the man and the dog. When the inferior temporal gyrus is stimulated, he describes "something which has happened to me before" but cannot say what it was.

Comment

This patient was reported by the neurosurgeon Wilder Penfield over 40 years ago. (The imaging technologies at his disposal were cerebral angiography and pneumoencephalography, not computerized tomography or magnetic resonance imaging, and there were few available anticonvulsants.) It had long been recognized that seizures of temporal lobe origin could consist of illusions, hallucinations, or memories. Penfield showed that such subjective experiences can be reproduced by direct cortical stimulation. Stimulating the primary visual cortex produces flashes of light or simple geometric shapes; stimulating temporal and occipital lobe visual association areas produces formed hallucinations, particularly people. Similarly, stimulating the primary auditory cortex produces simple noises; stimulating temporal lobe auditory association areas produces voices or music. Hallucinations can be simultaneously visual and auditory, and they are sometimes clearly identified from past experience. Sometimes, as in this patient, a memory is experienced but cannot be described. In other patients ictal memory phenomena consist of *déjà vu* (already seen), a weird sense of familiarity in an unfamiliar environment.

When we hear the name of a familiar person or piece of music, we do not actually see the person or hear the music. Epileptic memories, by contrast, can be frankly hallucinatory; they are, however, more fragmentory and static than hallucinations encountered in psychiatric illness. Voices can be identified, but what is being said usually cannot, and visual images are incomplete and, unlike a dream, without a plot. They are thus more like snapshots than tape recordings of past experiences.

Experiential auras of this sort are reproduced by stimulation of limbic structures—in particular, the hippocampus and the amygdala as well as temporal lobe neocortex—and, not surprisingly, they often have strong emotional content (see Case 71). That stimulation of a small number of neurons can produce such a vivid and intrusive recall of a past experience is consistent with parallel distributed processing (PDP) models of cognition. In PDP a perception or a recollection is represented by the particular pattern of excitation and inhibition in a network of neuronal groups widely scattered over isocortex and the limbic system. In normal experience a pattern representing a past experience can be triggered by stimulation of any of its components (eg, visual, auditory, or emotional); in focal epilepsy, spontaneous firing within or adjacent to a neuronal group participating in the pattern will similarly trigger a memory, a percept, or both.

The stereotypy of *epileptic experiential auras* is explained in terms of Hebb's rule: When neuron A repeatedly excites neuron B, subsequent synaptic excitation of neuron B by neuron A becomes increasingly efficient. Such synaptic plasticity probably also explains why complex experiential phenomena are rarely produced by electrical stimulation of the temporal lobe in nonepileptics. Presumably over time repeated epileptic discharges have triggered particular PDP network patterns sufficiently to strengthen their specific connections. In a broad sense, learning has occurred.

SELECTED REFERENCES

Bancaud J, Brunet-Bourgin F, Chauvel P, Halgren E: Anatomical origin of déjà vu and vivid memories in human temporal lobe epilepsy. Brain 1994;117:71.

Hallgren E, Chauvel P: Experiential phenomena evoked by human brain electrical stimulation. Adv Neurol 1992;65:87.

Mesulam M-M: From sensation to cognition. Brain 1998;121:1013.

Penfield W, Jasper H: *Epilepsy and the Functional Anatomy of the Human Brain.* Little, Brown, 1954.

► CASE 73

A 75-year-old right-handed college graduate becomes forgetful. She has increasing difficulty remembering people's names and often forgets minor events, misses appointments, and misplaces objects. On examination, she is well-groomed and socially appropriate, with normal spontaneous speech. She correctly identifies where she is and the month and year, but 5 minutes after correctly repeating three unrelated words, she can recall only one of them and then only by selecting it from a list. Speech comprehension is normal, and she correctly names objects she is shown, but she is abnormally hesitant at generating words of a single category (eg, animals or clothing). Asked to describe similarities between two words (eg, automobile and bicycle), she tends to give differences instead, and she has difficulty adding and subtracting numbers larger than 10. Attempts to copy simple geometric designs are clumsy and oversimplified. Findings on her physical and neurological examinations are otherwise normal.

Computerized tomography shows moderate cerebral atrophy, with widened cortical sulci and enlargement of the lateral and third ventricles. Magnetic resonance imaging coronal sections show bilateral shrinkage of her hippocampi. Single-photon emission computerized tomography reveals maximal reductions of blood flow over the posterior parietal and temporal cerebral cortices bilaterally. Metabolic and toxicological studies to exclude treatable causes of dementia are normal.

Over the next few years her mental state progressively worsens. Her speech becomes increasingly hesitant as a result of word-finding difficulty, and she often seems unable to grasp what is said to her. Unless observed, she tends to wander off, and it is evident that she does not know the correct year or her own age. Requiring a home aide, she sometimes displays paranoid delusions—for example, accusing the aide of hiding her belongings—and there are outbursts of agitation. Grooming becomes neglected, and she has difficulty using eating utensils. Six years after onset of symptoms, she is admitted to a nursing home, where her speech becomes reduced to monosyllables and she stops walking. Prior to her death from pneumonia she sits motionless in a chair without any evident awareness of her surroundings.

At autopsy there is diffuse cerebral atrophy most marked in the prefrontal and temporoparietal cortex and the hippocampus, with markedly reduced numbers of large neurons and moderate astrocytosis. Severe neuronal loss also affects the nucleus basalis of Meynert, the locus coeruleus, and the brain stem raphe nuclei. Scattered throughout the cerebral cortex are numerous senile plaques; many neurons, particularly those of the hippocampus, entorhinal cortex, and amygdala, contain neurofibrillary tangles.

Comment

The prevalence of *Alzheimer disease* is age dependent; it affects 1–4% of people aged 65–70 years and 22% (or more) of people aged 85–90 years. This patient's clinical course is typical, and the progression of her symptoms reflects, to a degree, the anatomical distribution of her cerebral pathology.

Two histological features define the pathology of Alzheimer disease (Figure 16–4). Neurofibrillary tangles are cytoplasmic accumulations within neurons of silver-staining fiber-like strands, which at electron microscopy consist of

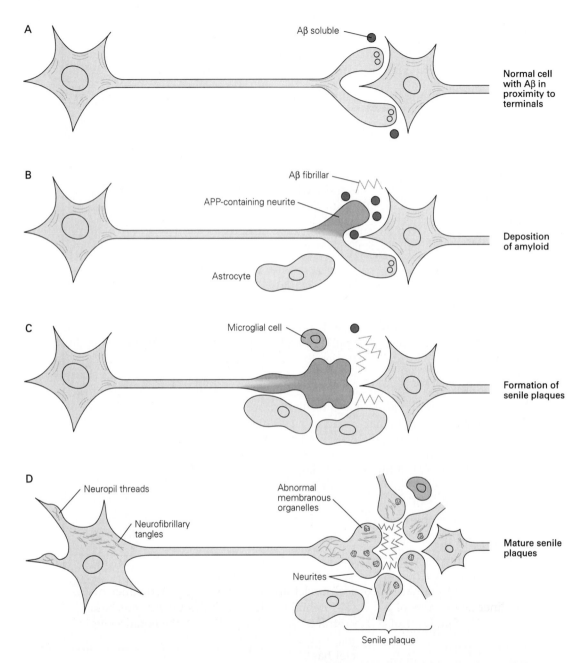

Figure 16–4. Neuronal pathology in Alzheimer disease. Neurofibrillary tangles in the cell body consist of paired helical filaments containing tau protein, a component of normal microtubules. Senile plaques consist of degenerating neuronal and glial processes surrounding a central core of Aβ amyloid protein, derived from proteolytic cleavage of amyloid precursor protein (APP). **A.** Normal neuron. **B–D.** Neurons in Alzheimer disease. (Reproduced with permission from Kandel ER, Schwartz JH, Jessell TM. 1999. *Principles of Neural Science,* 4th ed. New York: McGraw-Hill.)

straight or paired helical filaments. Neurofibrillary tangles are composed principally of phosphorylated tau, a protein normally associated with microtubules (see Case 77). Senile or neuritic plaques are silver-staining deposits of amorphous material surrounded by degenerating nerve and glial processes; electron microscopy and histological stains reveal the material to be an amyloid. (The term refers to a group of different fibrillary proteins that accumulate extracellularly in a β-pleated sheet conformation.) In Alzheimer disease the amyloid, called Aβ, is a 39- to 43-amino acid peptide that forms following proteolytic cleavage of a larger 695- to 770-amino acid transmembrane protein called amyloid precursor protein (APP).

Disease severity correlates more with neurofibrillary tangles than with senile plaques, and the parts of the brain most affected early in the disease are the hippocampus and the posterior parietotemporal cerebral cortex. The earliest symptom, therefore, is usually impaired memory with or without impaired word finding, calculation, and spatial manipulation. Memory impairment at first involves recent, usually trivial, events. With progression, more significant experiences, both recent and remote, are forgotten; retrograde amnesia can go back decades. There is disorientation to time and place but not, until the end stages, to person (self-identity).

Human memory is organized into several functional types, and in Alzheimer disease it is *episodic memory* (remembering *what,* ie, specific events in time) that is affected earliest and most severely. Less impaired are *working memory* (the ability to hold pieces of information in consciousness long enough to use them in performing cognitive tasks) and *semantic memory* (remembering familiar objects or facts). Usually preserved until late in the course of illness is *procedural memory* (remembering *how,* eg, the use of tools).

Early in the course most patients have relatively preserved social behavior, but over time poor judgment, delusions, restlessness, and agitation become increasingly severe. Inattentiveness and indifference may progress to akinetic mutism. The specific structures responsible for these behavioral abnormalities are obviously uncertain in a disease with such widespread pathology, but the fact that the earliest and most severe pathological abnormalities in Alzheimer disease involve limbic and associative areas, not primary motor or sensory areas, accounts for the conspicuous absence in these patients of prominent weakness or sensory toss. Alertness is also preserved until terminally.

Three additional subcortical nuclei are also affected by Alzheimer disease, cholinergic neurons of the basal forebrain (which includes the nucleus basalis of Meynert, a thin layer of cells ventral to the globus pallidus), the noradrenergic locus coeruleus (in the upper pons), and the serotonergic raphe nuclei (in the upper brain stem). Each of these nuclei has widespread projections to the cerebral cortex and limbic structures. There is also selective loss of certain neuropeptides in the cerebral cortex, including somatostatin and cholecystokinin. The contribution of these neurotransmitter and neuromodulator deficiencies to the symptoms of Alzheimer disease is uncertain, but, analogous to dopamine replacement in Parkinson disease (see Case 35), cholinomimetic drugs have been tried. Results have been marginal at best.

The cause (or causes) of Alzheimer disease is unknown, as is the role of genetics in cases of late onset. First-degree relatives of patients with late-onset Alzheimer disease have a fourfold increased risk of getting the disease. Intriguing clues have been obtained from studies of the much less prevalent forms of early-onset autosomal dominant familial Alzheimer disease (FAD). As of 1998 three separate candidate genes had been identified. The first followed the observation that patients with Down syndrome invariably develop Alzheimer pathological changes during middle age, with dementia then superimposed on their preexisting mental retardation. Down syndrome is trisomy 21, and chromosome 21 is the site of the APP gene. Several mutations of this gene have been identified in families with early-onset FAD, suggesting a pathogenic role for β-amyloid (Aβ) (Figure 16–5), but if Aβ is toxic, the mechanism is unknown. Moreover, APP mutations account for only 5–10% of published early-onset FAD pedigrees.

Far more common as a cause of early-onset FAD are mutations on chromosome 14 for a gene encoding a transmembrane protein called presenilin-1 (PS-1) and on chromosome 1 for a gene encoding a transmembrane protein called presenilin-2 (PS-2). The normal functions of APP, PS-1, and PS-2 are unknown; overexpression of the presenilins in transfected cells reportedly increases susceptibility to apoptosis (programmed cell death). Evidence suggests that the presenilins normally influence the processing of APP and that presenilin gene mutations lead to abnormal enzymatic cleavage of APP and the production of toxic Aβ.

In addition to these mutations, which imply causation, the age of onset of Alzheimer disease is modulated by the apolipoprotein E (Apo E) gene on chromosome 19. Compared with the e2 and e3 alleles of Apo E, the e4 allele confers earlier onset of disease and more rapid progression in both familial and sporadic cases. Two e4 alleles, moreover, carry a greater risk than one e4 allele. The biological basis of this association is unknown.

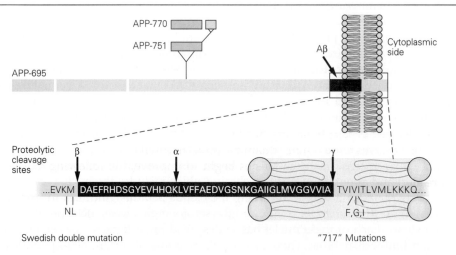

Figure 16–5. Transmembrane amyloid precursor protein (APP) exists in three principal isoforms of 695, 751, and 770 amino acids, each of which contains an Aβ fragment. APP can be cleaved at different sites by different secretase enzymes. Extracellular α cleavage occurs within the Aβ region, and so amyloidogenic Aβ protein is not formed. Intramembranal γ cleavage and extracellular β cleavage result in the production of amyloidogenic Aβ. Mutations of the APP gene prevent α cleavage, allowing increased production of amyloidogenic Aβ, which by uncertain mechanisms appears to be neurotoxic. Missense mutations resulting in substitution at residue 717 of isoleucine, glycine, or phenylalaline for normal valine and, as reported in two related Swedish families, double mutations resulting in substitution at residues 670 and 671 of asparagine-leucine for normal lysine-methionine are shown. (Reproduced with permission from Kandel ER, Schwartz JH, Jessell TM. 1999. *Principles of Neural Science,* 4th ed. New York: McGraw-Hill. Adapted with permission from Thinakaran G, et al. 1996. Endoproteolysis of presenilin I and accumulation of processed derivatives *in vivo.* Neuron 17:180.)

SELECTED REFERENCES

Cummings JL, Kaufer D: Neuropsychiatric aspects of Alzheimer's disease: The cholinergic hypothesis revisited. Neurology 1996;47:876.

Francis PT, Palmer AM, Snape M, Wilcock GK: The cholinergic hypothesis of Alzheimer's disease: A review of progress. J Neurol Neurosurg Psychiatry 1999;66:137.

Levy-Lahad E, Bird TD: Genetic factors in Alzheimer's disease: A review of recent advances. Ann Neurol 1996;40:829.

Martin JB: Molecular basis of the neurodegenerative disorders. N Engl J Med 1999; 340:1970.

Morrison JH, Hof PR: Life and death of neurons in the aging brain. Science 1997;278:412.

Price DL, Sisodia SS: Mutant genes in familial Alzheimer's disease and transgenic models. Annu Rev Neurosci 1998;21:479.

▶ CASE 74

A homeless middle-aged man is brought to an emergency room having been found sitting on the sidewalk in a daze. Blood pressure is 120/80 mm Hg lying and 90/60 mm Hg standing, with pulse rate increasing from 100 to 120/minute. Temperature is normal. He is lethargic, tending to close his eyes if not stimulated, and markedly inattentive, limiting cognitive assessment. Speech consists of monosyllabic answers to questions, and there is little spontaneous motor activity. He gives the incorrect year and says he is at home, but he does identify himself by name. Eye movements are restricted and disconjugate; there is reduced horizontal gaze in either direction with complete loss of abduction on the left, plus a lesser degree of upward gaze paresis. Pupils are normal. Within the limits of testing, strength appears normal, and arm and leg movements display neither tremor nor dysmetria; gait and stance, however, are broad based and ataxic. Sensory examination is impossible except for pinprick, which he appears to feel throughout. Tendon reflexes are symmetrically present in the arms and knees and absent at the ankles.

Computerized tomography reveals mild bilateral enlargement of the lateral ventricles and diffuse widening of the cerebral sulci. Cerebrospinal fluid is normal. He receives intravenous thiamine (plus multivitamins), and within a few hours his abducens and gaze palsies begin to improve; the following day he is more alert and attentive.

Over the next 2 weeks, receiving thiamine daily, he continues to improve. Examination then reveals a full range of eye movements, but with coarse bilateral nystagmus on lateral gaze to either direction. His gait is steadier, but he still cannot walk tandem. He is now alert, attentive, and cooperative, but there is a severe disturbance of memory. He gives the year as 1970 and the President as Reagan, and although able to repeat three unrelated words, he is unable to recall them after 5 minutes or to select them from a list. He recognizes that he is in a hospital but is unaware of why he is there, yet he declares that his memory is "fine." Minutes after being examined, he has no recollection of the encounter and if queried tends to fabricate plausible events. His memory of past experience is also impaired, but in a spotty fashion, with a tendency to report events in the wrong order. Verification is limited, but he appears reliable in describing his childhood, and he acknowledges many years of heavy ethanol use.

Over the next year his amnesia does not improve, but his confabulations gradually disappear, and he admits that his memory is not normal.

Comment

Wernicke-Korsakoff syndrome, encountered most often in alcoholics and caused by thiamine deficiency, is a two-phased illness. Wernicke syndrome consists of the triad of altered mentation, abnormal eye movements, and ataxia of gait and stance. The mental symptoms evolve over days or weeks to a global confusional state, with varying degrees of lethargy, inattentiveness, decreased spontaneous speech, abulia, impaired memory, and disordered perception. Without treatment there is progression to stupor, coma, and death. With treatment (thiamine, plus other nutritional supplements) ophthalmoparesis clears (often with residual lasting nystagmus), gait ataxia improves, and mental symptoms either clear or, as with this patient, evolve into Korsakoff syndrome, which differs from Alzheimer dementia (see Case 73) in that the mental abnormality is nearly restricted to impaired memory.

Like Alzheimer patients early in the course of illness, Korsakoff patients are alert, attentive, and behaviorally appropriate, but unlike Alzheimer patients, Korsakoff patients often have normal language function, calculating ability, and problem-solving skills. (Korsakoff's original patient continued to play chess but could not then recall having done so.) They are also more likely to lack insight into their impairment—*anosognosia*—and early in the course of illness often display *confabulation*—a filling of unremembered time with fabricated experiences that might have occurred in the past, but not during the period in question.

Like early Alzheimer patients, Korsakoff patients have normal *procedural memory*—they do not forget how to drive a car or use tools. In contrast to Alzheimer patients, they tend to have normal *working memory* (retention over 30 seconds or so) and *semantic memory* (memory for facts, concepts, and language). Their combined anterograde and retrograde disturbance indicates abnormalities of both memorization and retrieval, and it is *episodic memory*—for specific events in time—that is devastated. Psychometric testing does reveal abnormalities not explained by pure memory loss, but from a functional standpoint, Korsakoff syndrome is an amnestic disorder.

Severe amnesia similar to Korsakoff syndrome follows bilateral damage to the inferior medial temporal lobes, particularly the hippocampi. In Wernicke-Korsakoff disease, however, pathological changes affect the thalamus (particularly the dorsomedial nucleus and medial pulvinar), the hypothalamus (particularly the mammillary bodies), the midbrain (particularly the periaqueductal areas), and the pons and medulla (particularly the abducens and medial vestibular nuclei); there is also Purkinje cell loss in the cerebellar vermis. Brain stem and cerebellar lesions explain the disordered eye movements and ataxia. More controversial are attempts to explain the mental abnormalities, including amnesia.

Via the fornix, the mammillary bodies receive projections from the hippocampus; mammillary body damage might therefore be expected to result in memory impairment. Autopsies, however, reveal severe mammillary body destruction in alcoholic patients whose memory appeared to be normal (Figure 16–6). More consistently correlating with amnesia is damage to the medial dorsal nucleus of the thalamus (Figure 16–7). Also described is depletion of cholinergic neurons of the basal forebrain. The global confusional state of Wernicke syndrome, on the other hand, has occurred without visible thalamic or basal fore-

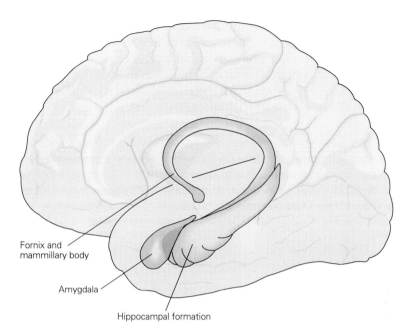

Fornix and
mammillary body

Amygdala

Hippocampal formation

Figure 16–6. The major output pathway of the hippocampal formation is the fornix, which projects to the mammillary body in the medial hypothalamus. Although the hippocampus plays a crucial role in memory consolidation, mammillary body damage does not correlate well with the amnestic disorder of alcoholic-nutritional Korsakoff syndrome. (Reproduced with permission from Martin JH. 1996. *Neuroanatomy Text and Atlas,* 2nd ed. Stamford, CT: Appleton & Lange.)

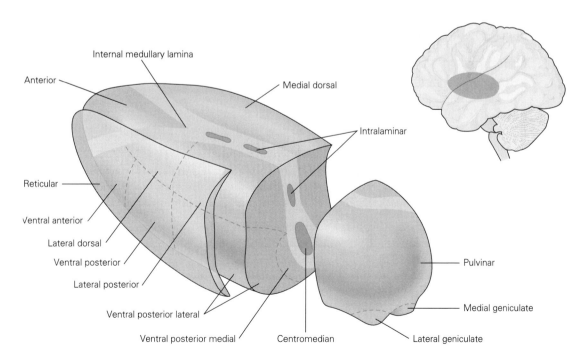

Internal medullary lamina

Anterior

Medial dorsal

Intralaminar

Reticular

Ventral anterior

Lateral dorsal

Ventral posterior

Lateral posterior

Pulvinar

Ventral posterior lateral

Medial geniculate

Ventral posterior medial

Centromedian

Lateral geniculate

Figure 16–7. Major nuclei of the thalamus. In alcoholic-nutritional Korsakoff syndrome, memory impairment correlates best with damage to the medial dorsal nucleus. (Reproduced with permission from Kandel ER, Schwartz JH, Jessell TM. 1991. *Principles of Neural Science,* 3rd ed. Norwalk, CT: Appleton & Lange.)

brain lesions and may be the result of cerebral thiamine depletion. At present clinical-pathological correlation in amnesia resulting from thiamine deficiency, in contrast to amnesia resulting from structural hippocampal damage, is speculative and uncertain. It is possible that ethanol itself, by causing up-regulation of glutamate *N*-methyl-D-aspartate (NMDA) receptors and excitotoxicity (see Case 59), contributes directly to cognitive impairment.

SELECTED REFERENCES

Kopelman MD: Frontal dsyfunction and memory deficits in the alcoholic Korsakoff syndrome and Alzheimer-type dementia. Brain 1991;114:117.

Squire LR: Declarative and nondeclarative memory: Multiple brain systems supporting learning and memory. J Cog Neurosci 1992;4:232.

Victor M, Adams RD, Collins GH: *The Wernicke-Korsakoff Syndrome,* 2nd edition. F.A. Davis, 1989.

Von Cramon DY, Hebel N, Schuri U: A contribution to the anatomical basis of thalamic amnesia. Brain 1985;108:993.

▶ CASE 75

Over the past year a 45-year-old lawyer has had a change in personality. His wife says that he first became irritable and short-tempered and then increasingly impulsive and suspicious. He began dressing sloppily, and his work was marked by ill-considered decisions. Social interactions have been compromised by sexual advances toward younger women and persecutory delusions regarding his friends. He has lost his job and become withdrawn and despondent. Over the past few weeks his wife has also noticed that he seems restless and fidgety and often drops objects.

The patient's mother died in her early 60s and his maternal grandfather in his late 60s, each after a progessive illness that began like the patient's and lasted a dozen or so years.

On examination he is alert but easily distracted. He describes himself as depressed and blames his occupational and social deterioration on others. Memory is moderately impaired; he is oriented to time and place but can recall only two of three words after 5 minutes, even with prompting. Language, including reading and writing, is normal, as is simple calculation, although he is dysarthric and manipulates a pen clumsily. Involuntary movements include frequent blinking, intermittent facial grimacing, and rapid, brief, irregular, asymmetric movements of his arms and legs, greatest distally. He has difficulty maintaining tongue protrusion and a tightly closed fist. Eye movements demonstrate delayed initiation of saccades and jerkiness of pursuit. Other cranial nerves, strength, muscle tone, sensation, and reflexes are normal.

Computerized tomography (CT) reveals enlarged lateral ventricles, particularly frontally, reflecting atrophy of the head of the caudate nucleus. Genetic study identifies over 60 repeats of the trinucleotide cytosine-adenine-guanine (CAG) near the tip of the short arm of chromosome 4.

Comment

Huntington disease is a progressive hereditary disorder that usually begins in adult life and is characterized by abnormal behavior, dementia, and chorea. Either altered mentation or abnormal movements characterize the onset of the disease; both features are usually present within a few months or years. Unlike Alzheimer disease or Korsakoff syndrome, personality change is a prominent early feature; there may be grandiosity, paranoid delusions, depression, outbursts of violence, or frank hallucinatory psychosis. The movement disorder can begin as simply clumsiness or fidgetiness. Choreic movements are less jerky than myoclonus and less stereotypic than tics (see Cases 37 and 76), and patients often convert them into seemingly purposeful movements to mask their involuntary nature. With progression, impaired memory and dementia become evident, but, in contrast to Alzheimer disease, language function is preserved. By the terminal stages, rigidity and dystonia replace chorea, and most patients die akinetic and mute after 10 to 15 years.

Pathologically the most affected structure in Huntington disease is the striatum, with the caudate nucleus more involved than the putamen. Caudate atrophy produces a characteristic ballooning of the lateral ventricle on CT or magnetic resonance imaging.

There are two broad categories of striatal neurons. Interneurons, variably expressing acetylcholine, γ-aminobutyric acid (GABA), or somatostatin, have axons that remain within the striatum. Projection neurons, expressing GABA plus encephalin, substance P, or other peptides, terminate on the external segment of the globus pallidus (GPe), the internal segment of the globus pallidus (GPi), the substantia nigra pars compacta (SNc), and the substantia nigra pars reticularis (SNr) (see Figure 12–26). In Huntington disease there is a predictable temporal sequence of neuronal degeneration: striato-SNc, followed by striato-GPe and striato-SNr, then followed by striato-GPi and GABA interneurons. The early loss of inhibitory striatal projections to GPe would be consistent with the appearance of chorea; decreased GABA inhibition of GPe results, indirectly, in increased thalamic inflow to the motor cortex and hyperkinesia. Later loss of inhibitory striatal projections to GPi would account for the disappearance of chorea; decreased inhibition of GPi results, directly, in decreased thalamic inflow to the motor cortex and hypokinesia (see Figure 12–27). In animal experiments intrastriatal injections of N-methyl-D-aspartate receptor agonists reproduces this pattern of neuronal degeneration, suggesting an excitotoxic mechanism of degeneration in Huntington disease.

Neuronal loss also occurs in other brain regions, particularly layer 3 of the cerebral cortex. Probably both caudate and cerebral damage contribute to the behavioral and cognitive symptoms of Huntington disease. In contrast to the putamen, which receives projections particularly from motor, premotor, and primary sensory cerebral cortex and, via GPi and thalamus, projects to premotor, primary motor, and supplementary motor cortex, the caudate receives projections from posterior parietal and frontal lobe motor association cortex as well as from temporal lobe limbic areas and projects, again via GPi and thalamus, to prefrontal, orbitofrontal, and anterior cingulate cortex.

Unlike Parkinson disease, Huntington disease is not symptomatically improved by adminstration of receptor agonists, including GABAergic agents. Haloperidol, a dopamine antagonist, can reduce chorea and psychotic symptoms, but a long-term complication of neuroleptic medications is tardive dyskinesia, a choreiform movement disorder. (In patients lacking a clear history, the differential diagnosis of altered mentation and abnormal movements always includes schizophrenia plus iatrogenic dyskinesia.) Dopamine agonists make the chorea of

Huntington disease worse, a predictable observation, for chorea is a commonly encountered side effect in parkinsonian patients receiving such agents. These pharmacological effects further demonstrate that whether caused by striatal or subthalamic damage (see Case 36), chorea is the neurophysiological opposite of bradykinesia.

The genetic abnormality in Huntington disease is extra copies of the repeating trinucleotide CAG on the p16.3 region of chromosome 4 coding for a protein called huntingtin. CAG codes for glutamine, and the excess polyglutamine of huntingtin increases its binding to other proteins. Huntingtin is present in all brain neurons and in some peripheral tissues. Why Huntington disease has such restricted neuropathology is unknown. One possibility is that huntingtin reacts with a cell-specific protein to cause disease. A candidate huntingtin-binding protein, called HAP-1, is expressed in regions of the brain most affected in Huntington disease. Energy metabolism is defective in Huntington disease brains, and in one pathogenic scenario huntingtin bound to HAP-1 impairs mitochondrial oxidative phosphorylation, predisposing neurons to cell death by excitotoxicity. Consistent with this proposal is the observation that the polyglutamine stretch of not only huntingtin but also of the abnormal proteins of three other CAG-repeat diseases—spinocerebellar ataxia type 1, X-linked bulbospinal muscular atrophy, and dentatorubropallidoluysian atrophy—binds to glyceraldehyde-3-phosphate dehydrogenase, an enzyme essential for glycolysis.

As in other trinucleotide repeat disorders (see Case 18), the CAG repeat is unstable in gametes and in successive generations may shorten or, more often, lengthen. Longer repeats lead to earlier onset and more severe disease, accounting for *anticipation*, the tendency of these diseases to appear earlier over successive generations. Huntington disease in childhood more often begins with rigidity and bradykinesia than with chorea and progresses to death in less than 10 years.

SELECTED REFERENCES

Albin RL: Selective neurodegeneration in Huntington's disease. Ann Neurol 1995;38:835.
Huntington G: On chorea. Med Surg Rep 1872;26:320.
Huntington's Disease Collaborative Research Group: A novel gene containing a trinucleotide repeat that is expanded and unstable on Huntington's disease chromosomes. Cell 1993;72:971.
Shapira AHV: Mitochondrial function in Huntington's disease: Clues for pathogenesis and prospects for treatment. Ann Neurol 1997;41:141.
Tabrizi SJ, Cleeter MWJ, Xuereb J, et al: Biochemical abnormalities and excitotoxicity in Huntington's disease brain. Ann Neurol 1999;45:25.

▶ CASE 76

Since the age of 7, a 20-year-old man has suffered involuntary movements and vocalizations. Beginning with facial grimacing and jerky head turning, the movements were initially considered habit spasms. Over the ensuing years involuntary movements continued, involving both cranial and limb muscles and, although stereotypic for months at a time, would wax and wane in severity and disappear in one part of his body only to reappear in another. The movements are sudden, rapid, and repetitive. In addition he experiences involuntary vocalizations, at first consisting of throat clearing and grunts and then progressing to loud snorting, barking, and uncontrollably shouting stereotypic phrases, particularly obscenities. Both his motor and his vocal tics are preceded by a psychic compulsion that he feels powerless to resist. In social settings he is able voluntarily to suppress his tics for brief periods, but eventually he has to excuse himself and, removed from the observation of others, vent his pent-up urges in a torrent of gesticulations and shouts. In addition, he often cannot help imitating either the facial expressions or speech inflections of people he is with, and he often compulsively reaches out to touch them, fully aware that he is creating embarrassment. The urge to touch or manipulate sometimes extends to inanimate objects, including fire.

Since childhood, his mother has had mild compulsive behavior and motor tics but no vocalizations.

Neurological examinations over the years have shown no abnormalities except for motor and vocal tics. Magnetic resonance imaging (MRI) at age 17 was normal. Haloperidol in low doses dampens his movements and vocalizations but does not obliterate them.

Comment

Tics are rapid repetitive stereotypic movements that range from simple brief jerks resembling myoclonus to complex coordinated motor activity. Commonly encountered in small children, they nearly always clear within a few weeks or months. In *Tourette syndrome* multiple motor and vocal tics persist with a waxing-waning course and a tendency for one type of tic to replace or be added to another. Severely affected subjects have nearly continuous jerkings and gesticulations and are unemployable because of shouted obscenities (*coprolalia*). Complex motor tics can be self-destructive, for example, chewing the lips or pushing a sharpened pencil into the ear. Antisocial behavior and inappropriate sexual activity (eg, exposing oneself) are also encountered.

A hereditary disorder, Tourette syndrome is transmitted in autosomal dominant fashion with mixed penetrance. Considerable differences in severity are often observed among members of the same family, including identical twins.

To call the movements involuntary is to miss a fascinating neuropsychiatric aspect of Tourette syndrome. Subjects move or shout because of an irresistible urge to do so. To them the tics are not strictly involuntary even though they are resisted. Tourette patients often display obsessive-compulsive behavior; they experience recurrent or persistent ideas, images, or impulses, and they perform complex behaviors as the result of an irresistible subjective compulsion. Moreover, within the same family some members have only tics and others have only obsessive-compulsive behavior, suggesting that Tourette syndrome and obsessive-compulsive disorder are variations of the same basal ganglia-limbic disturbance.

Tourette symptoms are usually responsive to the dopamine antagonist haloperidol, suggesting relative dopamine excess. Postmortem studies have been unrevealing or inconsistent, but an MRI study revealed reduced striatal volume, and in identical twins with Tourette syndrome of different severity, the right caudate nucleus was significantly smaller in the more severely affected twin. Moreover, in another study of monozygotic twins concordant for Tourette syndrome but discordant for severity, there was abnormally increased D_2 dopamine receptor binding in the head of the caudate nucleus but not in the putamen, and binding was greatest in the more severely affected of each twin pair.

The extensive direct and indirect connections of the caudate with associative and limbic structures (see Case 75) make neurotransmitter disturbance within that part of the striatum a plausible explanation for the extraordinary psychic and motor abnormalities of Tourette syndrome. Consistent with that hypothesis is the observation that surgical ablation of the cingulate gyrus (which, via the globus pallidus and thalamus, receives indirect projections from the caudate) relieves symptoms of Tourette syndrome.

SELECTED REFERENCES

Coffey BJ, Park KS: Behavioral and emotional aspects of Tourette syndrome. Neurol Clin North Am 1997;15:277.

Hyde TM, Stacey ME, Coppola R, et al: Cerebral morphometric abnormalities in Tourette's syndrome: A quantitative MRI study of monozygotic twins. Neurology 1995;45:1176.

Singer HS: Neurobiology of Tourette syndrome. Neurol Clin North Am 1997;15:357.

Wolf SS, Jones DW, Knable MB, et al: Tourette syndrome: Prediction of phenotypic variation in monozygotic twins by caudate nucleus D_2 receptor binding. Science 1996; 273:1225.

▶ CASE 77

A 57-year-old high school teacher undergoes a change in personality. Her classroom performance is increasingly unprepared and disorganized, and her mood shifts unexpectedly from inappropriate jocularity to irritability. A married woman with three children, she has recently made embarrassing sexual solicitations to different students, leading to suspension from her job. She is abnormally friendly with strangers and tends to wander into neighbors' homes.

On examination 2 years after the onset of symptoms she is somewhat disheveled and inappropriately facetious and uninhibited, at one point stroking the examiner's cheek. She also tends to imitate the examiner and to repeat his words. Lacking insight into her behavior, she denies there is any problem. She is alert but distractible, and her cooperation is intermittently interrupted by outbursts of hilarity. Speech is fluent without paraphasias, and she has normal speech comprehension and ability to name objects. She repeats seven digits forward and five backward. Oriented to time and place, she recalls two of three unrelated words after 5 minutes, recognizing the third from a list. She correctly copies simple geometric diagrams, for example, intersecting pentagons. Performance is poor on tests of executive function, for example, the ability to maintain or to shift sets in solving problems, to inhibit habitual responses, to alternate between different tasks, and to generate a list of words beginning with a particular letter. Except for the presence of snout and bilateral grasp reflexes, there are no other neurological abnormalities.

Magnetic resonance imaging shows mild frontal atrophy bilaterally. Single-photon emission computerized tomography reveals markedly decreased blood flow in both frontal lobes. Other laboratory tests relevant to dementia, including metabolic studies and tests for syphilis and human immunodeficiency virus, are normal.

Over the next several years she becomes increasingly withdrawn, and her speech becomes sparse and stereotypic. Memory and general cognitive abilities progressively deteriorate, and emotional lability and impulsiveness are replaced by abulia (psychomotor slowing and emotional indifference) and finally akinetic mutism.

Comment

The frontal lobes, comprising more than one third of the cerebral cortex, consist of the precentral cortex (the motor cortex, Brodmann area 4), the premotor cortex (Brodmann area 6, plus the supplementary motor area and the pars opercularis), and the prefrontal (limbic) cortex. Covering three surfaces—lateral, medial, and orbitofrontal—the prefrontal cortex has extensive connections—afferent, efferent, or both—with auditory, visual, and somatosensory association cortices, striatum, thalamus, hypothalamus, midbrain, amygdala, hippocampus, and other limbic areas. Predictably, frontal lobe damage produces a wide array of behavioral and cognitive symptoms. Over time three well-recognized frontal lobe syndromes were manifested by the present patient.

First, she exhibited impaired executive function. She could no longer plan or carry out her usual activities in a coherent goal-directed fashion. On neuropsychological testing she displayed difficulty adapting strategies for learning tasks, and once a particular strategy was adapted, she could not change to a new strategy to accommodate a new set of rules. Disturbed motor programming was evident in sequential, alternating, and reciprocal motor tasks.

Second, she exhibited a marked change in personality, becoming emotionally shallow and impulsive; irritability alternated with facetiousness, and she became disinhibited and inappropriate in her personal appearance and her social interactions. Sexual indiscretion led to dismissal from her job, yet she lacked insight into what was happening to her. During examination she behaved facetiously and distractedly, and her tendency to imitate speech and gestures reflected enslavement to environmental cues.

Disturbed long-term planning and inappropriate emotional responses were described a century and a half ago in Phineas Gage, a New England railroad foreman who, following an accident in which an iron spike traversed his frontal lobes, changed from a responsible member of his community to an occupational incompetent and a social misfit. Conflicting speculation over the fundamental nature of such symptoms continues to the present day. Some investigators associate the executive dysfunction with damage to the dorsolateral convexity of the prefrontal cortex and the emotional disturbance with damage to the orbitofrontal cortex. Each of these two regions participates in separate but parallel anatomic loops, from prefrontal cortex to caudate to substantia nigra and globus pallidus to thalamic ventral anterior and dorsomedial nuclei and back to prefrontal cortex. Perhaps relevant to the emotional disturbance associated with frontal lobe damage, the orbitofrontal cortex, but not the dorsolateral convexity, has extensive reciprocal connections to the amygdala and hippocampus.

Of note is that early in the course of her illnesss the patient's memory, language function, constructional skills, and praxis were only mildly impaired. Over time, however, more obvious cognitive decline ensued, and she then progressed to a third frontal lobe syndrome, namely *abulia* (literally lack of will), referring to blunting of emotional responses and slowing of mental and motor responses. Abulia is associated with mediofrontal lobe damage, including the supplementary motor area (bilateral damage produces bilateral motor neglect—see Case 32) and the cingulate gyrus (bilateral damage produces emotional indifference, including response to pain).

Snout and grasp reflexes are sometimes referred to as frontal release signs. Seen in newborns (in whom they confer an obvious survival advantage), they disppear early in life, presumably the result of normal inhibition by frontal lobe structures. The actual anatomy underlying these reflexes remains uncertain, however.

The disease process affecting this patient is probably one of the *frontal* or *frontotemporal dementias,* a poorly understood group of degenerative disorders. These include Pick disease, characterized histologically by ballooned neurons and cytoplasmic inclusions, as well as other pathologically distinct forms. They differ from Alzheimer disease not only histologically but in their predominant involvement of the frontal or frontotemporal lobes. As a consequence, in contrast to most cases of Alzheimer disease, altered behavior, with impaired regulation of personal conduct, emotional blunting, and loss of insight, is the most prominent early symptom of frontotemporal dementias, and impaired memory, language function, spatial orientation, and praxis may follow only years later; in addition, the frontal and frontotemporal dementias tend to appear before age 65, probably accounting for dementia in about 20% of people below that age.

Frontotemporal dementia, sometimes with additional features of parkinsonism (see Case 35) or motor neuron disease (see Case 26), is often familial, with autosomal dominant transmission. In 1998 affected families were shown to have mutations on chromosome 17q21–22 affecting the gene for tau protein, normally present in microtubules (see Cases 29 and 73). Both exonic and intronic mutations of the tau gene have been described in such families, resulting in neuronal (and glial) filamentous inclusions of abnormal tau protein and a variety of behavioral abnormalities. Disorders in which tau protein appears to play a pathogenic role are collectively referred to as *taupathies.*

SELECTED REFERENCES

Cummings JL: Frontal-subcortical circuits and human behavior. Arch Neurol 1993;50:873.

Devinsky O, Morrell, MJ, Vogt BA: Contributions of the anterior cingulate cortex to behavior. Brain 1995;18:297.

Hutton M, Lendon CL, Rizzu P, et al: Association of missense and 5'-splice-site mutations in *tau* with the inherited dementia FTDP-17. Nature 1998;393:702.

Mendez MF, Cherrier M, Perryman KM, et al: Frontotemporal dementia versus Alzheimer's disease: Differential cognitive features. Neurology 1996;47:1189.

Neary D, Snowden JS, Gustafson L, et al: Frontotemporal lobar degeneration. A consensus on clinical diagnostic criteria. Neurology 1998;51:1546.

Smith EE, Jonides J: Storage and executive processes in the frontal lobes. Science 1999;283:1657.

Spillantini MG, Goedert M: Tau protein pathology in neurodegenerative diseases. Trends Neurosci 1998;21:428.

Vogel G: Tau protein mutations confirmed as neuron killers. Science 1998;280:1524.

▶ CASE 78

A 17-year-old high school student, always considered by his classmates to be a loner, becomes increasingly withdrawn. Although he has never had a girlfriend, he has participated in social activities, but he now avoids them. His previously average school performance deteriorates, and he frequently skips classes altogether. His parents observe that he spends hours at a time sitting in his room doing nothing. In sessions with a school counselor he gives no reason for his changed behavior, denying depression or interpersonal difficulties. After several months of persistent withdrawal and apathy, he develops delusions that certain classmates are seeking to harm him, and he appears to be conversing with a hallucinated voice.

On examination he is alert but inattentive, seeming to ruminate in his own thoughts. His speech is sparse and lacking in affective tone, his responses are tangential and often nonsequitur, and he describes hearing voices that are talking about him perjoratively and are plotting to kill him. Within the limits of testing, he appears fully oriented, with normal memory, language function, and spatial manipulation.

Hospitalized, he is treated with haloperidol, and over the next few weeks his delusions and hallucinations clear. He remains emotionally blunted, however, evidencing no pleasure at his improvement and expressing little interest in returning to school. His conversation continues to display tangentiality and often stops unexpectedly in mid-sentence. He spends much of his time uncommunicative and preoccupied with his own thoughts.

Comment

Affecting 1% of people worldwide, *schizophrenia* is the most mysterious of all neurological diseases. The term, coined by Bleuler over 70 years ago, refers to a split, or dissociation, of emotion from cognition. Since then, in the absence of predictable biological markers, diagnostic criteria have repeatedly changed; currently required by the *Diagnostic and Statistical Manual of Mental Disorders*, 4th edition (*DSM-IV*) is "psychosis"—a break with reality—as manifested by "delusions, prominent hallucinations, marked loosening of associations, catatonic behavior, or flat or grossly inappropriate affect." These symptoms must last at least a week, preceded or followed by at least 6 months of "deterioration in work, social relations, or self-care." The *DSM-IV* criteria exclude transient psychotic states such as cocaine or phencyclidine (angel dust) intoxication and do not address the question of whether the several schizophrenic subtypes—simple, catatonic, disorganized (hebephrenic), paranoid, and mixed—are facets of a single diagnostic entity or whether, in fact, schizophrenia should be considered a descriptive term for a number of different genetic and acquired disorders.

Schizophrenic symptoms have traditonally been divided into negative (eg, flatness of affect) and positive (eg, hallucinations). In recent years a threefold clustering has gained favor, consisting of psychotic symptoms (hallucinations, delusions, bizarre behavior), cognitive impairment (disordered thinking, with inappropriate emotional expression, tangentiality, fragmentation of ideas, looseness of associations, incoherence, and neoligisms), and negative symptoms (restricted affect, reduced emotional range, poverty of speech and spontaneous movement, curbing of interests, decreased sense of purpose, and social withdrawal). During childhood many schizophrenic patients display subtle disturbances in associative thinking, emotional responsiveness, and social interaction, and psychometric testing of asymptomatic subjects genetically at risk for schizophrenia often reveals subtle abnormalities of attention, executive function, and memory. The defining symptoms of schizophrenia, however, reflect a disordered perception of the inner self in relation to the outside world. Patients describe *depersonalization,* a feeling of separation between body and mind, and *derealization,* a sense of environmental unreality.

Controversial is the relative importance of genetic and environmental factors in schizophrenia. Concordance is 40–50% for monozygotic twins and 10% for dizygotic twins and siblings, and linkage has been reported (but not, as yet, replicated) between schizophrenia and chromosomes 5, 6, and 22. As in other common disorders such as hypertension and alcoholism, multiple genes probably play a role. There is also an increased prevalence of gestational and birth complications in schizophrenic patients. Each of these genetic and environmental risk factors is consistent with the concept of schizophrenia as a disorder of brain development. So are imaging and morphological studies, which reveal enlargement of the lateral and third ventricles, decreased volume of the amygdala, hippocampus, and thalamus, and structural abnormalities of the superior temporal gyrus, anterior cingulate gyrus, and prefrontal white matter. In schizophrenic patients, positron emission tomography reveals that blood flow in the prefrontal cortex does not increase during psychometric tests that normally activate the frontal lobes.

Some investigators believe that the fundamental impairment in schizophrenia is a defect in working memory—the ability to hold a mental representation online long enough to perform cognitive operations on it. Disruption of working memory would make it difficult to respond to external stimuli flexibly, which would then inappropriately drive behavior. In primates, including humans, the dorsolateral prefrontal cortex, through reentrant circuits to and from other brain areas, plays a key role in working memory. In schizophrenics functional imaging reveals decreased activity of this area during delayed reponse tasks requiring spatial information to be held online. Consistent with these observations are neuropathological studies demonstrating loss of neuropil in the prefrontal cortex of schizophrenics.

Dopamine-blocking neuroleptic drugs such as haloperidol and the phenothiazines reduce psychotic symptoms in the majority of schizophrenic patients; they are considerably less effective with negative symptoms. The clinical potency of these drugs correlates with their affinity for D_2-dopamine receptors, normally abundant in the cingulate gyrus, the caudate nucleus, the nucleus accumbens (ventral striatum), and the amygdala. Reduced numbers of γ-aminobutyric acid (GABA)ergic inhibitory interneurons in the cingulate gyrus of schizophrenics have been reported; the efficacy of dopamine blockade might be related to an abnormally increased density of dopamine receptors on the GABAergic interneurons that remain.

The brain has four functionally separate dopamine systems (Figure 16–8).

1. The tuberoinfundibular system projects from the arcuate nucleus of the hypothalamus and inhibits prolactin secretion; damage to this system results in galactorrhea and amenorrhea.
2. The nigrostriatal system projects from the substantia nigra pars compacta to the caudate nucleus and putamen; damage to this system results in parkinsonism (see Case 35).
3. The mesolimbic system projects from the ventral tegmental area (VTA) of the midbrain to limbic structures that include the nucleus accumbens, parts of the

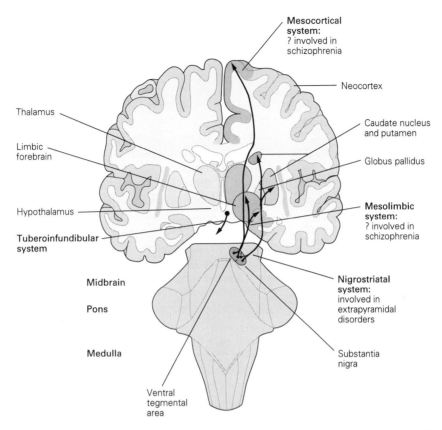

Figure 16–8. The brain has four dopamine systems: the tuberoinfundibular, the nigrostriatal, the mesolimbic, and the mesocortical. (Reproduced with permission from Kandel ER, Schwartz JH, Jessell TM. 1999. *Principles of Neural Science*, 4th ed. New York: McGraw-Hill.)

amygdala and hippocampus, the lateral septal nuclei, and the orbitofrontal cortex and cingulate gyrus. This system, known as the reward circuit, is essential for the subjective effects of many psychotropic drugs; animals with implanted electrodes will continuously stimulate the VTA, and animals with ablation of the VTA will no longer self-administer drugs such as cocaine (which in humans produces an acute schizophrenic-like paranoid psychosis).

4. Finally, the mesocortical dopaminergic system projects from the VTA to the neocortical prefrontal lobe; damage to this system results in disordered motivation, impaired executive function, and abnormal social behavior.

Animal studies reveal interesting interactions between the mesolimbic and mesocortical systems; specifically, lesioning of the mesocortical system results in overactivity of the mesolimbic system. A current hypothesis is that the negative symptoms of schizophrenia result from a hypoactive mesocortical system; loss of normal inhibition by the mesocortical system results in a hyperactive mesolimbic system, accounting for psychotic symptoms (Figure 16–9). The primary event, damage to the mesocortical system, occurs early in development, either from genetic predisposition or gestational injury, but this damage does not cause obvious

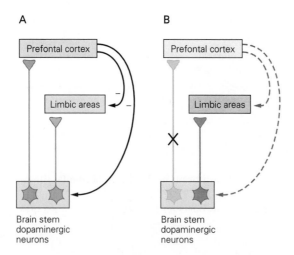

Figure 16–9. A. Normal state. **B.** A proposed neuroanatomical model of schizophrenia. A primary defect in the meso-cortical dopaminergic (DA) system causes both frontal lobe hypofunction and, because there is then loss of frontolim-bic inhibitory feedback, hyperactivity of the dopaminergic mesolimbic system. Frontal lobe hypofunction might under-lie schizophrenic negative symptoms. Limbic hyperactivity might underlie schizophrenic positive (psychotic) symptoms. (Reproduced with permission from Kandel ER, Schwartz JH, Jessell TM. 1999. *Principles of Neural Science*, 4th ed. New York: McGraw-Hill. Adapted with permission from Weinberger DR. 1987. Implications of normal brain development for the pathogenesis of schizophrenia. Arch Gen Psychiatry 44:660.)

symptoms until adolescence or young adulthood, a period of crucial mesocortical maturation.

Early parenting appears to have little to do with the later appearance of schizophrenia; children of schizophrenic parents reared by adoptive parents have the same risk for developing the disease as those reared by their biological parents. The normal stresses of adolescence are a plausible trigger for symptomatic onset, however.

That schizophrenia is probably more than a disorder of D_2-dopamine receptors was suggested by the response of symptoms to newer classes of antipsychotic drugs. For example, clozapine binds to D_1-, D_2-, and D_4-dopamine receptors as well as to 5-hydroxytryptamine type 2 (5-HT_2) receptors, and unlike D_2-receptor blockers such as haloperidol, it has a very low incidence of parkinsonian side effects. Moreover, allelic variation of a gene on chromosome 13 coding for the serotonin 5-HT_{2A} receptor confers risk for schizophrenia. Clozapine is somewhat more effective than haloperidol in reducing positive schizophrenic symptoms, and it increases glutamate efflux in the nucleus accumbens. In monkeys performing working memory tasks, clozapine increases the activity of prefrontal neurons at the principal sulcus, an area critical for the performance of such tasks. However, the antipsychotic efficacy of clozapine appears to be largely the result of D_2-receptor blockade; the lower incidence of extrapyramidal side effects is the result of reduced binding at basal ganglia receptors compared to limbic receptors.

Phencyclidine, which reproduces both negative and positive symptoms of schizophrenia, blocks *N*-methyl-D-aspartate (NMDA)-type glutamate receptors. It also impairs working memory in animal models. Attempts to treat schizophrenia with NMDA agonists have been unsuccessful; not surprisingly, seizures are a common side effect of such drugs. For reasons unclear—and somewhat paradox-ically—brain glutamate levels increase sharply in brains of animals receiving phencyclidine, and a novel approach to schizophrenia pharmacotherapy involves regionally selective agents that block glutamate activity. The efficacy of such drugs would be consistent with the idea that reduced activity of GABAergic in-hibitory interneurons leads to a net increase in glutamatergic output from af-fected limbic and cortical regions in schizophrenic brains.

SELECTED REFERENCES

Andreasen NC: Linking mind and brain in the study of mental illness: A project for a sci-entific psychopathology. Science 1997;275:1586.
Benes F: Is there a neuroanatomic basis for schizophrenia? An old question revisited. Neu-roscientist 1995;1:104.
Carpenter WT, Buchanan RW: Schizophrenia. N Engl J Med 1994;330:681.
Harrison PJ: The neuropathology of schizophrenia. A critical review of the data and their interpretation. Brain 1999;122:593.
Maghaddam B, Adams B: Reversal of phencyclidine effects by a group II metabotropic glutamate receptor agonist in rats. Science 1998;281:1349.
Sedrall G, Farde L: Chemical brain anatomy in schizophrenia. Lancet 1995;346:743.
Williams J, Spurlock G, McGuffin P, et al: Association between schizophrenia and T102C polymorphism of the 5-hydroxytryptamine type 2a receptor gene. Lancet 1996;347:1294.

▶ CASE 79

For several months a 53-year-old lawyer has experienced increasing insomnia and fatigue. Formerly enthusiastic and energetic in her work and social activities, she finds that neither work nor play provides pleasure or satisfaction any longer, and she feels tired all the time. She tends to awaken in the early morning, unable to return to sleep, and loss of appetite has led to weight loss. Trivial matters pre-cipitate inappropriate worry or irritability, and she complains of difficulty con-centrating and poor memory. Nagging low back pain and constipation are addi-tional preoccupations.

On examination she is alert, attentive, and cooperative, but her speech is slow, halting, and monotonous, and her facial expression registers sadness. Occa-sional smiles seem forced and artificial. She complains of loss of energy and tiredness. When specifically queried, she acknowledges that she might be de-pressed but can identify no precipitating cause. She denies suicidal ideation. Al-though her responses are delayed and reveal a paucity of content, there are no gross abnormalities of memory, language function, or cognition, and although she expresses hopelessness over her inability to function, she is not delusional and denies hallucinations. Her examination reveals no other abnormalities, and workup fails to reveal any occult medical or neurological illness.

Treatment is begun with a tricyclic antidepressant drug. Two weeks later her symptoms begin to improve, and for the next several months she returns to her former level of work and social activity. A year after the onset of her symptoms her behavior abruptly changes. She becomes unusually talkative and hyperac-tive, sleeping only 4 or 5 hours nightly and displaying increased appetite and sexual interest. At work she describes ambitious and daring plans, but her per-formance is erratic and more impulsive than creative. One afternoon she appears in her local liquor store describing an elaborate but incoherent scheme to control the world's population. Her mood is expansive, but attempts to break into her ramblings produce irritability or brief bursts of anger. She appears to be experiencing auditory hallucinations. Although she allows herself to be examined, memory and cognition cannot be assessed; there are no other neurological abnormalities.

She receives parenteral haloperidol and the following day is considerably calmer and more grounded to reality. Lithium carbonate is begun in divided oral doses. Over the next several months, taking both lithium carbonate and a tricyclic antidepressant, she is again functional at work and home.

Comment

Depression and mood swings are a universal human experience, and suicidal depression can follow a devastating experience (reactive depression). Depression is part of a normal grief reaction, and it can be a symptom (ie, not simply a psychological response) of many medical and neurological diseases, including stroke, multiple sclerosis, Huntington disease, and Parkinson disease. In *endogenous depression* the symptoms cannot be explained by underlying medical illness or adverse life events. In such patients symptoms often wax and wane unpredictably. Recurrent bouts of severe depression constitute *unipolar* disease. When there are bouts of mania as well as depression, the illness is referred to as *bipolar* (*manic-depressive disorder*).

If untreated, first attacks of depression or mania usually last a few months, and more than half of such patients experience one or more recurrences. The core features of *major depression* are dysphoria, inability to experience pleasure (anhedonia), and loss of interest; variably present are insomnia or hypersomnia, increased or decreased appetite, psychomotor slowing, anxiety or agitation, fatigue or loss of energy, feelings of guilt or worthlessness, difficulty concentrating, complaints of impaired memory or thinking, hypochondriacal preoccupation, and suicidal ideation. Some patients become frankly delusional or even hallucinatory (depressive psychosis), and psychomotor retardation may reach the point of catatonia. By contrast, mania ranges from an infectious effervescence to a delusional hallucinatory psychosis with ideational fragmentation resembling acute schizophrenia (see Case 78). In other words, depression and mania are polar opposites—grotesque extremes of the normal fluctuations in mood that color the psychic life of nearly everybody.

The anatomical and physiological basis of normal and abnormal affective tone is unknown but surely involves limbic structures, including the Papez circuit (cingulate–hippocampus–mammillary bodies–anterior thalamus–cingulate) and the reward circuit (ventral tegmental area of midbrain–nucleus accumbens–prefrontal cortex), as well as other hypothalamic nuclei, insular and anterior temporal cortex, amygdala, and dorsomedial nucleus of the thalamus. Of uncertain significance are observations in stroke patients that right frontal damage produces indifference or euphoria whereas left frontal damage produces anxiety or depression. Moreover, in right-handed people left cerebral lesions cause aphasia, yet such patients are usually able to recognize the emotional tone of speech (eg, sad, glad, or mad); by contrast, nonaphasics with right cerebral damage often fail to recognize the emotional tone of speech.

Patients experiencing major depression have decreased blood flow and metabolism in the dorsolateral prefrontal, medial prefrontal, and posterior parietal cortices; with treatment, flow improves in frontal but not parietal regions. Conversely, blood flow and metabolism in depressed patients are increased in parts of the orbitofrontal cortex as well as in the amygdala, the mediodorsal nucleus of the thalamus, and the nucleus accumbens, with returns toward normal during remission.

The response of depressive symptoms to drugs such as monoamine oxidase inhibitors and tricyclic antidepressants, which increase the availability of norepinephrine and serotonin at forebrain synapses, implicates these systems in depressive illness, and indeed concentrations of 3-methoxy-4-hydroxyphenylglycol (a metabolite of norepinephrine) and 5-hydroxyindoleacetic acid (a metabolite of serotonin) are reduced in some—but not all—depressed patients (Figures 16–10 and 16–11). A high proportion of patients receiving the noradrenergic tricyclic antidepressant desipramine relapse when their brain catecholamines are depleted but not when their brain tryptophan is depleted. A similarly high proportion of patients receiving the serotonin reuptake inhibitor fluoxetine relapse when their brain tryptophan is depleted but not when their brain catecholamines are depleted. The noradrenergic and serotonin systems thus appear to independently stimulate a common downstream system involved in mood control.

Lithium carbonate is effective in treating acute mania and, as maintenance therapy, in preventing recurrences of either mania or depression. Lithium disrupts the G-protein/phosphoinositide second messenger system by blocking the enzyme that converts inositol phosphate to inositol, causing accumulation of inositol triphosphate; whether this action has anything to do with its efficacy in bipolar disease, however, is unknown.

The anticonvulsants sodium valproate and carbamazepine also dampen the manic and depressive swings of bipolar illness, but it is not known how their basic pharmacological properties (involving axonal sodium conductance and additionally, in the case of valproate, indirect GABA agonism) render them effective. Similarly, electroconvulsive therapy (ECT), which can rapidly relieve symptoms of either depression or mania, does so by obscure mechanisms. (In rats, chronic ECT leads to increased levels of 5-HT$_2$ receptor binding sites in the frontal cortex.)

Psychological stress causes release of substance P in the amygdala, and clinical studies suggest that substance P antagonists have antidepressant effects. Such studies have been confounded by placebo effect, however.

Several weeks are often required for antidepressant drugs to relieve symptoms, suggesting that they might act through genetic transcription factors. One hypothesis holds that depression is related to regional reductions in the expression of brain-derived neurotrophic factor (BDNF) and that antidepressant drugs, acting through the transcription factor cyclic-AMP response element binding protein (CREB), turn on the gene for BDNF.

Both unipolar and bipolar disease are genetically influenced. Concordance for bipolar disease is 72% among monozygotic twins and 14% for dizygotic twins. For monopolar disease concordance is 40% for monozygotic twins and 11% for dizygotic twins. Gene mapping studies have been inconsistent, suggesting multiple disorders with polygenetic influences. Linkage has been reported between manic-depressive illness and markers on chromosomes 6, 11, 18, 21, and X. In one family, allelic variation in the gene coding for a serotonin transporter conferred a sevenfold risk of developing depressive illness.

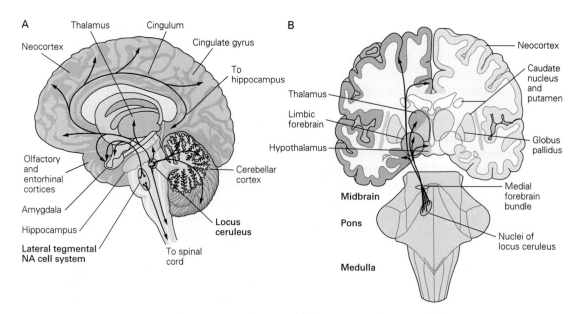

Figure 16–10. The major noradrenergic (NA) pathways originate in the locus ceruleus and lateral tegmentum of the brain stem and project to the forebrain, cerebellum, and spinal cord. **A.** Sagittal view. **B.** Coronal view. (Reproduced with permission from Kandel ER, Schwartz JH, Jessell TM. 1999. *Principles of Neural Science,* 4th ed. New York: McGraw-Hill. Adapted with permission from Heimer L. 1995. *The Human Brain and Spinal Cord,* 2nd ed. New York: Springer-Verlag.)

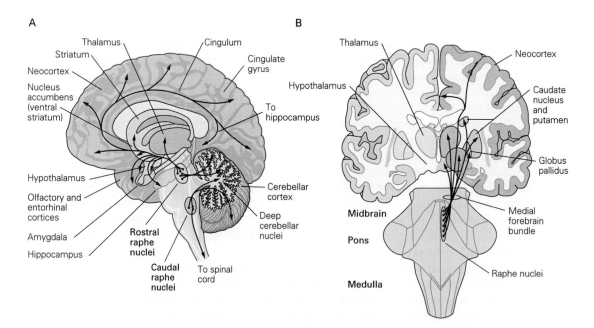

Figure 16–11. The major serotonergic pathways originate in the raphe nuclei of the brain stem and project to the forebrain and spinal cord. **A.** Midsagittal section. **B.** Coronal section. (Reproduced with permission from Kandel ER, Schwartz JH, Jessell TM. 1999. *Principles of Neural Science,* 4th ed. New York: McGraw-Hill. Adapted with permission from Heimer L. 1995. *The Human Brain and Spinal Cord,* 2nd ed. New York: Springer-Verlag.)

SELECTED REFERENCES

Drevets WC: Functional neuroimaging studies of depression: The anatomy of melancholia. Annu Rev Med 1998;49:341.

Duman RS, Heninger GR, Nestler EJ: A molecular and cellular theory of depression. Arch Gen Psychiatry 1997;54:597.

Green AI, Mooney JJ, Posner JA, Schildkraut JJ: Mood disorders: Biochemical aspects. In: Kaplan HI, Sadock BJ (eds): *Comprehensive Textbook of Psychiatry*, 6th edition (pp. 1089–1102). Williams & Wilkins, 1995.

Kramer MS, Cutler N, Feighner J, et al: Distinct mechanism for antidepressant activity by blockade of central substance P receptors. Science 1998;281:1640.

MacKinnon DF, Jamison KR, DePaulo JR: Genetics of manic depressive illness. Annu Rev Neurosci 1997;20:355.

Ogilrie AD, Battersby S, Bubb VJ, et al: Polymorphism in serotonin transporter gene associated with susceptibility to major depression. Lancet 1996;346:731.

Winokur G, Coryell W, Keller M, et al: A prospective follow-up of patients with bipolar and primary unipolar effective disorder. Arch Gen Psyshictry 1993;50:457.

Index

Note: A *t* following a page number indicates tabular material and an *f* following a page number indicates an illustration.

ISBN 0-8385-8117-X

9 780838 1179

90000

THE BODY BUILDER'S KITCHEN

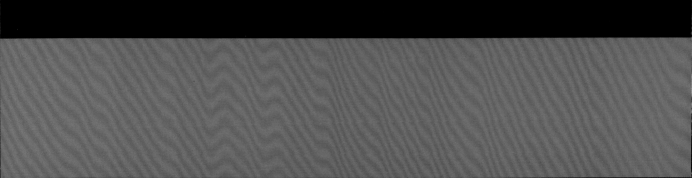

THE BODY BUILDER'S KITCHEN

ERIN STERN

CONTENTS

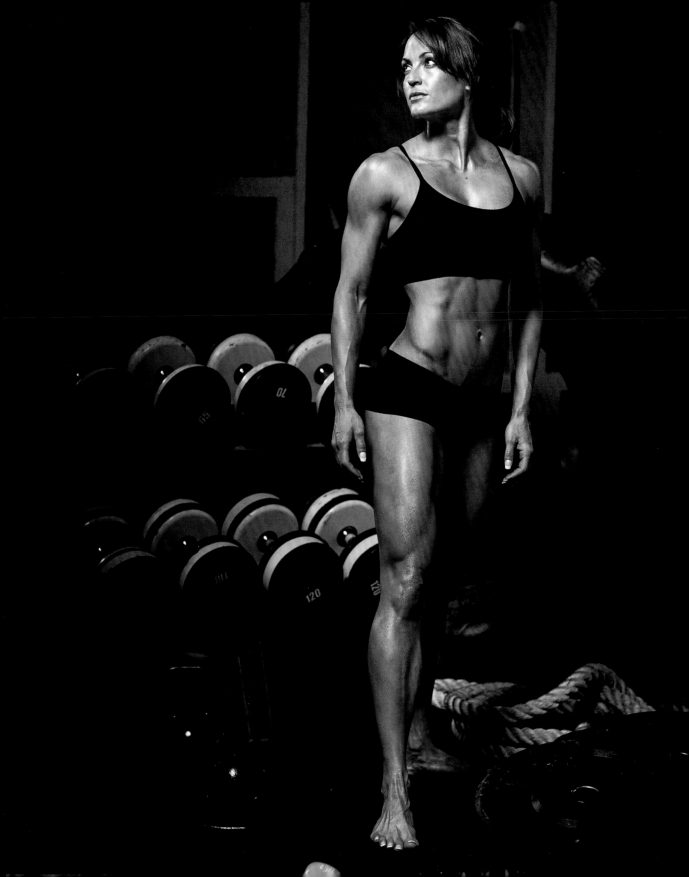

WELCOME TO THE BODYBUILDER'S KITCHEN!

When I first started training for physique competitions, I quickly realized that I couldn't follow the standard food pyramid any longer. Simply watching my overall caloric intake wasn't helping me get leaner or gain muscle. I began to research different eating styles and meal plans that included higher amounts of protein in the form of whole foods. I also learned that when we eat can be just as important as what we eat.

This book is intended to give you a foundation of recipes and meal plans to help you develop a nutrition plan that works for you, and features 100 recipes that have given me successful results. I believe that for a recipe to be successful, it must hit certain nutritional thresholds, but it also must be delicious and easy to make. So, each recipe in this book uses a minimal amount of ingredients, all of which can be found in any grocery store. Every recipe also includes key macronutrient totals for calories, protein, carbohydrates, and fat.

It's not enough to just have recipes, though. These recipes are applied in five of my favorite meal plans that will help you achieve any training goal. I think that a meal plan should be easy to follow, and we're more likely to stick with something if it isn't tedious and monotonous, so each plan is simple and gives you exactly the information you need to follow the plan each day. I include basic nutrition tips and tricks that make meal planning and meal substitutions a snap, and I've included easy-to-remember guidelines for determining macronutrient combinations and timing your meals.

I hope this book helps streamline your search for simple, delicious recipes that will take the guesswork out of setting your nutrition goals, and that it helps you find an eating plan that is right for your body. Don't be afraid to experiment with the different plans, or even to build your own plan. Whatever you do, stick with it, don't quit, and eventually you will begin to see the results you want!

Train hard ya'll!

Erin Stern

THE ESSENTIALS

Just as any house is built by laying the foundation first, the body is built first through an understanding of how to train, how to eat, and how our bodies use the food we eat to build muscle and burn fat. This chapter lays the framework for defining your goals, eating right, and choosing a meal plan that will get the results you're seeking.

THE SCIENCE OF TRAINING AND NUTRITION

Bodybuilding isn't just about lifting heavy things in the gym. It's actually a precise science that requires not only hard work in the gym, but eating the proper nutrients, and timing the delivery of those nutrients to optimize the gains your body is capable of achieving. Getting strong and ripped also requires hard work in the kitchen!

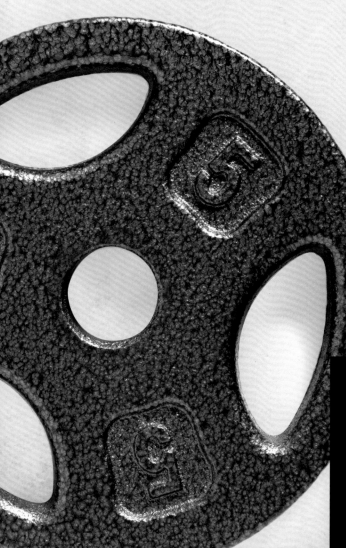

THE ROLE OF TRAINING

Every successful bodybuilder will tell you that in order to achieve a strong, ripped physique, you have to start by training hard and training consistently in the gym. Simply put, the harder you work, the stronger and more defined you will become. But how does that happen, and where do you start?

When we train, whether it be by pushing our bodies through strength training or through cardio training, we create physical stress that requires our bodies to heal and rebuild. The stress imposed on our muscles actually creates tiny micro tears in the muscle fibers, and those tears happen to be why we're sore after a hard training session, but they're also a sign that our bodies are becoming stronger. Our bodies have to heal that damage, and the healing response is to not only repair the existing damaged muscle fibers, but also to build brand new muscle tissue that eventually results in us growing stronger and bigger. This amazing regenerative process is why we're able to progressively lift more and heavier weight, and to see the steady improvement in our physiques that we're seeking.

Training hard is a critical component in achieving the physique you desire, but it takes time and effort, along with careful planning both in the gym and in the kitchen. Start first by defining your goals. Are you wanting to get stronger and add bulk? Or, are you looking to trim excess fat and show off the muscle you've worked so hard to attain? Whatever your goal may be, it starts with creating a program that includes disciplined training and a precise nutrition program, both designed to maximize the benefits of your hard work. In short, as a bodybuilder there are no shortcuts to success, but as an old saying goes, the master of anything was once a beginner, so start your long-term success by developing a comprehensive training and nutrition plan. Whatever your goal may be, the hard work will be worth the effort in the end!

THE BENEFITS

The benefits of building a strong body through a carefully planned training and nutrition program are immeasureable. Here are just a few.

IMPROVED STRENGTH It's no secret that strength training, along with proper nutrition, burns body fat and produces strong, lean muscle to make us better able to perform virtually any task, no matter the age.

THE ROLE OF NUTRITION

While many people might think a strong physique is just about working hard in the gym, what they may not realize is that nutrition plays a critical role in changing the body's composition. Proper bodybuilding nutrition involves choosing the right types of foods for the right meals, along with consuming the right number of calories to meet your body's daily needs. If you meet these needs, you'll eventually be able to redefine your silhouette to your liking—not just bulk up or lose fat.

But bodybuilding nutrition isn't just about cutting calories, it's about eating the right balance of calories each day so your body can repair existing muscle and build new muscle fibers. This means your body needs a slight surplus of calories each day to use as fuel for energy and recovery. Some fad diets might have you running a caloric deficit, and while this might encourage weight loss, it has no effect on improving body composition, and it could actually result in a loss of muscle mass. Calorie restriction can also cause your metabolism to slow down, and significantly reduce energy levels. Controlling caloric intake to deliver the proper amount of calories so the body has the energy it needs to function and heal is the only proper approach.

Your body also needs the right balance of key macronutrients to heal and grow stronger. These macronutrients, which include protein, carbohydrates, and healthy fats, can help your body maximize its ability to repair, rebuild, and grow stronger. Timing is also important. By eating the right combinations of these key macronutrients at strategic intervals throughout the day, we can help our bodies heal and grow even faster.

IMPROVED SELF-ESTEEM How we look has a direct impact on how we feel about ourselves. If we look good physically, and we feel good physically, then naturally we'll feel better about ourselves.

MORE LEAN BODY MASS The more muscle you have, the higher your metabolism, which means the body works harder to burn calories and keep you lean.

FEWER INJURIES Strength training and nutrition makes our bodies stronger, strengthens our bones and connective tissues, and improves our balance.

IMPROVED BRAIN FUNCTION AND MOOD Science has proven that exercise and proper nutrition both have a direct impact on improving brain function, as well as improving sleep and bettering mood.

BODYBUILDING NUTRITION BASICS

Your body is a complex system, and how you feed and fuel it has a direct impact on how effective your training can be. As a bodybuilder, there are several important processes to understand and manage in order to maximize your body's full potential for growing lean, strong muscle, and burning off excess body fat.

CONTROLLING CALORIES

Calories are essentially units of energy contained in the foods we eat, and our bodies convert those units into the energy it needs to function and heal. By controlling the number of calories you consume, and monitoring when you consume them, you can maximize the benefits from the foods you eat.

Think of your body as a furnace that needs a fairly constant supply of wood in order to keep burning. Feeding the furnace a steady flow of wood will keep the furnace burning at a level where it's not burning too hot, or being starved for fuel. Our bodies work much the same way. Eating an excess of calories can result in extra fuel that goes unused, and is eventually stored in your body as fat. Eating too few calories may mean you will not have the energy you need to perform, and hence your body is starved of the fuel it needs to function at peak efficiency. Eating just the right amount of calories at a steady pace throughout the day will mean you'll have the fuel you need to power through workouts and perform at your best. This is why eating 5 to 6 smaller meals over the course of the day helps keep your metabolic fire burning at a more consistent level, and your metabolism plays a role in this process. Metabolism is the rate and efficiency at which our bodies convert calories to energy, and while there are metabolic factors that are somewhat out of your control, including age, genetics, and current physical condition, how you train and how you eat can have a significant impact on how efficiently your body uses the fuel that you put into it.

Our bodies also have to work harder to convert certain types of food to energy, a phenomenom known as the Thermic Effect of Food (TEF). Through TEF, because our bodies have to work even harder to metabolize proteins, our metabolism kicks into an even higher gear when we eat protein-rich foods. Conversely, when we eat foods that are high in simple carbohydrates, our bodies burn through the nutrients much more quickly and don't have to work as hard to process the calories, so the benefits of TEF aren't fully realized. By eating foods that our bodies have to work the hardest to burn, the "furnace" burns hotter and requires more fuel. If our bodies have to work harder to burn the fuel we feed them, our metabolism kicks into a higher gear.

MANAGING MACROS

What we eat is just as important as how much we eat, and at the heart of every bodybuilding nutrition program are three core macronutrients that every bodybuilder needs to manage: carbohydrates, fats, and protein. Together, these nutrients form the nutritional foundation our bodies need to fuel workouts, heal damaged muscle tissue, and replenish cells. They're essential to keep us healthy and functioning at peak performance, and to build muscle and burn fat.

While simply controlling caloric intake can help with weight loss, eating the proper ratios of these key macronutrients is the real key to losing fat and gaining—and maintaining—lean, strong muscle. What type of combination should we eat prior to a workout? A macro ratio emphasizing protein and complex carbohydrates will deliver a formula of muscle-building nutrients and slow-burning energy that together will provide the perfect fuel for an effective training session. What type of macro ratio is ideal after a workout? A ratio high in protein and good fats will give our bodies a post-workout formula that emphasizes the rebuilding of new muscle tissue, while supplying a potent nutrient boost that will help rebuild damaged muscle tissue and replenish nutrient-starved cells.

Consuming the wrong combinations of macros can have an adverse effect on training, as well. Eating meals that combine large amounts of carbohydrates with high amounts of fats can result in overloading our bodies with too many calories that we can't burn through. This can result in our bodies storing the excess nutrients and calories as body fat.

TIMING NUTRIENTS

We know that what we eat is important to building a strong body, but when we eat is almost as important. Think of every meal, and every meal plan, as a formula which requires not only eating the right ratios of macronutrients, but eating those ratios at the precise times your body needs them the most. This concept, called nutrient timing, involves strategically planning which nutrients you eat before, after, and in between workouts, so you can help your body maximize the benefits from your food and your workouts. By strategically planning your macro intake around performance, recovery, and nourishment, you can reach your training goals faster because you'll be maximizing your body's ability to utilize the right nutrients when it needs them the most.

PRE-WORKOUT TIMING

When we're trying to gain muscle, it's necessary for our bodies to synthesize more protein than we're breaking down, and to eat just enough calories to ensure our bodies have the fuel they need to build muscle without adding excess fat. Properly fueling the body about an hour before training is essential, and the optimum pre-workout macro combination will include a high level of complex carbs for sustained energy, high levels of protein to aid in the generation of muscle, but a relatively low level of fat.

Complex Carbs	Proteins	Fats
HIGH	HIGH	
		LOW

POST-WORKOUT TIMING

After a hard workout, our bodies need to maximize the benefits of training, but also reenergize and heal. Consuming faster-digesting simple carbohydrates, such as those from bananas and grapes, within an hour of training helps quickly replenish depleted energy stores. The optimum macro formula for a post-workout recovery meal will include high levels of simple carbs for quick recovery of glycogen, high levels of protein for muscle growth, and a moderate level of fat to aid in recovery. A particularly tough training day will deplete energy and amino acids stores even faster, and might require a slightly higher intake of protein and carbs.

Simple Carbs	Proteins	Fats
HIGH	HIGH	
		MEDIUM

BETWEEN WORKOUTS

Nutrient timing is also important when we're more sedentary. Our days should begin with a balanced ratio of complex carbohydrates, protein, and fats to give us a strong start and sustained energy. But while we may eat more calories during the day, we should taper our caloric intake at night, when our metabolism tends to slow down. At night there's less of a need to eat energy-rich foods, so the last snack of the day should be eaten 2 to 3 hours before going to sleep, and consist of a ratio that's high in protein, but low in carbs and fat. This will help reduce inflammation, improve recovery, and burn body fat.

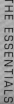

THE ESSENTIALS

THE CORE MACRONUTRIENTS

At the heart of any bodybuilder's nutrition plan are three core macronutrients: protein, carbohydrates, and fat. And while managing caloric intake is important, the real science behind bodybuilding nutrition begins with understanding these macros and their roles in your body's development so you can better plan your meals and optimize the benefits of the foods you eat.

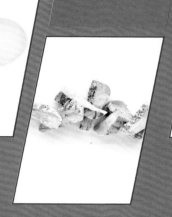

PROTEINS include eggs, chicken, fish, beef

PROTEIN

Protein is made up of amino acids and provides the foundation for building muscle and maintaining overall health. Protein's role in our bodies development is significant. It gives our cells structure, aids in tissue recovery, and contributes to the healthy production of hormones. It also increases satiety, and boosts our metabolism so our bodies can burn calories more efficiently. Protein is also the only macronutrient we're not able to store in our bodies, so a lack of dietary protein can potentially cause the body to start breaking down muscle tissue to use as energy, so it's important that we eat protein throughout the day, and in every meal. And while the average person may only need 50 to 60 grams of protein per day, a bodybuilder may need twice that amount.

The word protein, which is derived from ancient Greek, means "of prime importance," but not all forms of protein are optimal for muscle growth and maintenance. Complete proteins, which each contain around 21 amino acids, can be found in food sources such as lean meats, fish, eggs, and dairy products, and are the most complete and most efficient at building new muscle tissue.

Incomplete sources of protein contain fewer amino acids and are less efficient at giving us energy and building muscle. Many vegetarian protein sources, such as tofu and most legumes, are usually less complete and often require the supplementing of other protein sources to attain a complete amino acid profile in the body. This should be done with caution, however, as supplementing incomplete proteins with additional protein sources can have

the adverse effect of increasing carbohydrate and fat ratios beyond what our bodies need, and what remains unused can be stored in the body as fat.

Protein can also be consumed in the form of supplements, which may include powders, shakes, and bars. Supplements can bolster daily protein intake to help keep you full and fill in the gaps between meals, but they should not be considered as everyday replacements for natural protein sources. Supplements are just that—a supplement to a healthy, balanced meal plan, and their use should be limited to once per day, if possible.

Complete protein sources: eggs, turkey, chicken, beef, fish, shellfish, full-fat dairy, Greek yogurt, quinoa

Incomplete protein sources: legumes, tofu, rice, nuts, seeds

CARBOHYDRATES

Carbohydrates are the starches and sugars found in many food sources, such as fruits, vegetables, grains, and dairy products. They're essential for providing our bodies with energy, and are the body's primary go-to source for fuel. Our bodies convert carbohydrates into glycogen, which is stored in the muscles and liver until our bodies utilize it as fuel.

There are two types of carbohydrates, and both are important for our bodies. Simple carbohydrates, which come from food sources like fruit juices, corn syrup, sugar, as well as high-sugar fruits, are

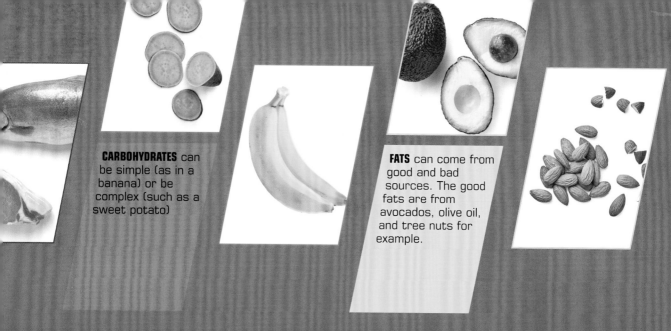

CARBOHYDRATES can be simple (as in a banana) or be complex (such as a sweet potato)

FATS can come from good and bad sources. The good fats are from avocados, olive oil, and tree nuts for example.

converted into energy very quickly by the body. Complex carbohydrates, which are higher in fiber and come from foods that include whole grains, legumes, sweet potatoes, and lower sugar fruits, are slower to digest and can provide slower, more sustained energy.

Which carbs you eat, and when you eat them, is important. When you're training hard, your body's glycogen stores tend to be depleted quickly, so it's important to have ample fuel in your body before a workout, as well as after a workout. Since complex carbohydrates provide energy that is more prolonged and sustained, it's ideal to eat a concentration of complex carbs before a workout so your body has ample energy stores to make it through a long workout. Simple carbohydrates are ideal for a post-workout refuel because they provide quick energy that will help replenish your body's glycogen stores quickly. One gram of carbohydrates provide our bodies with 4 calories of energy.

Simple carb sources: high-sugar fruits (watermelon, bananas, grapes), fruit juices, vegetables, sugar

Complex carb sources: whole grains, legumes, sweet potatoes, low-sugar fruits (kiwi, berries, citrus fruits)

FATS

Fats are essential for the development of a strong and healthy physique. They provide our bodies with energy, reduce inflammation, help transport essential fat-soluble vitamins to our cells, aid in maintaining healthy skin and hair, and aid in healthy cell function. One gram of fat provides our bodies with 9 calories of energy.

Good fats, often known as monounsaturated or polyunsaturated fats, come from sources that include foods like avocados, grass-fed butter, coconut oil, nuts, olive oil, and cold water, wild-caught fish. These fats are essential for the healthy functioning of our bodies, and for generating energy. They're also easier for the body to break down into fuel than less healthy fats.

Saturated fats are less healthy than good fats, and our bodies are less efficient at metabolizing them and turning them into energy. Saturated fats come primarily from sources such as some fatty red meats, and processed meats like ham and salami. As a general rule, including a small amount of saturated fat in the diet is okay, but it's best to limit the amount you consume.

Trans fats, on the other hand, are highly processed and found in fried foods, processed oils, some tropical oils, margarine, and other highly processed foods, and should be avoided altogether. They can cause spikes in cholesterol, high blood pressure, coronary artery disease, and inflammation. They're not good sources of energy, and because our bodies are not efficient at processing them, what's not processed by the body usually ends up stored as fat in the body's cells.

Good fat sources: avocados, tree nuts, olive oil, eggs, natural nut butters, flax seed, chia seed, oily fish (salmon, tuna), full-fat dairy

Bad fat sources: processed meats (ham, salami, bacon, hot dogs), deep-fried foods, margarine, commercially-made baked goods, partially hydrogenated vegetable oil, corn oil, sunflower oil

THE BULKING AND CUTTING PHASES

There are two primary dieting phases that are key to building a strong physique: bulking and cutting. If you think of bodybuilding in terms of sculpting, bulking is like adding clay to a sculpture—the overall shape is there, but the details may be difficult to see. Cutting, on the other hand, is like taking a chisel to the clay to reveal the distinct curves and aesthetic shape of the body. Each phase requires a unique nutritional approach to achieve the desired physical results.

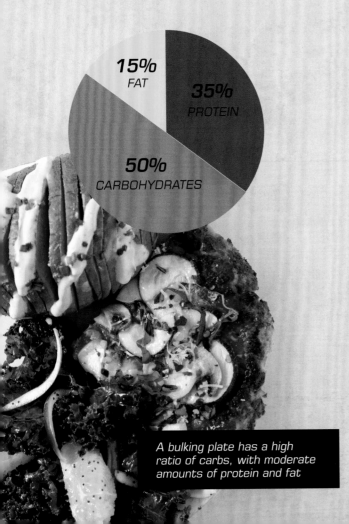

15%
FAT

35%
PROTEIN

50%
CARBOHYDRATES

A bulking plate has a high ratio of carbs, with moderate amounts of protein and fat

BULKING

Bulking isn't about eating burgers, pizza, and fries, it's about consuming a slight surplus of calories in conjunction with the right mix of properly timed macronutrients. The goal of the bulking phase is to gain muscle without gaining excessive body fat.

In bodybuilding, trainees typically do either a "clean" bulk, or a "dirty" bulk. A clean bulk will require consuming a small excess of calories, but it will encourage building muscle, rather than gaining fat, and is the best way to avoid the "fluffy" look of a layer of body fat over muscle. A dirty bulk typically utilizes any kind of food, including junk foods and supplements, in order to produce a calorie surplus that will build bulk as quickly as possible. A dirty bulk might add size quickly, but most of it likely will be in the form of fat, and the more fat that's added to a physique, the harder and longer the cut needs to be in order to get rid of it. Putting on more fat during the bulking phase also means you'll have to work harder and longer during the cutting phase to take it off. A clean bulk may take longer than a dirty bulk, but it will add more quality muscle and less fat, and in the end is the fastest and most reliable way to get strong and ripped. The goal of the bulking plan in this book is to produce a clean bulk, where excess calories are consumed in the form of whole foods, and are comprised mostly of protein and carbohydrates.

HOW IT'S DONE

One of the keys to the bulking phase is keeping the body in a state of protein synthesis, where it's utilizing sufficient protein supplies to build muscle, not break it down. To maintain protein synthesis during a clean bulk, your protein intake should be between 1 to 1.5g per pound of body weight to encourage the body to gain lean mass. Nutrient timing is also important. When you're in the bulking phase, your carbohydrate intake will be high before and after training, with slower-digesting complex carbohydrates being consumed before training, and faster-digesting simple carbohydrates being consumed after training. In a clean bulking plan, the macro ratios will average 15% fats, 50% carbohydrates, and 35% protein.

WHAT TO EXPECT

Depending on your level of lifting experience, a bulking phase may last from a few months to more than a year. If you're a seasoned lifter, a few months may be enough time to see small changes in your physique. If you're new to lifting, you may need more time in the bulking phase to allow your body to build a foundation of muscle that won't melt away once you enter the cutting phase.

CUTTING

The goal of the cutting phase is to trim the body of excess fat, while minimizing the loss of lean muscle. While bulking requires work in the weight room to build the muscle, cutting is achieved primarily in the kitchen through careful macronutrient manipulation.

During the cutting phase, the goal is to keep protein intake high, and to strategically plan carbohydrate-rich meals around the times when you're most active. This approach will give you the energy you need to continue to train with intensity, and still supply the nutrients necessary to replenish fuel stores in muscles for a better recovery. During this time, you'll be running a slight caloric deficit to encourage fat loss, which will reveal the hard-earned muscle that was created during the bulking phase. As opposed to the bulking phases, where you're consuming primarily carbs and protein in order to add muscle, the cutting phase is more about cutting calories and eating ample protein, while limiting carbohydrate and fat intake. During the cutting phase, your calorie intake will be decreased, and macro ratios average 20% fats/40% carbohydrates/40% protein.

HOW IT'S DONE

As opposed to buking, where you'll be utilizing a slight calorie surplus, the cutting phase involves utilizing a slight calorie deificit. This slight decrease in caloric intake will result in gradual fat loss, but excess deprivation during the cutting phase can lead to low energy levels and strong cravings, both of which can cause yo-yo dieting and rebounding after the cutting phase is complete. For this reason it's important to not let your calorie intake drop below your basal metabolic rate (BMR). BMR is the minimum number of calories that your body needs just to survive, and it's critical to keep your caloric intake above your BMR so your body doesn't enter a state of starvation, which means it could start burning muscle to use for energy.

WHAT TO EXPECT

The cutting phase should last from 1 to 2 months, and no more. Staying in a cutting phase for extended periods of time can potentially result in problems like yo-yo dieting, a decreased metabolic rate, and potentially the loss of valuable muscle mass. The good news is that your metabolic rate should be high after a bulk, so reducing overall caloric intake should create noticeable physique changes within just a couple of weeks of starting a cut. You can expect to lose one pound or less per week, but your measurements may change more drastically than that as you lose more from your waist and other areas where the body tends to store excess fat.

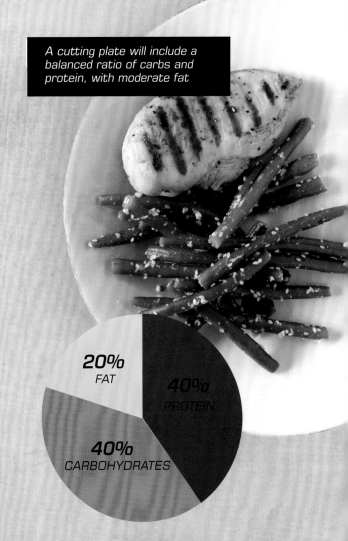

A cutting plate will include a balanced ratio of carbs and protein, with moderate fat

20% FAT

40% PROTEIN

40% CARBOHYDRATES

The two main challenges you may encounter in a cutting phase are increased hunger and a possible decrease in metabolism. You can combat these challenges by increasing lean protein and vegetable servings whenever you're feeling excessively hungry. It's difficult for the body to convert protein and vegetables to body fat, and protein has a satiating effect that will help keep any cravings to a minimum.

Another way to combat some of the challenges of a cutting phase is to trick your brain. It's important to remember that we eat with our eyes first, and it's satisfying to eat from a plate full of brightly colored vegetables and richly spiced, healthy foods, so keep the foods on the plate bright, vivid, and flavorful. Another trick is to try using a smaller plate, if the plate looks sparse, your brain may think you haven't had enough food and you may feel unsatisfied. However you do it, stick to your long-range plan and never starve yourself just to get quick results.

KETOGENIC DIETING, CARB CYCLING, AND CALORIE CYCLING

No single plan works for any one person, and there are different ways to achieve the ultimate goals of building muscle or cutting fat. Ketogenic dieting, carb cycling, and calorie cycling are three unique nutritional approaches that can be used in place of the traditional bulking and cutting methods, and all three will yield results.

KETOGENIC DIETING

Ketogenic dieting is a nutritional approach where the majority of calories come from eating dietary fat, while a moderate amount of calories come from protein and carbohydrate intake is very tightly restricted. A ketogenic plan is ideal for those who want to lose body fat, but may also be sensitive to carbohydrates. It's especially effective for those who need to lose 10% body fat or more.

On a ketogenic diet, the body is starved of carbohydrates, the body's normal preferred source of energy, and thus cannot produce a sufficient level of glucose to use as energy. In turn, the body begins to burn fat for energy, which produces a by-product called *ketones*, which are used for fuel in place of glucose. Once the body enters this phase, the resulting process is called *ketosis*. By keeping dietary fat intake high, protein intake moderate, and carbohydrate intake low, the body is encouraged to burn more fat for fuel. In a ketogenic plan, 60% of calories comes from fat, 30% from protein, and 10% or less from carbohydrates.

Note that an excess of ketones in the body can potentially result in a condition known as ketoacidosis, which is a potentially dangerous health condition. If you're considering a ketogenic approach to cutting, it's best to do your research and consult with your physician before doing so.

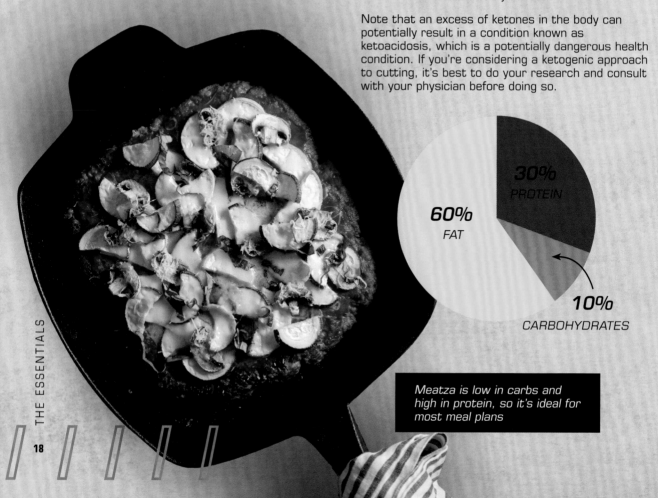

60% FAT

30% PROTEIN

10% CARBOHYDRATES

Meatza is low in carbs and high in protein, so it's ideal for most meal plans

CARB CYCLING

Carb cycling is the process of consuming a normal diet of carbohydrates and a sufficient number of calories for five days out of the week, while tightly restricting carbs for the remaining two days of the week. Carb cycling can help you build lean mass and burn body fat, without having to stick to a restrictive plan seven days a week. By going low carb two days a week, you'll restrict calories without slowing down your metabolism, and without feeling deprived.

On a carb cycling plan, protein intake will remain steady for all seven days to help keep you full, but your carbohydrate intake on low days will drop to 30 to 50 grams for the entire day. Low carb days should be scheduled for days off from the gym, or on lower intensity days, because your energy reserves won't be as high since you'll be consuming fewer carbs, which means your body will have less glucose to use as energy. If you're working out on a low day, the majority of your carbohydrate intake should occur just before and just after your training sessions to maximize the fuel your body has available for energy and recovery. Average caloric ratios for a carb cycling plan are 15% from fat, 45% from carbs, and 40% from protein on a normal day, and 30% from fat, 20% from carbs, and 50% from protein on low carbohydrate days.

CALORIE CYCLING

Calorie cycling is similar to carb cycling, but instead of restricting carbohydrates, you'll be restricting caloric intake for 2 days of the week, while following a balanced meal plan for the balance of the week. Calorie cycling is another way to trim body fat, while still keeping your protein intake at a level that is sufficient enough to build lean muscle and burn fat.

On low calorie days, both carbohydrates and fats are restricted, while protein intake either remains the same or is increased slightly. Increasing your protein intake by 2 to 3 ounces on the low calorie days will help improve satiety and decrease cravings. On a calorie cycling plan, the caloric ratios are 20% from fats, 40% from carbs, and 40% from protein on normal days, and 15% from fat, 25% from carbs, and 60% from protein on low calorie days.

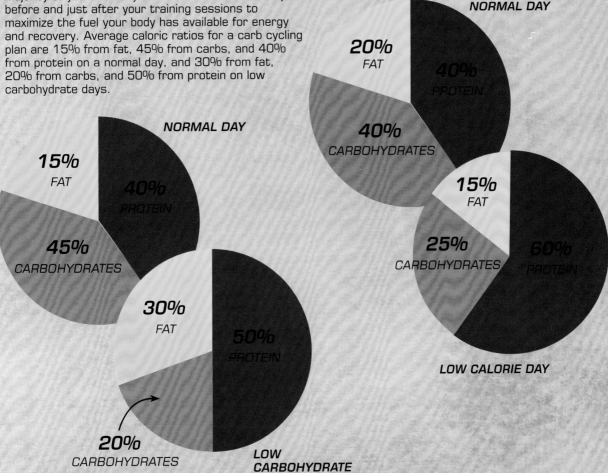

CARB CYCLING — NORMAL DAY: 15% FAT, 45% CARBOHYDRATES, 40% PROTEIN. LOW CARBOHYDRATE DAY: 30% FAT, 20% CARBOHYDRATES, 50% PROTEIN.

CALORIE CYCLING — NORMAL DAY: 20% FAT, 40% CARBOHYDRATES, 40% PROTEIN. LOW CALORIE DAY: 15% FAT, 25% CARBOHYDRATES, 60% PROTEIN.

GETTING STARTED

What works for one person may not work for the next, which is why successful meal planning often is a process of trial and error to find what works best. Follow these simple steps to choose a plan and get started, then make adjustments to develop the plan that works for you.

USING THE RECIPES

Each recipe includes total calories, helpful prep tips and variations, and a bar scale reflecting the amount of macronutrients contained in the recipe. One bar on the scale means the macronutrient content is low, two bars equals a moderate amount, and three bars indicates a high amount.

	HIGH	MEDIUM	LOW
FAT	15g and up	5.1g to 14.9g	5g or less
CARBOHYDRATES	25g and up	10.1g to 24.9g	10g or less
PROTEIN	25g and up	10.1g to 24.9g	10g or less

1

CHOOSE YOUR PLAN

Choose a plan that aligns with your goals and fits your lifestyle. The bulking and cutting plans are the most common plans and are good ways to begin. But if you have excess body fat and want to burn fat more quickly, the ketogenic plan might be the ideal way to start. The calorie cycling and carb cycling plans both offer alternatives that don't require sticking to the same formula every day of the week. Each meal plan averages between 1,300 and 2,000 calories per day, and is designed to be as simple as possible to follow, with the total calories and macro amounts listed, along with a detailed shopping list.

2

CALCULATE YOUR CALORIES

The default portion sizes in the recipes are designed for a moderately active person who weighs 150 pounds. Use these calculations to determine how to adjust the meal plans and recipes to meet your daily caloric needs:

LIGHTLY ACTIVE: Your weight x 12

MODERATELY ACTIVE: Your weight x 13

VERY ACTIVE: Your weight x 14

(Note that in order to stay above your BMR, you should never allow your daily caloric intake to drop below 70% of your daily caloric needs.)

THE ESSENTIALS

20

TIPS FOR SUCCESS

Focus on eating nutritious, calorie-dense foods *When eating for physique composition, the quality of the food matters. Opting for single ingredient, natural foods like boneless, skinless chicken breasts, fish, oats, brown rice, apples, bananas, avocados, nuts, spinach, onions, and cucumbers means you will always be eating a diet comprised primarily of foods that are both nutritious and filling.*

Eat protein with every meal (and fill your plate) *Simply adding a large handful of spinach, a full serving of lean chicken breast, and a full serving of brown rice to a plate will create a mountain of food that will keep you full for hours, and still total only around 300 calories. Always eating ample protein and a healthy volume of food at every meal means both your belly and your brain will feel satisfied because you're eating from a full plate that contains color and a satisfying mix of flavors.*

Keep a food log to track progress *If you're struggling to make progress, a food log can help identify where adjustments might be needed. Try a meal plan for a week, log your meals, and document how you feel at various points in the day. Are you hungry at particular times of the day, or feeling too full? How is your progress at the end of the week? Are you seeing the results you expected? Which foods made you feel the most satisfied? This feedback will help you fine tune your plan.*

Avoid the scale *Weighing yourself on a scale isn't what physique development is about. A scale only shows a number that reflects weight gain or loss—not improvements in body composition. Gauge your success by how you look and feel. If you feel good and like the way you look, you're doing it right!*

Enjoy a treat meal to crush cravings *An occasional treat meal can be effective in combatting metabolism slowdown and calming cravings. A treat meal typically contains ample protein, is low in fat, but is higher in carbs to help replenish glycogen stores that may have been depleted during an extended cutting phase. A treat meal might also include an extra dessert (if you're craving sweets), or a baked potato (if you're craving carbs). The idea is to crush the cravings and boost your metabolism, while still staying on track with your plan. Treat meals should be consumed no more than once a week.*

Be patient and don't quit! *If you find a plan isn't yielding the results you desire, or the changes aren't happening as quickly as you'd like, try making small, incremental adjustments before abandoning the plan. Some people naturally gain muscle or lose fat faster than others, so hang in there and don't quit!*

3

GET PREPARED

Plan your week carefully by knocking out your shopping and prepping your meals in advance, as much as possible. While a few of the recipes in this book are best eaten fresh, the majority of the recipes can be made in advance, portioned out, and stored in the refrigerator or freezer. By planning your meals in advance, you'll be better prepared to manage your meal plan. Also, take the time to plan your nutrient intake around your workouts. If you're cognizant about eating the right nutrients at the right times, your body will build more muscle and burn more fat in less time, and will recover from workouts faster.

4

TRACK YOUR PROGRESS

Try a plan for 1 to 2 weeks, then gauge your progress. Are you seeing results? Taking bi-weekly progress pictures is a helpful way to assess any changes in your body composition. If you find you're not gaining muscle mass, try increasing your protein intake. If you feel you're not burning the fat, try a slight decrease in the amount of calories you're consuming each day. If you find you're constantly hungry, slightly increase your protein intake with each meal. You can also add an occasional snack to help combat the cravings. The key is to stay flexible and make small adjustments as you move along.

THE ESSENTIALS

7-DAY BULKING MEAL PLAN

THE MACRO FORMULA
BREAKFAST: starchy carbs, protein
SNACK: fruit carbs, protein
LUNCH: carbs, protein
SNACK: carbs, protein
DINNER: low glycemic carbs, protein
SNACK: protein

	DAY 1	DAY 2	DAY 3
BREAKFAST	Southern Breakfast Casserole	Savory Apple Sage Turkey Sausages, Blueberry Muffins (2 servings)	Chicken and Polenta Breakfast Pizza
SNACKS	Oatmeal Raisin Cookie Shake	Blueberry Cheesecake Shake	Carrot Cake Shake
LUNCH	Grilled Southwestern Pork Medallions, Coconut Cayenne Smashed Sweet Potatoes, Rosemary Beefsteak Tomatoes	Tex-Mex Fajitas, Zesty Zoodles	Stuffed Florentine Chicken Breasts, Fluffy Basmati Rice
SNACKS	Egg White Custards (2 servings)	Paleo Protein Crackers, Greek Yogurt Hummus	Almond Butter and Oats Bars
DINNER	Bison and Portobello Sliders, Sweet Potato Medallions, Roasted Brussels Sprouts and Fennel	Slow Cooker Pulled BBQ Chicken, Cloud Bread, Herb-Roasted Vegetables	Muscle Building Meatloaf, Hasselb Sweet Potatoes, Wilted Spinach and Tomato Salad
SNACKS	Savory Rosemary Almond Bars	Golden Milk Shake	Baked Cheeseburger Bites
TOTAL CALORIES	1906	2012	1981
TOTAL FAT (grams)	52.1g	67.3g	49g
TOTAL CARBS (grams)	179g	161g	179g
TOTAL PROTEIN (grams)	189g	202g	168g

SHOPPING LIST

- **STARCHES:** old-fashioned oats, cornmeal, pre-rinsed white quinoa, basmati rice, brown rice, sweet potatoes (4, large), russet potatoes (4, large), 1 15oz (420g) can chickpeas, 1 15oz (420g) can pumpkin purée (not pumpkin pie filling), 1 15oz (420g) can black beans, 1 1lb (450g) bag frozen hash browns, no-sugar-added crispy brown rice cereal, gluten-free flour, corn tortillas (8, small)

- **PROTEINS:** large eggs (1 dozen), 3 32oz (950g) containers liquid egg whites, 1 32oz (950g) container Greek yogurt, 1 16oz (450g) container 1% cottage cheese, 5lbs (2.3kg) boneless, skinless chicken breasts, 2lbs (1kg) 99% lean ground turkey breast, 2lbs (1kg) sirloin steak, 1lb (450g) lean ground beef (92/8 lean-to-fat ratio), 2lbs (1kg) pork tenderloin, 1lb (450g) lean ground bison, 2 5oz (140g) cans tuna (packed in water), 2 5oz (140g) cans salmon (packed in water), ½lb (225g) sliced deli turkey, ½lb (225g) sliced deli ham, 1 7oz (200g) package low fat shredded mozzarella cheese

- **FRUITS AND VEGETABLES:** 1 10oz (285g) package frozen blueberries, naval oranges (2, medium), white onions (2, medium), 1lb (450g) fresh broccoli, 1 6oz (170g) bag fresh baby spinach, 1 12oz (340g) bag chopped kale, 1 10oz (285g) package frozen riced cauliflower or cauliflower (1 medium), green cabbage (2, medium), watermelon (1, small), cantaloupe (1, small), avocados (2, large), spaghetti squash (2, small), zucchini (2, medium), yellow squash (2, medium), beefsteak tomatoes (2, large), 1 pint (470ml) cherry tomatoes, 1lb (450g) fresh, young asparagus, 1lb fresh Brussels sprouts, fennel bulbs (2, medium), bananas (6, medium), 1lb fresh green beans, bell peppers (4, medium), portobello mushrooms (4, large), lemons (2, small), 1 16oz (450g) bag baby carrots, 1 10oz (285g) bag shredded carrots

- **OTHER:** coconut oil, whey protein powder, powdered stevia, unflavored almond milk, almond flour, powdered peanut butter, low-sodium chicken broth, natural almond butter, unsweetened cocoa powder, jarred minced garlic, no-sugar-added tomato sauce, heavy cream

DAY 4	DAY 5	DAY 6	DAY 7
Cottage Cheese and Cantaloupe Bowl	Keto Breakfast Burritos	Crustless Quiche, Blueberry Muffins	Pumped-Up Protein Pancake
Golden Milk Shake	Orange Creamsicle Shake	Grilled Balsamic Watermelon and Cheese	Elvis Shake
Coconut Curry Shrimp (2 servings), Curried Rice Pilaf	Sriracha Curry Coconut Chicken, Fluffy Basmati Rice	Southwestern Chicken Street Tacos, Spicy Black Beans and Quinoa	Meatza, Carb Cutter Twice-Baked Potatoes (2 servings)
Greek Yogurt Hummus, Quick and Easy Egg Bites	Quick and Easy Egg Bites (2 servings)	Gains Glazed Donuts	Lean Rice Crispy Treats (2 servings)
Vietnamese-Style Pork Tenderloin, Spicy Black Beans and Quinoa, Cauliflower Fried Rice	Ginger Beef Bok Choy Stir Fry, Coconut Cayenne Smashed Sweet Potatoes, Craveable Citrus Kale Salad	Stuffed Bell Peppers, Fluffy Basmati Rice	Spicy Salmon Burgers, Crunchy Avocado Salad, Lemony Grilled Asparagus
Quick and Easy Egg Bites (2 servings)	Baked Cheeseburger Bites	Carrot Cake Shake	Egg White Custards (2 servings)
2053	1837	1944	1888
36g	53.3g	38g	60.2g
160g	118g	199.1g	183.6g
255g	216g	192g	192.3g

7-DAY CUTTING MEAL PLAN

THE MACRO FORMULA

BREAKFAST: starchy carbs, protein
SNACK: fats, protein
LUNCH: carbs, protein
SNACK: carbs, protein
DINNER: fats, protein

	DAY 1	DAY 2	DAY 3
BREAKFAST	Pumped-Up Protein Pancake	Savory Apple Sage Turkey Sausages, Blueberry Muffins	Steamed Squash Custard
SNACKS	Quick and Easy Egg Bites	Greek Yogurt Hummus	Turkey and Veggie Roll-Up
LUNCH	Broth-Poached Snapper with Broccoli, Hasselback Sweet Potatoes	Tex-Mex Fajitas	Almond-Crusted Mustard Chicken, Sweet Potato Medallions
SNACKS	Key Lime Shake	Carrot Cake Shake	Hulk Shake
DINNER	Reverse-Seared Sirloin Steak, Roasted Cabbage Steaks, Curried Rice Pilaf	Ginger Soy Shrimp Skewers, Cauliflower Fried Rice, Crunchy Avocado Salad	Blackened Baked Tilapia, Lemony Grilled Asparagus, Fluffy Basmati Rice
TOTAL CALORIES	1449	1401	1473
TOTAL FAT (grams)	21.1g	36g	27g
TOTAL CARBS (grams)	149.1g	125.9g	156.5g
TOTAL PROTEIN (grams)	168.6g	118.4g	162.2g

SHOPPING LIST

- **STARCHES:** old-fashioned oats, pre-rinsed white quinoa, basmati rice, brown rice, sweet potatoes (6, large), russet potatoes (2, large), 1 15oz (420g) can chickpeas, 1 15oz (420g) can pumpkin purée (not pumpkin pie filling), 1 15oz (420g) can black beans

- **PROTEINS:** large eggs (1 dozen), 3 32oz (950g) containers liquid egg whites, 1 32oz (950g) container Greek yogurt, 1 16oz (450g) container 1% cottage cheese, 4lbs (1.8kg) boneless, skinless chicken breasts, 1 whole chicken (small, approximately 3lbs (1.4kg)), 1lb (450) medium shrimp (fresh or frozen), 1lb (450g) 99% lean ground turkey breast, 2lbs (1kg) sirloin steak, 1lb (450g) lean ground beef (2/8 lean-to-fat ratio), 1lb (450g) tilapia filets (fresh or frozen), 1lb (450g) cod filets (fresh or frozen), 1lb (450g) pork tenderloin, 2 5oz (140g) cans tuna (packed in water)

- **FRUITS AND VEGETABLES:** navel oranges (2 medium), white onions (2 medium), 1lb (450g) fresh broccoli , 1 16oz (450g) bag fresh baby spinach, 1 12oz (340g) bag chopped kale, 1 10oz (285g) bag frozen riced cauliflower or cauliflower (1 medium), cabbage (2, medium), acorn squash (2, medium), watermelon, (1, small), cantaloupe (1, small), avocado (1, medium), Granny Smith apple (1, medium), zucchini (2, medium), yellow squash (2, medium), beefsteak tomatoes (2, large), 1 pint (470ml) fresh cherry tomatoes, spaghetti squash (1, large), 1lb (450g) fresh asparagus, lemons (3, medium), limes (2, medium), bananas (4, medium), 1 16oz (450g) bag baby carrots, 1 10oz (285g) bag shredded carrots

- **OTHER:** coconut oil, whey protein powder, powdered stevia, unflavored almond milk, almond flour, powdered peanut butter, low-sodium chicken broth, natural almond butter, unsweetened cocoa powder, jarred minced garlic

DAY 4	DAY 5	DAY 6	DAY 7
Overnight Mocha Oats	Chicken and Polenta Breakfast Pizza	Crispy Rice Skillet	Cottage Cheese and Cantaloupe Bowl
Grilled Balsamic Watermelon and Cheese	Pumpkin and Oat Bars	Zesty Tuna Snack Bowl	Baked Cheeseburger Bites
Grilled Jerk Chicken Breasts, Spicy Black Beans and Quinoa, Roasted Cabbage Steaks	Grilled Southwestern Pork Medallions, Carb Cutter Twice-Baked Potatoes	Chicken Cacciatore, Fluffy Basmati Rice	White Chicken Chili, Herb-Roasted Vegetables
Elvis Shake	Grilled Balsamic Watermelon and Cheese	Orange Creamsicle Shake	No-Bake Cocoa and Oats Bars
Slow Cooker BBQ Pulled Chicken, Wilted Spinach and Tomato Salad, Cloud Bread	Chili Lime Salmon Pouches, Zesty Zoodles, Spicy Black Beans and Quinoa	Apple-Roasted Whole Chicken, Craveable Citrus Kale Salad, Sweet Potato Medallions	Broiled Cod with Charred Tomatillo Salsa, Rosemary Beefsteak Tomatoes, Coconut Cayenne Smashed Sweet Potatoes
1364	1324	1371	1336
29.6g	23.6g	13.9g	30.8g
156.5g	135.5g	142.1g	118.1g
160g	139g	161.7g	117.8g

7-DAY KETOGENIC MEAL PLAN

THE MACRO FORMULA

BREAKFAST: fats, protein
SNACK: fats, protein
LUNCH: fats, protein
SNACK: fats, protein
DINNER: fats, protein
SNACK: protein

	DAY 1	DAY 2	DAY 3
BREAKFAST	Smoked Salmon Avocado Boats	Keto Breakfast Burritos	Low-Carb Pancake (keto version)
SNACKS	Savory Rosemary Almond Bars	Paleo Protein Crackers	Quick and Easy Egg Bites
LUNCH	Spicy Stuffed Peppers	Broiled Greek Chicken Kebobs, Crunchy Avocado Salad	Ginger Soy Shrimp Skewers (keto version), Cauliflower Fried Rice, Cloud Bread
SNACKS	Guacamole Deviled Eggs	Golden Milk Shake	Coco-Choco Almond Shake
DINNER	Chili Lime Salmon Pouches, Crunchy Avocado Salad	Sriracha Curry Coconut Chicken (keto version), Cloud Bread	Stuffed Florentine Chicken Breasts, Wilted Spinach and Tomato Salad
SNACKS	Baked Cheeseburger Bites	Quick and Easy Egg Bites	Baked Cheeseburger Bites
TOTAL CALORIES	1597	1745	1713
TOTAL FAT (grams)	108.5g	110.3g	88.1g
TOTAL CARBS (grams)	48.2g	39.1g	54.8g
TOTAL PROTEIN (grams)	122.2g	151.6g	179.8g

SHOPPING LIST

- **Proteins:** large eggs (1 dozen), 3 32oz (950g) containers liquid egg whites, 1 32oz (950g) container fat-free Greek yogurt, 1 16oz (450g) container 1% cottage cheese, 3lbs (1.4kg) boneless, skinless chicken breasts, 1lb (450g) 99% lean ground turkey breast, 2lbs (1kg) sirloin steak, 1lb (450g) grass-fed ground beef, 2lbs (1kg) pork tenderloin, 1lb (450g) medium shrimp (fresh or frozen), 1/2lb (225g) deli ham (unsliced), 2lbs (1kg) pork roast, 1lb (450g) beef roast, 4oz (110g) smoked salmon, 1lb (450g) fresh salmon filets, 1 6oz (170g) package Canadian bacon, 2 5oz (140g) cans salmon (packed in water), 4 5oz (140g) cans tuna (packed in water), ½lb (225g) sliced deli turkey, 1 8oz (225g) package shredded mozzarella cheese

- **Fruits and vegetables:** white onions (2, medium), 1lb (450g) fresh broccoli, 1 16oz (450g) bag fresh baby spinach, 1 10oz (285g) package frozen riced cauliflower or cauliflower (1, medium), green cabbage (2, medium), avocados (4, large), zucchini (2, medium), yellow squash (2, medium), 1 pint (470ml) cherry tomatoes, portobello mushrooms (4, large), 1lb (450g) fresh Brussels sprouts, fennel bulbs (2, medium), lemons (2, medium), limes (2, medium)

- **Other:** coconut oil, almond flour, heavy cream, whey protein powder, powdered stevia, unflavored almond milk, powdered peanut butter, low-sodium chicken broth, natural almond butter, unsweetened cocoa powder, jarred minced garlic

DAY 4	DAY 5	DAY 6	DAY 7
Canadian Bacon and Egg Cups	Crustless Quiche (keto version)	Steak and Egg Burrito (keto version)	Southern Breakfast Casserole (keto version)
Paleo Protein Crackers	Savory Rosemary Almond Bars	Quick and Easy Egg Bites	Zesty Tuna Snack Bowl
White Chicken Chili (keto version)	Reverse-Seared Sirloin Steak, Roasted Cabbage Steaks	Spicy Salmon Burgers, Cloud Bread	Coffee-Rubbed Steaks, Rosemary Beefsteak Tomatoes
Baked Cheeseburger Bites	Golden Milk Shake	Baked Cheeseburger Bites	Choco-Cado Mousse, Quick and Easy Egg Bites
Vietnamese-Style Pork Tenderloin, Zesty Zoodles, Crunchy Avocado Salad	Muscle-Building Meatloaf, Cauliflower Fried Rice	Slow Cooker Rosemary Pot Roast, Roasted Brussels Sprouts and Fennel	Bison and Portabello Sliders (keto version)
Zesty Tuna Snack Bowl	Coco-Choco Almond Shake	Zesty Tuna Snack Bowl	Baked Cheeseburger Bites
1674	1681	1515	1615
100g	97.2g	84g	107g
50.3g	57g	33.3g	26.2g
153.7g	180g	192g	141g

7-DAY CALORIE CYCLING MEAL PLAN

THE MACRO FORMULA

(NORMAL DAYS)	(LOW CALORIE DAYS)
BREAKFAST: carbs, protein	**BREAKFAST:** carbs, protein
SNACK: carbs, protein	**SNACK:** carbs (half portion), protein
LUNCH: carbs, protein	**LUNCH:** carbs (half portion), protein
SNACK: fats, protein	**SNACK:** protein
DINNER: fats, protein, carbs	**DINNER:** fats, protein, carbs
SNACK: protein	

	DAY 1	DAY 2	DAY 3
BREAKFAST	Break-the-Fast Skillet	Pumpkin Pie Protein Bowl	Overnight Mocha Oats
SNACKS	Elvis Shake	No-Bake Almond and Oat Bars	Pumpkin and Oat Bars
LUNCH	Slow Cooker BBQ Pulled Chicken, Fluffy Basmati Rice, Rosemary Beefsteak Tomatoes	Grilled Jerk Chicken Breasts, Spicy Black Beans and Quinoa, Roasted Brussels Sprouts and Fennel	Almond-Crusted Mustard Chicken, Sweet Potato Medallions, Herb-Roasted Vegetab
SNACKS	Baked Cheeseburger Bites	Guacamole Deviled Eggs	Zesty Tuna Snack Bowl
DINNER	Spicy Stuffed Peppers, Zesty Zoodles, Sweet Potato Medallions	Ridiculously Easy Pork Roll-Ups, Craveable Citrus Kale Salad, Curried Rice Pilaf	Reverse-Seared Sirloin Steak, Fresh Veggie Stir Fry, Hasselback Sweet Potatoes
SNACKS	Guacamole Deviled Eggs	Quick and Easy Egg Bites	Lean Rice Crispy Treats
TOTAL CALORIES	1662	1688	1660
TOTAL FAT (grams)	47.6g	54.5g	39.6g
TOTAL CARBS (grams)	156.4g	143g	175.2g
TOTAL PROTEIN (grams)	135.6g	159.1g	155g

SHOPPING LIST

- **STARCHES:** old-fashioned oats, pre-rinsed white quinoa, basmati rice, brown rice, sweet potatoes (8, large), russet potatoes (2, large), 1 15oz (420g) can chickpeas, 1 15oz (420g) can pumpkin purée (not pumpkin pie filling), 1 15oz (420g) can black beans, 1lb (450g) bag frozen hash browns, no-sugar-added crispy brown rice cereal

- **FRUITS AND VEGETABLES:** 1 12oz package frozen blueberries, navel oranges (1, medium), white onions (2, medium), 1lb (450g) fresh broccoli, ½lb (225g) bok choy, 1 16oz (450g) bag fresh baby spinach, 1 12oz (340g) bag frozen chopped kale, 1 10oz (285g) package frozen riced cauliflower or cauliflower (1, medium), green cabbage (2, medium), watermelon (1, small), avocado (1, large), spaghetti squash (2, small), zucchini (2, medium), yellow squash (2, medium), beefsteak tomatoes (2, large), lemons (2, medium), 1 pint (470ml) cherry tomatoes, 8oz (225g) button mushrooms, spaghetti squash (1, large),

1lb (450g) fresh asparagus, 1lb (450g) fresh Brussels sprouts, fennel bulbs (2 medium), bananas (6, medium), 1lb (450g) fresh green beans, bell peppers (4, large), 1 16oz (450g) bag baby carrots

- **PROTEINS:** large eggs (1 dozen), 3 32oz (950g) containers liquid egg whites, 1 32oz (950g) container Greek yogurt, 1 16oz (450g) 1% cottage cheese, 5lbs (2.3kg) boneless, skinless chicken breasts, 2lbs (1kg) 99% lean ground turkey breast, 2lbs (1kg) sirloin steak, 1lb (450g) lean ground beef (92/8 lean-to-fat ratio), 1lb (450g) tilapia filets (fresh or frozen), 1lb (450g) medium shrimp (fresh or frozen), 2lbs (1kg) pork tenderloin, 2 5oz (140g) cans tuna (packed in water), ½lb (225g) sliced deli turkey, 1 8oz (225g) package low fat shredded mozzarella cheese

- **OTHER:** coconut oil, whey protein powder, powdered stevia, unflavored almond milk, almond flour, powdered peanut butter, low-sodium chicken broth, natural almond butter, unsweetened cocoa powder, jarred minced garlic

DAY 4 (LOW CALORIE)	DAY 5	DAY 6	DAY 7 (LOW CALORIE)
Savory Apple Sage Turkey Sausages	Baked Banana and Oat Bars	Savory Breakfast Oatmeal	Low-Carb Pancake
Key Lime Shake	Grilled Balsamic Watermelon and Cheese	Orange Creamsicle Shake	Turkey and Veggie Roll-Up
Almond-Crusted Mustard Chicken, Baked Zucchini Fries	Coconut Curry Shrimp, Curried Rice Pilaf	Grilled Southwestern Pork Medallions, Coconut Cayenne Smashed Sweet Potatoes	Pan-Seared Chicken Breasts, Fluffy Basmati Rice, Cauliflower Fried Rice
Quick and Easy Egg Bites	Paleo Protein Crackers	Pumpkin and Oat Bars	Chocolate Protein Snack Mug
Blackened Baked Tilapia, Roasted Cabbage Steaks, Fluffy Basmati Rice	Spaghetti Squash and Meatball Boats, Spicy Black Beans and Quinoa	Coffee-Rubbed Steak, Wilted Spinach and Tomato Salad, Carb Cutter Twice-Baked Potatoes	Broiled Greek Chicken Kebobs, Lemony Grilled Asparagus, Coconut Cayenne Smashed Sweet Potatoes
(no snack)	Cocoa and Oat Bars	Quick and Easy Egg Bites, Choco-Cado Mousse	(no snack)
1352	1582	1572	1331
33.2g	38g	29g	23g
90.2g	160.3g	148g	123.4g
179g	160.5g	176.9g	161g

7-DAY CARB CYCLING MEAL PLAN

THE MACRO FORMULA

(NORMAL DAYS)	(LOW CARB DAYS)
BREAKFAST: carbs, protein	**BREAKFAST:** fats, protein
SNACK: carbs, protein	**SNACK:** protein
LUNCH: carbs, protein	**LUNCH:** fats, protein
SNACK: fats, protein	**SNACK:** fats, protein
DINNER: carbs, protein	**DINNER:** fats, protein
SNACK: protein	**SNACK:** protein

	DAY 1	DAY 2	DAY 3
BREAKFAST	Breakfast Hash	Steamed Squash Custard	Pumpkin Pie Bowl
SNACKS	Oatmeal Raisin Cookie Shake	Carrot Cake Shake	Grilled Balsamic Watermelon and Cheese
LUNCH	Pan-Seared Chicken Breasts, Hasselback Sweet Potatoes, Wilted Spinach and Tomato Salad	Reverse Seared Sirloin Steak, Spicy Black Beans and Quinoa	Tex-Mex Fajitas
SNACKS	Quick and Easy Egg Bites	Chocolate Protein Snack Mug	Blueberry Cheesecake Shake
DINNER	Bison and Portobello Sliders, Lemony Grilled Asparagus, Sweet Potato Medallions	Meatza, Craveable Citrus Kale Salad, Coconut Cayenne Smashed Sweet Potatoes	Grilled Southwestern Pork Medallions, Herb-Roasted Vegetables, Carb Cutter Twice-Baked Potatoes
SNACKS	Guacamole Deviled Eggs	Paleo Protein Crackers	Greek Yogurt Hummus
TOTAL CALORIES	1589	1704	1657
TOTAL FAT (grams)	48g	38.5g	30.5g
TOTAL CARBS (grams)	147.6g	161.2g	220g
TOTAL PROTEIN (grams)	158.8g	180g	162.1g

SHOPPING LIST

- **STARCHES:** old-fashioned oats, pre-rinsed white quinoa, basmati rice, brown rice, sweet potatoes (8, large), russet potatoes (2, large), 1 15oz (420g) can chickpeas, 1 15oz (420g) can pumpkin purée (not pumpkin pie filling), 1 15oz (420g) can black beans, corn tortillas (8, small), 1lb (450g) bag frozen hash brown potatoes, no-sugar-added crispy brown rice cereal

- **PROTEINS:** Large eggs (1 dozen), 2 32oz (950g) containers liquid egg whites, 1 32oz (950g) container fat-free Greek yogurt, 1 16oz (450g) container 1% cottage cheese, 4lbs (1.8kg) boneless, skinless chicken breasts, 2lbs (1kg) 99% lean ground turkey breast, 2lbs (1kg) sirloin steak, 1lb (450g) lean ground bison, 1lb (450g) salmon filets, 3lbs (1.4kg) pork tenderloin, 2lbs (1kg) pork roast, 1lb (450g) medium shrimp (fresh or frozen), ½lb (225g) sliced deli turkey, 1 8oz (225g) package low fat shredded mozzarella cheese, 2 5oz (140g) cans tuna (packed in water)

- **FRUITS AND VEGETABLES:** 1 12oz (340g) package frozen blueberries, naval oranges (1, medium), white onions (2, medium), 1lb (450g) fresh broccoli, 1 16oz (450g) bag fresh baby spinach, 12oz (340g) fresh kale, ½lb (225g) fresh bok choy, 8oz (225g) button mushrooms, 1 10oz (285g) package frozen riced cauliflower or cauliflower (1, medium), green cabbage (2, medium), watermelon (1, small), avocado (2, medium), zucchini (2, medium), yellow squash (2, medium), 1 pint (470ml) cherry tomatoes, spaghetti squash (1, medium), 1lb (450g) fresh asparagus, 1lb (450g) fresh Brussels sprouts, fennel bulbs (2, medium), bananas (3, medium), 1lb (450g) fresh green beans, acorn squash (4, medium), 1 16oz (450g) bag baby carrots, lemons (3, medium)

- **OTHER:** coconut oil, whey protein powder, powdered stevia, unflavored almond milk, almond flour, powdered peanut butter, low-sodium chicken broth, jarred minced garlic, unsweetened cocoa powder

DAY 4 (LOW CARB)	DAY 5	DAY 6	DAY 7 (LOW CARB)
Keto Breakfast Burrito	Cottage Cheese and Cantaloupe Bowl	Break-the-Fast Skillet	Keto Breakfast Burrito
Guacamole Deviled Eggs	Orange Creamsicle Shake	Elvis Shake	Golden Milk Shake
Slow Cooker Pork Roast, Roasted Cabbage Steaks	Slow Cooker BBQ Pulled Chicken, Carb Cutter Twice-Baked Potatoes, Wilted Spinach and Tomato Salad	Vietnamese-Style Pork Tenderloin, Spicy Black Beans and Quinoa, Fresh Veggie Stir Fry	Ridiculously Easy Pork Roll-Ups, Cauliflower Fried Rice
Zesty Tuna Snack Bowl	Greek Yogurt Hummus, Paleo Protein Crackers	Turkey and Veggie Roll-Up	Baked Cheeseburger Bites
Muscle-Building Meatloaf, Roasted Cabbage Steaks	Ginger Soy Shrimp Kebobs, Fresh Veggie Stir Fry, Curried Rice Pilaf	Chicken Hobo Dinner, Snappy Sesame Green Beans, Fluffy Basmati Rice	Chili Lime Salmon Pouches, Zesty Zoodles
Savory Rosemary Almond Bars	Quick and Easy Egg Bites	Zesty Tuna Snack Bowl	Egg White Custards
1452	1694	1658	1466
80g	35.4g	27.1g	71g
46.7g	171g	186.3g	38.6g
143.7g	175.6g	189g	166.4g

BREAKFASTS

It's the most important meal of the day, and these breakfast recipes will help energize your body and fuel you through the morning. All averaging around five ingredients each, these recipes are simple and feature a wide variety of flavors and ingredients you can find at any supermarket. And each is designed not only to please your palate, but also to provide the proper macronutrients necessary to help you reach your goals.

This recipe, featuring hints of garlic and ginger, is an enticing mix of textures and flavors that will help knock out carb cravings. Egg whites provide satiating protein and bind the crispy rice with sweet pops of peas. Liquid aminos aid tissue repair and add a more savory flavor than plain table salt.

CRISPY RICE SKILLET

Makes	2 servings	Serving size	½ skillet	Prep time	10 minutes	Cook time	15 minutes

INGREDIENTS

2 cups liquid egg whites

½ tsp ground ginger

⅛ tsp red pepper flakes

1 tsp liquid aminos

1 cup frozen peas

2 tbsp finely chopped scallions (green parts only)

1 tsp minced garlic

1 cup cooked basmati rice

DIRECTIONS

1 Preheat the broiler to low. In a large bowl, make the egg mixture by whisking together the egg whites, ginger, red pepper flakes, and liquid aminos. Add the peas to the bowl, and stir well to combine. Set aside.

2 Spray a medium cast iron skillet with non-stick cooking spray and preheat over medium heat. Add the scallions and garlic, and cook for 2 to 3 minutes until soft and fragrant.

3 Increase the heat to medium-high, add the rice to the skillet, and use a wooden spoon to spread it into a thin, even layer. Toast for 1 to 2 minutes. Use the wooden spoon to press the rice into the skillet and toast for an additional 1 to 2 minutes, or until the rice is brown and crispy.

4 Reduce the heat to low. Pour the egg mixture evenly over the toasted rice. Cook for 4 to 5 minutes, then transfer the skillet to the oven. Broil for 2 to 3 minutes, or until the egg whites are set. Serve hot.

NUTRITION FACTS

per serving

CALORIES
278

TOTAL FAT
0.5g

TOTAL CARBS
32.1g

PROTEIN
33.9g

PREP TIPS / Any variety of leftover rice will work well for this recipe.

Store in an airtight container in the refrigerator for up to 5 days.

CHANGE IT UP

For a crunchier texture, substitute 1 cup chopped carrots for the peas. Macros per serving will be 249 calories, 0.5g fat, 28.3g carbs, and 30.8g protein.

STEAMED SQUASH EGG CUSTARD

Decedent, creamy, and rich, this satisfying breakfast treat is loaded with vitamins, resistant starch carbs, and muscle-building protein, and it also makes a beautiful presentation. The egg whites cook inside the squash and take on a custard-like consistency, while earthy spices add warmth.

Makes **4** servings | Serving size **1** squash | Prep time **10** minutes | Cook time **45** minutes

INGREDIENTS

4 medium acorn squash

4 cups liquid egg whites

4 tbsp coconut milk

1 tbsp powdered stevia

1 tsp ground cinnamon

1 tsp pumpkin pie spice

DIRECTIONS

1 Using a sharp knife, carefully cut a large hole around the stem of each squash. Remove the stems and reserve for later, and use a spoon to scoop out and discard the seeds.

2 Fill the bottom of a large pot with 1 inch (2.5cm) water. Place a steaming tray in the pot, cover, and heat the water on medium-low until just simmering.

3 In a large bowl, combine the egg whites, coconut milk, stevia, cinnamon, and pumpkin pie spice. Mix well.

4 Pour equal amounts of the egg mixture into each squash. Place the stems back on the squash and place them upright in the pot. Cover, and steam for 45 minutes.

5 Using tongs, carefully remove the squash from the pot and transfer to a plate. Allow to cool slightly before serving.

PREP TIPS // *Make these ahead for a quick and easy breakfast when you're in a rush. Just reheat in the microwave on high for 2 to 3 minutes.*

Store in an airtight container in the refrigerator for up to 6 days.

CHANGE IT UP
For a more savory flavor, omit the stevia, cinnamon, and pumpkin pie spice, and add 1 tsp minced garlic, ½ tsp ground black pepper, and ½ tsp salt to the filling.

NUTRITION FACTS

per serving

CALORIES

268

TOTAL FAT

0.3g

TOTAL CARBS

33.1g

PROTEIN

32.7g

BREAKFASTS

This hearty breakfast dish features a savory blend of spicy turkey, sweet potatoes, and earthy spinach, as well as a balanced serving of lean protein, complex carbohydrates, and healthy fats. A soft-cooked egg perched on top adds creaminess, as well as an extra boost of protein.

NUTRITION FACTS

per serving

CALORIES
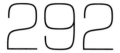
292

TOTAL FAT
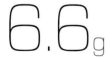
6.6g

TOTAL CARBS
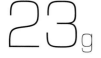
23g

PROTEIN

35g

BREAKFAST HASH

Makes 4 servings	Serving size	¼ of the hash with 1 egg	Prep time 15 minutes	Cook time 25 minutes

INGREDIENTS

1 medium white onion, diced

1 lb (450g) ground turkey breast

1 tsp ground cumin

1 tsp red pepper flakes

1 tsp paprika

1 tsp salt

2 medium sweet potatoes, peeled and cut into ½-inch (1.25cm) cubes

2 cups fresh baby spinach

4 medium eggs

DIRECTIONS

1 Preheat the broiler to low. Spray a medium cast iron skillet with coconut oil cooking spray and place over medium heat.

2 Add the onion to the skillet. Cook until soft and translucent, stirring frequently. Add the turkey breast, cumin, red pepper flakes, paprika, and salt. Stir well to combine, using a wooden spoon to break up the ground turkey. Cook for 6 to 8 minutes, stirring frequently, until the turkey is browned. Transfer to a large bowl and set aside.

3 Add the sweet potatoes to the skillet and cook for 8 to 10 minutes, or until soft. Add the spinach and cook for an additional 1 to 2 minutes, or until wilted. Add the turkey and onions back to the skillet. Mix well.

4 Make 4 divots in the hash and carefully crack an egg into each divot. Place the skillet in the oven and broil for 5 to 7 minutes, or until the eggs are set and the hash is lightly browned. Serve hot.

PREP TIPS *You can save money and prep time by buying frozen diced sweet potatoes. Make sure to thaw them in the refrigerator 1 day before using.*

Portion out the servings and store in separate airtight containers in the refrigerator for up to 5 days.

CHANGE IT UP

You can substitute 1lb (450g) diced chicken breast for the ground turkey breast. The macros will be the same.

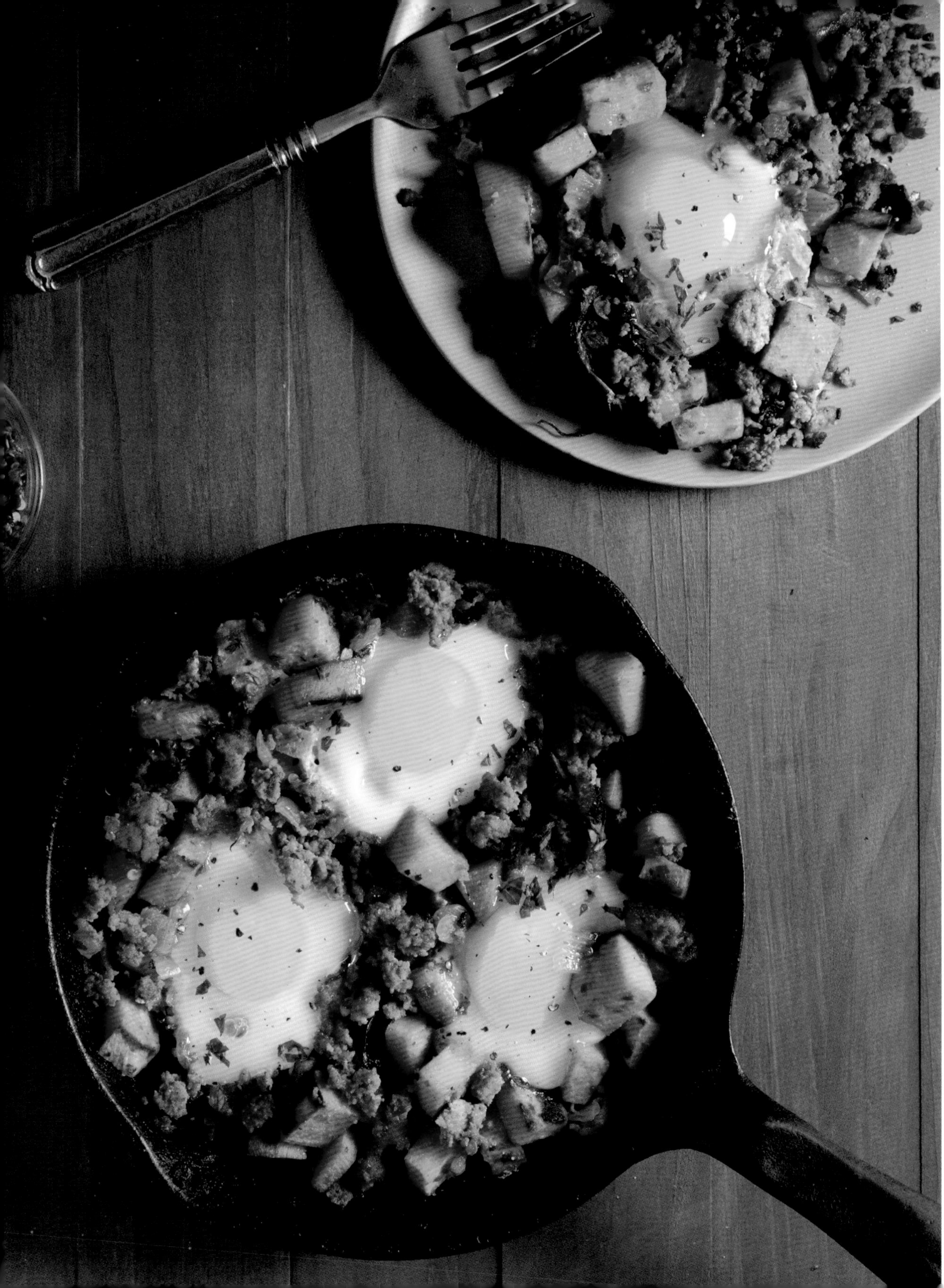

Fluffy and slightly chewy, this pancake is low in carbs and high in fiber. Almond flour adds a nutty flavor and healthy fats, which can help keep you feeling full. This pancake cooks quickly in a hot pan, and can be topped with any no-calorie pancake syrup for a sweet breakfast treat!

NUTRITION FACTS

per serving

CALORIES
275

TOTAL FAT
9.8g

TOTAL CARBS
13.5g

PROTEIN
33.5g

LOW-CARB PANCAKE

| Makes | 1 serving | Serving size | 1 pancake | Prep time | 15 minutes | Cook time | 12 minutes |

INGREDIENTS

1 cup liquid egg whites

⅓ cup unsweetened almond milk

½ tsp vanilla extract

2 tbsp coconut flour

⅛ cup almond flour

½ tsp baking powder

¼ tsp ground cinnamon

½ tsp powdered stevia

2 tbsp no-calorie pancake syrup (optional)

DIRECTIONS

1 In a medium bowl, combine the egg whites, almond milk, and vanilla extract. Stir well. In a separate medium bowl, combine the coconut flour, almond flour, baking powder, cinnamon, and stevia. Mix well.

2 Make the batter by adding the wet ingredients to the dry ingredients. Mix well, and allow the batter to thicken for 10 minutes.

3 Spray a medium skillet with non-stick cooking spray and preheat over medium-high heat. Pour the batter into the hot pan, and cook until the edges are set and bubbles appear on the surface. Flip, and cook for 1 additional minute. Transfer the cooked pancake to a plate.

4 Drizzle with the syrup (if using). Serve warm.

PREP TIPS *Double or triple this recipe for a quick and easy breakfast option.*

Store in an airtight container in the refrigerator for up to 6 days, or in the freezer for up to 2 months.

CHANGE IT UP

Make a pumpkin pancake by substituting ½ tsp pumpkin pie spice for the cinnamon.

To make this keto, top with 1 tbsp almond butter. This will add 98 calories, 9g fat, 3g carbs, and 2g protein per serving.

PUMPED-UP PROTEIN PANCAKE

Makes 1 serving | **Serving size** 1 pancake | **Prep time** 10 minutes | **Cook time** 12 minutes

We eat with our eyes first, and at just 300 calories this giant, protein-packed pancake will fill an entire plate and help crush those morning hunger pangs! The egg whites help boost the protein to 30g per serving, while the coconut flour and oats add fiber to help keep you full.

INGREDIENTS

1 cup liquid egg whites

½ cup old-fashioned oats

1 tbsp coconut flour

½ tsp ground cinnamon

½ tsp baking powder

2 tbsp no-calorie pancake syrup (optional)

DIRECTIONS

1 In a medium bowl, combine the egg whites, oats, coconut flour, cinnamon, and baking powder. Mix well, and allow to thicken for 5 to 10 minutes.

2 Spray a medium skillet with non-stick cooking spray and preheat over medium heat.

3 Add the batter to the hot pan, cover, and cook for 10 to 12 minutes. Transfer the cooked pancake to a plate.

4 Drizzle with the syrup (if using). Serve warm.

NUTRITION FACTS
per serving

CALORIES
300

TOTAL FAT
3.7 g

TOTAL CARBS
36 g

PROTEIN
30 g

CHANGE IT UP
Try substituting ½ cup quinoa flakes or 6oz (160g) cooked sweet potato for the oats. The macros will be very similar.

PREP TIPS
The batter can be made ahead of time and stored in the refrigerator for up to 2 days.

Store the cooked pancakes in an airtight container in the refrigerator for up to 5 days.

Baking these boats enhances the silky texture and slightly sweet flavor of the avocado, which contrasts nicely with the buttery smoked salmon. Pairing the avocado and salmon with an egg, spicy chipotle powder, and earthy dill creates the perfect keto-friendly breakfast.

SMOKED SALMON AVOCADO BOATS

Makes	2 servings		Serving size	1 boat		Prep time	10 minutes		Cook time	17 minutes

INGREDIENTS

1 large avocado, halved lengthwise, seed removed

2oz (55g) smoked salmon, chopped

2 medium eggs

⅛ tsp chipotle powder

Pinch of salt

Pinch of ground black pepper

2 tsp chopped fresh dill

DIRECTIONS

1 Preheat the oven to 425°F (218°C). Line an 8 x 8in (20 x 20cm) baking dish with aluminum foil.

2 Using a small spoon, carefully scoop out enough flesh from each avocado half to form a well large enough to hold half of the salmon and one egg.

3 Place the avocado halves in the baking dish, flesh-side up. Carefully crack one egg into each well.

4 Season each avocado half with equal amounts of the salt, pepper, and chipotle powder. Bake for 15 to 17 minutes, or until the egg whites are set but the yolk is still soft.

5 Transfer the boats to a serving plate and top each with 1oz (25g) salmon and 1 tsp dill. Serve hot.

PREP TIPS // You can double this recipe for easy meal prep.
Store in an airtight container in the refrigerator for up to 3 days. To reheat, place on a baking sheet in a 250°F (121°C) oven for 10 to 12 minutes.

NUTRITION FACTS

per serving

CALORIES
267

TOTAL FAT
21.1 g

TOTAL CARBS
5.9 g

PROTEIN
15.6 g

CHANGE IT UP

Replace the salmon with 1oz (25g) lean ground beef, and omit the dill. The macros will be about the same.

If you don't have fresh dill, sprinkle ⅛ tsp dried dill over each boat before baking.

SAVORY APPLE SAGE TURKEY SAUSAGES

Makes	4 servings	Serving size	2 patties	Prep time	10 minutes	Cook time	10 minutes

Pair this classic sweet and savory flavor combination with oats or eggs for a hearty, high-protein breakfast. You can also toss these in a wrap for lunch, or eat them on the go for a satisfying snack. Lean turkey is high in protein, and apple provides a sweet balance to the more savory flavors.

INGREDIENTS

1lb (450g) ground turkey breast

¼ cup liquid egg whites

2 tbsp chopped fresh sage

1 small Granny Smith apple, cored, peeled, and finely chopped

1 tsp sea salt

½ tsp ground black pepper

½ tsp allspice

DIRECTIONS

1 In a large bowl, combine the turkey breast, egg whites, sage, apple, sea salt, black pepper, and allspice. Mix well to combine. (Be careful not to overmix, which can make the sausages rubbery.) Form the mixture into 8 equal-sized patties.

2 Spray a large skillet with non-stick cooking spray and place over medium-high heat. Cook the patties for 4 to 5 minutes per side, until both sides are browned.

3 Reduce the heat to medium-low, cover, and steam for 4 to 5 minutes, or until the internal temperature reaches 160°F (71°C).

4 Transfer the patties to a paper towel to drain. Serve hot.

NUTRITION FACTS

per serving

CALORIES

151

TOTAL FAT

1.1g

TOTAL CARBS

6.5g

PROTEIN

29.6g

CHANGE IT UP

Make Southwestern sausages by omitting the sage, apple, and allspice, and adding ¼ cup salsa and ½ tsp chili powder to the filling.

For a distinctive Ethiopian flavor, substitute ½ tsp Berbere seasoning for the allspice.

PREP TIPS

You can double this recipe for easy meal prep.

Store the cooked patties in an airtight container in the refrigerator for up to 3 days, or in the freezer for up to 2 months.

Creamy, spicy, a little crunchy—and ready in less than an hour! This dish has the flavors of fall, the feel of comfort food, and the protein you need to get your day going. The fiber in the pumpkin, mixed with the slower-digesting protein in Greek yogurt will help you feel full for longer.

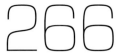

NUTRITION FACTS

per serving

CALORIES
266

TOTAL FAT
5.9g

TOTAL CARBS
30.9g

PROTEIN
25.7g

PUMPKIN PIE BOWL

Makes | 1 serving | Serving size | 1 bowl | Prep time | 10 min + 30 min | Cook time | none

INGREDIENTS

1 6oz (170g) container plain 2% Greek yogurt

½ cup canned pumpkin purée (not pumpkin pie mix)

½ tsp powdered stevia

½ tsp ground cinnamon

½ tsp ground ginger

¼ cup puffed brown rice cereal

¼ cup fresh strawberries, thinly sliced

DIRECTIONS

1 In a medium bowl, combine the Greek yogurt, pumpkin purée, stevia, cinnamon, and ginger. Mix well to combine.

2 Top with the brown rice cereal and strawberry slices. Cover tightly with plastic wrap and place in the refrigerator to chill for at least 30 minutes before serving.

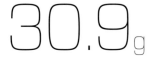

PREP TIPS *This bowl can be made ahead of time and stored in the refrigerator for up to 6 days. Add the toppings just before you're ready to eat.*

CHANGE IT UP

You can substitute cooked sweet potato for the pumpkin purée. Make sure to thoroughly mash the sweet potato before combining it with the other ingredients.

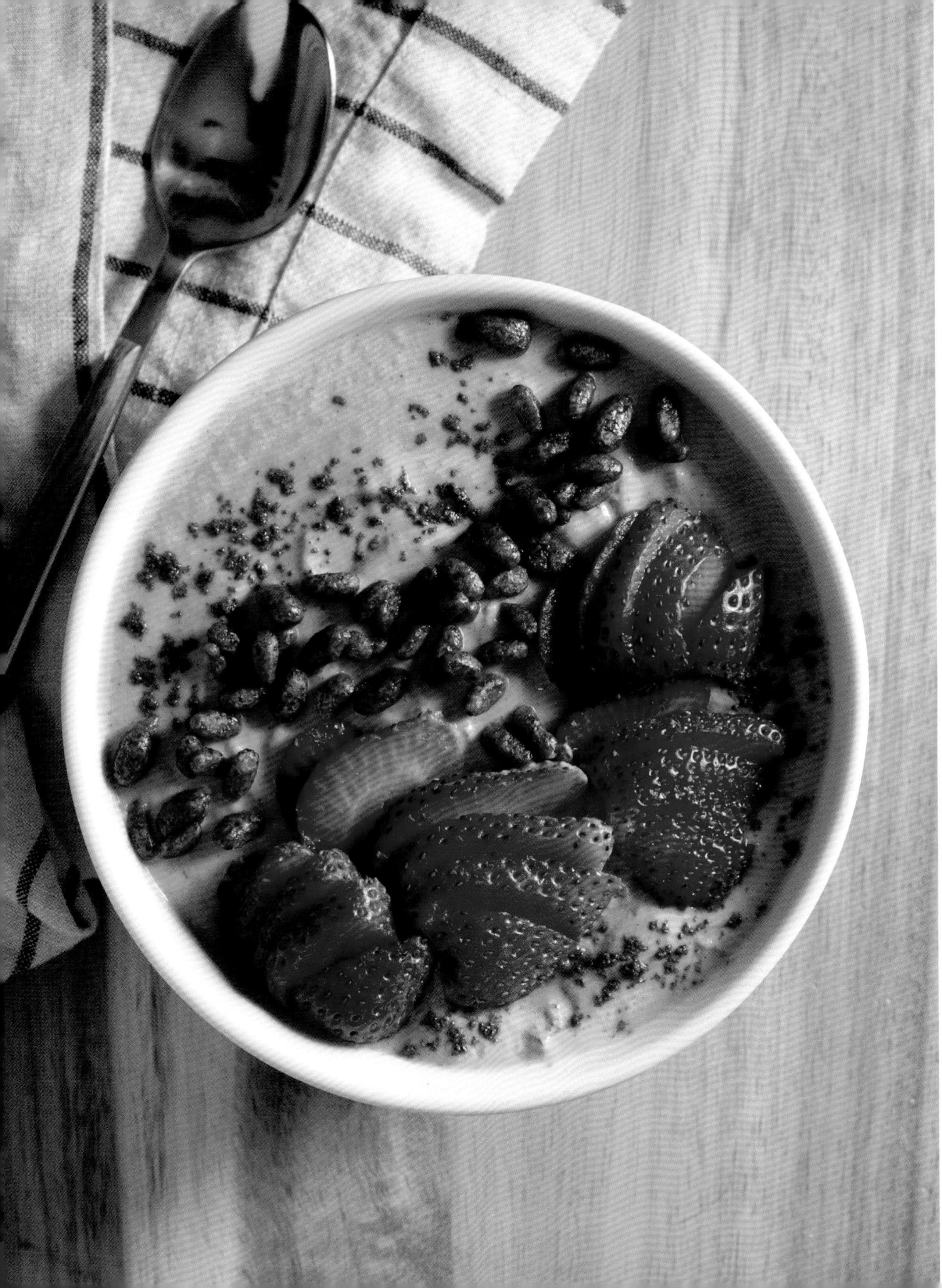

Breakfast is an essential meal for maintaining a healthy body weight. These oats offer complex carbohydrates and fiber to keep you full and energize your mornings. Chia seeds promotes satiety, and coffee will boost metabolism and give you a spark of energy to get your day going.

NUTRITION FACTS

per serving

CALORIES
300

TOTAL FAT
5.7g

TOTAL CARBS
43g

PROTEIN
24.2g

OVERNIGHT MOCHA OATS

| Makes | 1 serving | Serving size | 1 jar | Prep time | 15 min + 8 hours | Cook time | none |

INGREDIENTS

½ cup old-fashioned rolled oats

1 tbsp chia seeds

1 tbsp unsweetened cocoa powder

1 tbsp powdered stevia

½ cup plain nonfat Greek yogurt

⅓ cup pasteurized liquid egg whites

¼ cup brewed coffee, cold

DIRECTIONS

1 In a 12-ounce (340g) glass jar, combine the oats, chia seeds, cocoa powder, and stevia. Stir well to combine.

2 Add the Greek yogurt, egg whites, and coffee. Tightly seal the jar and shake until all ingredients are well incorporated.

3 Refrigerate for a minimum of 8 hours to allow the oats to soften. Serve chilled.

PREP TIPS *For meal prep, these can be made ahead and stored in the refrigerator for up to 5 days.*

Eat these cold or hot. To reheat, place in a microwave-safe bowl and microwave on high for 1 minute.

CHANGE IT UP

For a little more spice, add ½ tsp ground cinnamon.

Make coco-mocha oats by substituting 2 tbsp unsweetened coconut for the chia seeds. The calories will remain the same, but the fat will increase by 2g, and the carbs will decrease by 5g.

BAKED BANANA AND OAT BARS

Makes **4** servings | Serving size **1** bar | Prep time **10** minutes | Cook time **30** minutes

These yummy bars, featuring sweet bananas and hearty old-fashioned oats, will provide quick and sustained energy to keep you going throughout the morning. Whey protein and egg whites boost the protein, and also hold these bars together nicely, making them easy to eat on the go.

INGREDIENTS

2 medium ripe bananas, mashed

1 cup liquid egg whites

¼ cup unsweetened vanilla almond milk

1 tsp vanilla extract

1½ cups old-fashioned rolled oats

½ cup vanilla whey protein powder

1 tsp baking powder

DIRECTIONS

1 Preheat the oven to 350°F (177°C). Spray an 8 x 8in (20 x 20cm) baking dish with non-stick cooking spray.

2 In a medium bowl, combine the bananas, egg whites, almond milk, and vanilla extract. Mix well. In a separate large bowl, combine the oats, protein powder, and baking powder. Mix well.

3 To make the batter, add the wet ingredients to the dry ingredients. Stir well to combine.

4 Pour the batter into the baking dish and bake for 28 to 30 minutes, or until the top is golden brown. Cut into four equal-sized bars.

NUTRITION FACTS

per serving

CALORIES
281

TOTAL FAT
2.7 g

TOTAL CARBS
34.6 g

PROTEIN
30.1 g

CHANGE IT UP

Try substituting strawberry or chocolate protein powders for the vanilla protein powder.

For a more decadent flavor, add ⅓ cup powdered peanut butter. This will add 45 calories, 1.5g fat, 2.7g carbs, and 5g protein per serving.

PREP TIPS _You can double this recipe for easy meal prep._

Store in an airtight container in the refrigerator for up to 6 days, or in the freezer for up to 2 months.

This Southern-inspired casserole is lean on calories, but will keep you full and is loaded with flavor. Ground turkey packs in the protein, while grits and light cheddar cheese add essential carbs for your workouts. Green onions give it all a pop of color and a fresh, bright kick.

| Makes | 4 servings | | Serving size | 1 slice | | Prep time | 20 minutes | | Cook time | 27 minutes |

NUTRITION FACTS

per serving

CALORIES
331

TOTAL FAT
3.7 g

TOTAL CARBS
35.1 g

PROTEIN
37.5 g

INGREDIENTS

1 cup instant dry grits

1 tsp salt

1lb (450g) lean ground turkey breast

1 tsp dried sage

1 tsp dried thyme

½ tsp marjoram

½ tsp red pepper flakes

½ cup liquid egg whites

½ cup finely chopped green onion (green ends only)

¼ cup light cheddar cheese

DIRECTIONS

1 Preheat the oven to 375°F (191°C). Spray a 9 x 9in (23 x 23cm) baking dish with non-stick cooking spray.

2 In a medium stock pot, bring 4 cups of water to a boil. Add the grits and salt, and bring just to a boil. Reduce the heat to low and cook for 5 minutes, stirring frequently.

3 Spray a medium skillet with non-stick cooking spray and place over medium heat. Add the turkey, sage, thyme, marjoram, and red pepper flakes. Cook for 4 to 5 minutes, stirring frequently.

4 In a large glass bowl, combine the seasoned turkey, cooked grits, egg whites, green onions, and cheddar cheese. Mix well to combine. Spoon the mixture into the prepared baking dish.

5 Bake for 25 to 27 minutes, or until the casserole is lightly browned. Cut into four equal-sized slices. Serve hot.

PREP TIPS *Tightly seal the slices in plastic wrap and store in the refrigerator for up to 6 days. Eat cold, or reheat on a baking sheet in a 250°F (121°C) oven for 15 minutes.*

CHANGE IT UP

Make it keto by replacing the grits with 4 tbsp unsalted butter, replacing the liquid egg whites with 8 large eggs, and reducing the ground turkey from 1lb (450g) to ½lb (225g). Macros will be 326 calories, 23.4g fat, 0.8g carbs, and 27.5g protein per serving.

KETO BREAKFAST BURRITOS

Makes	1 serving	Serving size	2 burritos	Prep time	10 minutes	Cook time	15 minutes

INGREDIENTS

4 1oz (25g) slices lean deli ham (97% fat free, preferably)

2 large eggs

10 thin asparagus stalks, ends trimmed, and chopped into ½-inch (1.25cm) pieces

¼ cup shredded cheddar cheese

DIRECTIONS

1 Preheat the oven to 400°F (204°C). Spray a small non-stick frying pan with non-stick cooking spray and place over medium heat.

2 Crack the eggs into the pan and add the asparagus pieces. Cook for 4 to 5 minutes, stirring occasionally, until the eggs just begin to set. Sprinkle the cheese over top of the eggs and cook for 1 additional minute, or until the cheese is melted. (Do not stir.)

3 Make the wraps by placing two slices of ham side-by-side on a plate, overlapping the edges just slightly. Repeat with the remaining slices. Divide the filling into two equal portions and spoon onto each of the wraps. Grasp the ends of each wrap and gently roll into bundles.

4 Spray an 8 x 8in (20 x 20cm) baking dish with non-stick cooking spray, and place the wraps in the dish. Bake for 6 to 8 minutes, or until the ham is lightly browned and the cheese starts to bubble. Serve hot.

CHANGE IT UP

If you don't prefer asparagus, you can substitute ¼ cup sliced fresh button mushrooms and ¼ cup diced tomato. The macros will be about the same.

PREP TIPS

You can double or triple this recipe for easy meal prep. To ensure proper portions, weigh the cooled filling on a scale before adding the filling to each ham wrap.

Store in an airtight container in the refrigerator for up to 5 days.

Fresh eggs, crunchy asparagus, and gooey cheddar cheese are all wrapped in lean ham in these low-carb alternatives to traditional breakfast burritos. Asparagus adds a wonderful crunch as well as essential nutrients like vitamin K and folate. You won't miss the tortilla!

NUTRITION FACTS

per serving

CALORIES

318

TOTAL FAT

20.5g

TOTAL CARBS

2.2g

PROTEIN

29.7g

BREAKFASTS

Just a hint of parmesan cheese adds a decadent flavor to this low-carb take on a traditional breakfast quiche. Egg whites and milk offer muscle-building protein, seasonal vegetables help keep you full, and antioxidant-rich spices add flavor without adding unnecessary calories.

NUTRITION FACTS

per serving

CALORIES
196

TOTAL FAT
4.1g

TOTAL CARBS
11.2g

PROTEIN
29.1g

CRUSTLESS QUICHE

Makes 2 servings | **Serving size** 1 slice | **Prep time** 10 minutes | **Cook time** 35 minutes

INGREDIENTS

1 cup yellow squash, thinly sliced

1 cup zucchini, thinly sliced

1 large bell pepper, seeded and thinly sliced

2 tsp minced garlic

1 tbsp dried thyme

1½ cups liquid egg whites

¾ cup 1% milk

¾ tsp salt

½ tsp ground black pepper

¼ cup grated parmesan cheese

DIRECTIONS

1 Preheat the oven to 350°F (177°C). Spray a large skillet with non-stick cooking spray and place over medium heat. In a large bowl, combine the egg whites, milk, salt, black pepper, and parmesan cheese. Mix until well incorporated. Set aside.

2 Add the squash, zucchini, bell pepper, garlic, and thyme to the pan, and cook until the vegetables are slightly softened, about 5 to 6 minutes. Set aside.

3 Spray an 8-inch (20cm) pie dish with non-stick cooking spray. Spoon the vegetables into the pie dish, and carefully pour the egg and milk mixture over top of the vegetables.

4 Place the pie dish on a baking sheet and bake for 30 to 35 minutes, or until the center is set. Slice into two equal-sized portions. Serve warm.

PREP TIPS

Unflavored almond milk can be used in place of 1% milk.

Save time by microwaving the vegetables on high for 4 to 6 minutes, stirring frequently. Total baking time will be reduced to 20 to 25 minutes.

Tightly wrap the individual slices in plastic wrap and store in the refrigerator for up to 6 days.

CHANGE IT UP

Make it keto by replacing the egg whites with 6 large eggs, replacing the milk with ¼ cup heavy whipping cream, and adding ½ cup grated Parmesan cheese. The macros per serving will be 225 calories, 16.6g fat, 3.4g carbs, and 15.6g protein.

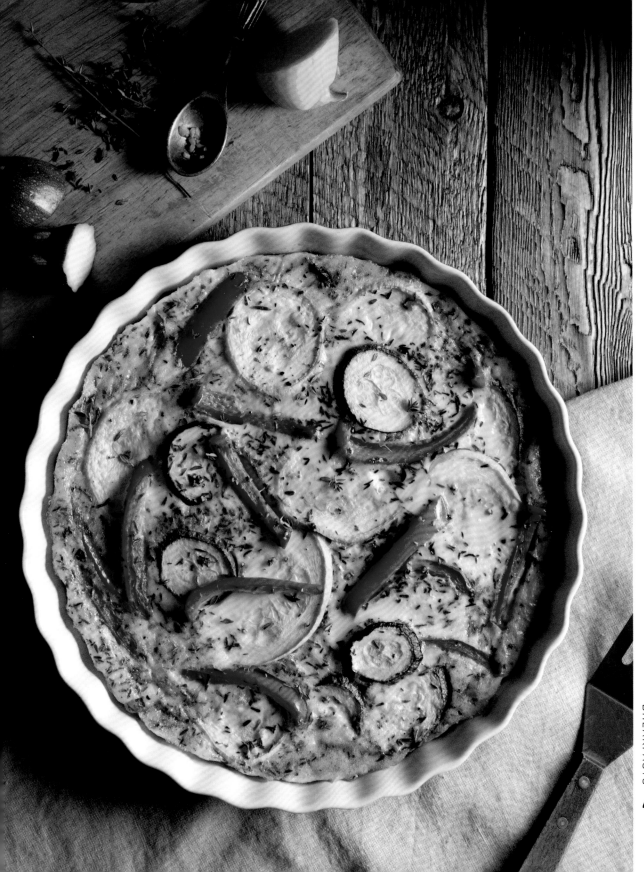

These oats take on a savory spin when topped with fiery sriracha scrambled eggs. Sesame seeds add crunch, while scallions add bright pops of flavor. The oats pack complex carbohydrates and soluble fiber, while the egg whites help keep you full and provide muscle-building protein.

NUTRITION FACTS

per serving

CALORIES
275

TOTAL FAT
3g

TOTAL CARBS
27g

PROTEIN
34g

SAVORY BREAKFAST OATMEAL

Makes	1 serving	Serving size	1 bowl	Prep time	10 minutes	Cook time	10 minutes

INGREDIENTS

1 cup low-sodium chicken broth

½ cup old-fashioned rolled oats

1 cup liquid egg whites

2 tsp sriracha hot chili sauce

1 scallion, thinly sliced

½ tsp sesame seeds

Pinch of salt

DIRECTIONS

1 Spray a small saucepan with non-stick cooking spray and place over medium-high heat. Add the chicken broth and oats, bring just to a boil. Reduce the heat to low and simmer for 5 minutes, stirring occasionally.

2 While the oats cook, spray a small skillet with non-stick cooking spray and place over medium heat. Add the egg whites and cook until the whites are nearly cooked through, then add the sriracha sauce and stir to evenly distribute. Continue cooking until the whites are firm, stirring occasionally.

3 Transfer the cooked oats to a serving bowl and top with the eggs. Sprinkle the scallions and sesame seeds over top, and season with a pinch of salt. Serve hot.

PREP TIPS *This also can be prepared in the microwave. Add the oats and chicken broth to a microwave-safe bowl, and cook on high for 2 to 3 minutes, stirring every 30 to 45 seconds.*

Store the egg and oatmeal mixture in an airtight container in the refrigerator for up to 4 days. Top with the sesame seeds and scallions just before serving.

CHANGE IT UP

For a different flavor and an extra probiotic boost, omit the sriracha and add 2 tbsp kimchi to the bowl after the oats and eggs are cooked. This will add about 15 calories per serving.

CANADIAN BACON AND EGG CUPS

Makes 6 servings | Serving size 1 cup | Prep time 10 minutes | Cook time 20 minutes

These portable bacon and egg cups are a quick and satisfying breakfast treat. Canadian bacon has a similar flavor profile to regular bacon, but contains more protein and less fat. Eggs are rich in healthy monounsaturated and polyunsaturated fats, and will help keep you full for longer.

INGREDIENTS

6 large eggs

12 slices nitrate-free Canadian bacon

Pinch of salt

Pinch of ground black pepper

DIRECTIONS

1 Preheat the oven to 350°F (177°C). Spray a large muffin tin with non-stick cooking spray. Place 2 slices of Canadian bacon into each tin and shape them into cups.

2 Crack one egg into each cup, and season with equal amounts of salt and black pepper.

3 Bake for 18 to 20 minutes, or until the centers of the eggs are set and firm. (For creamier yolks, bake just until the centers of the yolks are set.) Serve warm.

NUTRITION FACTS

per serving

CALORIES

264

TOTAL FAT

12.6g

TOTAL CARBS

2.8g

PROTEIN

34.6g

CHANGE IT UP

For a zestier flavor, add 1 tbsp grated parmesan cheese to the top of each cup before baking. This will add 20 calories, 1g fat, 2g carbs, and 1g protein to each serving.

Spice it up! Top each cup with a slice of fresh jalapeno. This has no impact on the macros.

PREP TIPS

Store in an airtight container in the refrigerator for up to 6 days, or in the freezer for up to 2 months.

To reheat unfrozen cups, place on a baking sheet in a 250°F (121°C) oven for 10 to 12 minutes.

Sweet, juicy cantaloupe is the vessel for this protein-packed treat. Cottage cheese adds creaminess and contains casein, which helps make it a slower digesting protein. Slivered almonds add crunch and healthy fats, while warming cinnamon helps regulate blood sugar levels.

COTTAGE CHEESE AND CANTALOUPE BOWL

Makes **2** servings | Serving **size** **1** bowl | **Prep time** 10 minutes | **Cook time** none

INGREDIENTS

1 small cantaloupe

2 cups 1% cottage cheese

2 tbsp slivered almonds

⅛ tsp ground cinnamon

DIRECTIONS

1 To create the bowls, slice the cantaloupe in half crosswise, and use a spoon to scoop out the seeds of each half.

2 Add 1 cup cottage cheese to each cantaloupe bowl and top each with 1 tbsp slivered almonds and a pinch of cinnamon. Serve immediately.

NUTRITION FACTS

per serving

CALORIES
314

TOTAL FAT
6.7 g

TOTAL CARBS
32 g

PROTEIN
31.9 g

PREP TIPS // This is best prepared and served immediately.

Tightly wrap any unprepared cantaloupe in plastic wrap and store in the refrigerator for up to 2 days.

CHANGE IT UP

For a sweeter flavor, sprinkle 1 tsp powdered stevia over top of each bowl.

For a nuttier flavor, substitute 2 tbsp pumpkin seeds for the slivered almonds. The macros will remain the same.

CHICKEN AND POLENTA BREAKFAST PIZZA

Makes	4 servings	Serving size	1 slice	Prep time	10 minutes	Cook time	35 minutes

The crust of this pizza is made from polenta, a coarsely ground corn meal which contains complex carbs that will help keep you fueled throughout the day. Cooking the polenta in chicken broth imparts a rich, savory taste, which is accented by lean chicken breast, spinach, and mushrooms.

INGREDIENTS

1 cup dried polenta

3 cups low-sodium chicken broth

1 tsp salt

1lb (450g) ground chicken breast

1 tsp garlic powder

1 tsp dried oregano

2 cups fresh baby spinach

1 cup button mushrooms, thinly sliced

DIRECTIONS

1 Preheat the oven to 425°F (218°C). In a large saucepan over high heat, bring the chicken broth to a boil. Reduce the heat to medium and gradually add the polenta to the pan, whisking constantly. Add ½ tsp salt and continue to whisk until the polenta starts to thicken.

2 Spray an 8 x 8in (20 x 20cm) baking dish with non-stick cooking spray. Spread the polenta mixture evenly across the prepared baking dish. Bake for 28 to 30 minutes.

3 While the crust is baking, spray a large skillet with non-stick cooking spray and place over medium heat. Add the ground chicken, and season with the garlic powder, oregano, and the remaining ½ tsp of salt. Cook for 8 to 10 minutes, stirring occasionally, and using a wooden spoon to break up the chicken.

4 Add the spinach and mushrooms to the pan. Cook for an additional 2 to 3 minutes, stirring constantly, until the spinach is wilted, the mushrooms are soft, and all of the liquid has cooked off.

5 Top the baked crust with the chicken, mushroom, and spinach mixture, making sure the mixture is evenly distributed across the crust. Place the pizza in the oven and bake for 4 to 5 minutes, or until the toppings are lightly browned. Cut into four equal-sized slices. Serve hot.

PREP TIPS

Store in an airtight container in the refrigerator for up to 3 days. To reheat, place on a baking sheet in a 250°F (121°C) oven for 15 minutes.

The unbaked crust can be prepared ahead of time. Tightly seal in plastic wrap and store in the refrigerator for up to 4 days.

NUTRITION FACTS

per serving

CALORIES
295

TOTAL FAT
3.2 g

TOTAL CARBS
33.1 g

PROTEIN
30.1 g

Store-bought muffins may be convenient, but they're loaded with fat and sugar. This simple version pumps up the protein, while giving you the goodness of whole-grain oats and antioxidant-rich blueberries. A touch of butter gives just enough flavor and moisture to make these muffins feel like a treat!

BLUEBERRY MUFFINS

Makes 12 servings | **Serving size** 1 muffin | **Prep time** 10 minutes | **Cook time** 25 minutes

NUTRITION FACTS

per serving

CALORIES
135

TOTAL FAT
5.2 g

TOTAL CARBS
14.1 g

PROTEIN
8.7 g

INGREDIENTS

1 cup old-fashioned rolled oats

⅔ cup gluten-free or all purpose flour

½ cup vanilla whey protein powder

1 tsp ground cinnamon

1 tsp baking powder

1 tsp baking soda

¼ cup powdered stevia

⅓ cup liquid egg whites

1 cup unsweetened applesauce (preferably cinnamon flavored)

¼ cup butter, softened

¾ cup unsweetened almond milk

1 tsp vanilla extract

1 cup fresh blueberries

DIRECTIONS

1 Preheat the oven to 400°F (204°C). Spray a large muffin tin with non-stick cooking spray.

2 In a large bowl, combine the oats, flour, protein powder, cinnamon, baking powder, baking soda, and stevia. Mix well.

3 In a separate medium bowl, combine the egg whites, applesauce, butter, almond milk, and vanilla extract. Mix well.

4 Make the batter by adding the wet ingredients to the dry ingredients, and mixing until the ingredients are just incorporated. Gently fold in the blueberries, being careful not to crush them. Fill each muffin tin cup to two-thirds full with the batter.

5 Bake for 20 to 25 minutes, or until a toothpick inserted into the middle comes out clean. Serve warm.

PREP TIPS / *Store in an airtight container at room temperature for up to 4 days, or in the refrigerator for up to 1 week. To freeze, tightly wrap individual muffins in plastic wrap and freeze for up to 2 months.*

CHANGE IT UP

Strawberries, raspberries, or blackberries also will work well with this recipe, and won't impact the macros.

Add 1 tbsp unsweetened cocoa powder to the batter for a chocolate kick that adds only a few extra calories.

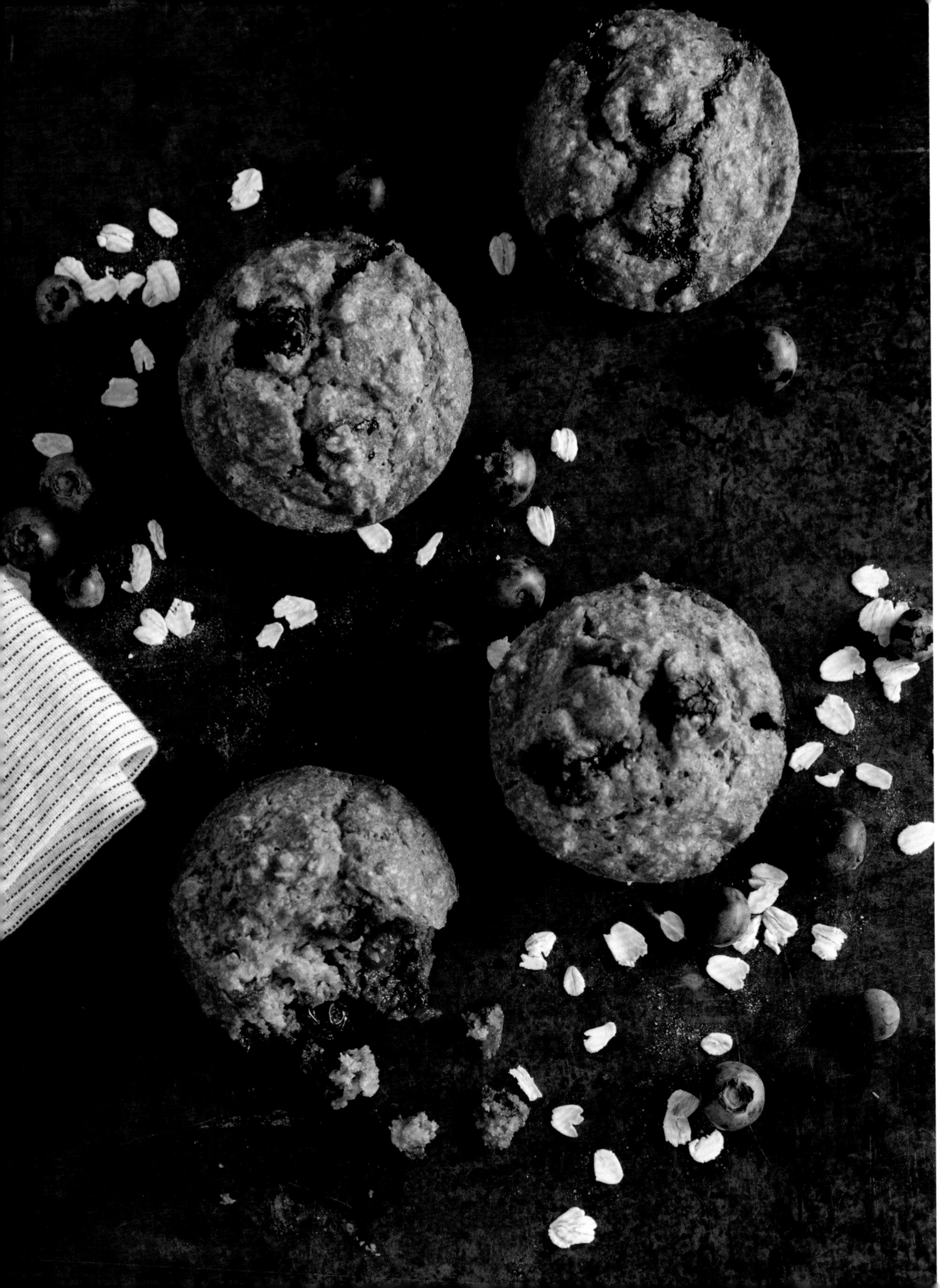

This hearty breakfast skillet is incredibly satisfying. Browning the potatoes and onions in a cast iron skillet imparts a beautiful golden color and rich flavor, and just a touch of almond milk keeps the egg whites soft and fluffy. Tomato adds a pop of color and a potent nutrient boost.

NUTRITION FACTS

per serving

CALORIES
225

TOTAL FAT
0.3g

TOTAL CARBS
30.6g

PROTEIN
23.1g

BREAK-THE-FAST SKILLET

Makes	4 servings	Serving size	1 slice	Prep time	10 minutes	Cook time	35 minutes

INGREDIENTS

3 cups liquid egg whites

2 tbsp plain unsweetened almond milk

1 20oz (560g) package frozen shredded hash brown potatoes, thawed

½ cup diced onion

1 tsp salt

1 tsp garlic powder

1 tsp dehydrated bell pepper flakes

1 large tomato, cut crosswise into ¼-inch (.5cm) slices

DIRECTIONS

1 Preheat oven to 350°F (177°C). In a medium bowl, combine the egg whites and almond milk, and stir well to combine. Set aside.

2 Spray a large cast iron skillet with coconut oil spray and place over medium heat. Add the potatoes, onion, salt, garlic powder, and bell pepper flakes. Cook for 8 to 10 minutes, stirring frequently, until the potatoes begin to brown and the onions become soft and translucent.

3 Pour the egg white and almond milk mixture over top of the potatoes and onions. Stir gently. Place the tomato slices over top.

4 Bake for 20 to 25 minutes, or until the middle is set and firm. Cut into four equal-size slices. Serve warm.

PREP TIPS // *Tightly wrap the individual slices in plastic wrap and refrigerate for up to 5 days. To reheat, place in an oven-safe dish and bake in a 250°F (121°C) oven for 10 minutes.*

CHANGE IT UP

For a Southwestern flavor, add ½ tsp chili powder, ½ tsp paprika, and ½ tsp cumin to the potatoes, and substitute ¼ cup salsa for the almond milk.

STEAK AND EGG BURRITO

Makes 1 serving | Serving size 1 burrito | Prep time 5 minutes | Cook time 12 minutes

This low carb burrito features an egg wrap, instead of a tortilla, and is perfect for a quick, on-the-go breakfast. Patience in cooking the egg is the key to creating a perfect wrap. Top with any lean protein and a scoop of salsa, and you'll have a protein-packed breakfast in minutes!

INGREDIENTS

2 extra large eggs

Pinch of salt

Pinch of ground black pepper

2oz (55g) flank steak, thinly sliced

Pinch of garlic powder

1 tbsp salsa

DIRECTIONS

1 Spray a medium skillet with non-stick cooking spray. In a medium bowl, combine the eggs, pinch of salt, and pinch of black pepper. Whisk until the ingredients are well combined.

2 Add the eggs to the skillet and cook over medium-high heat for 4 to 5 minutes, or until the edges are set. Using a spatula, carefully flip the eggs and cook for an additional 3 to 4 minutes, or until the eggs are fully set. Remove the wrap from the skillet and place on a plate.

3 Add the flank steak to the skillet, season with salt, black pepper, and garlic powder, and cook for 2 to 3 minutes, or until the steak is well done.

4 Top the egg wrap with the steak and salsa, and gently fold the edges in to form a burrito. Serve warm.

CHANGE IT UP

Make it keto by adding one quarter of a sliced avocado, ¼ tsp chipotle powder, and a squeeze of lime juice. This will add about 70 calories and 7g fat per serving.

Substitute 1 tbsp pico de gallo or 1 tbsp creamy dijon mustard for the salsa.

PREP TIPS

You can substitute equal amounts of any leftover lean protein for the steak.

The egg wraps can be made ahead of time and stored in the refrigerator for up to 4 days. To store, layer the wraps in parchment paper then tightly seal in plastic wrap.

NUTRITION FACTS

per serving

CALORIES
276

TOTAL FAT
16.2g

TOTAL CARBS
3g

PROTEIN
26.5g

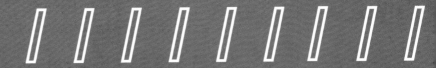

ENTRÉES

In terms of nutrition, lunch and dinner can be just as important as breakfast. Whether you want to maintain, lean down, or gain muscle, it's important to properly fuel your body throughout the day. The entrées in this chapter are big on flavor, but also rich in protein to help keep you full, and help your body burn calories while building new muscle.

It's time to stop eating the same boring chicken recipes! Searing the chicken breasts in this dish helps seal in the juices, and the spinach, sun-dried tomatoes, and gooey mozzarella all burst with flavor. At less than 200 calories per serving, this recipe is a muscle-making winner!

STUFFED FLORENTINE CHICKEN BREASTS

Makes 4 servings | Serving size 5oz (140g) | Prep time 15 minutes | Cook time 25 minutes

NUTRITION FACTS
per serving

CALORIES
193

TOTAL FAT
5g

TOTAL CARBS
7g

PROTEIN
30g

INGREDIENTS

3 boneless, skinless chicken breasts, or approximately 1lb (450g)

½ tsp salt

½ tsp ground black pepper

½ tsp garlic powder

½ cup chopped sun-dried tomatoes

½ cup chopped fresh baby spinach

½ cup light shredded mozzarella cheese

DIRECTIONS

1 Preheat oven to 350°F (177°C). Lightly spray a medium cast iron skillet with non-stick cooking spray and place over medium-high heat.

2 Add the chicken breasts to the skillet and season with the salt, pepper, and garlic powder. Cook for 1 to 2 minutes per side, or until lightly browned.

3 Remove the skillet from the heat and allow the breasts to rest in the skillet for 5 minutes. Once the breasts are cool enough to handle, transfer to a cutting board and create pockets for the fillings by slicing halfway through each breast lengthwise, being careful not to slice completely through the breasts.

4 Stuff each breast with equal amounts of the spinach, tomatoes, and cheese, and secure by inserting a toothpick through each breast. Transfer the breasts back to the skillet and bake for 20 minutes. The chicken is done when the juices run clear and the internal temperature reaches 165°F (74°C). Serve hot.

PREP TIPS Store in an airtight container in the refrigerator for up to 5 days.

CHANGE IT UP
For a spicier twist, sprinkle small pinches of red pepper flakes and dried oregano over each chicken breast before baking.

BISON AND PORTOBELLO SLIDERS

Makes 2 servings | *Serving size* 2 sliders | *Prep time* 30 minutes | *Cook time* 15 minutes

INGREDIENTS

1 lb (450g) lean ground bison, preferably 92/8 lean-to-fat ratio

¼ cup liquid egg whites

2 tbsp dried onion flakes

1 tsp garlic powder

½ tsp salt

½ tsp ground black pepper

4 tbsp no-sugar-added ketchup (optional)

For the portobello buns

8 large portobello mushrooms

½ tsp salt

½ tsp ground black pepper

½ tsp garlic powder

DIRECTIONS

1 Preheat the grill to medium. In a large bowl, combine the ground bison, egg whites, onion flakes, garlic powder, salt, and black pepper. Mix until the ingredients are well incorporated. With wet hands, shape the mixture into 8 even-sized patties. Set aside.

2 Rinse the mushrooms and pat dry with a paper towel. Remove the stems and place on a flat surface, gill-sides up. Season with the salt, black pepper, and garlic powder.

3 Place the mushrooms on the grill, gill-sides up, and grill for 3 minutes. Flip and grill for an additional 2 to 3 minutes. Transfer to a paper towel to drain, gill-sides down.

4 Place the bison patties on the grill, and cook for 4 to 5 minutes per side. Transfer to a plate and allow to rest for 5 minutes. Assemble the sliders by placing a bison patty between two portobello buns. Top each slider with 1 tbsp ketchup (if using). Serve warm.

PREP TIPS *Store the burgers in an airtight container in the refrigerator for up to 5 days. Store the portobello buns in a separate airtight container for up to 4 days. Assemble just before serving.*

CHANGE IT UP

Make these keto by replacing the lean ground bison with ground bison with an 80/20 lean-to-fat ratio, and replacing the egg whites with one large egg. The macros per serving will be 288 calories, 22.2g fat, and 21.6g protein.

Lean ground bison lends richness to these bite-sized burgers, and Portobello buns add rich flavor without adding loads of carbs. Dried onion flakes help bind the patties so they're easier to shape, flip, and serve, and the egg whites add more protein and help keep the burgers juicy.

NUTRITION FACTS

per serving

CALORIES
212

TOTAL FAT
9 g

TOTAL CARBS
9.1 g

PROTEIN
27 g

Lime adds wonderful vibrancy and a gorgeous touch of color to this dish. Chili and cilantro pair perfectly with the buttery flavor of the salmon, which is high in protein and rich in omega-3 fatty acids, which have numerous health benefits. Parchment paper makes prep and clean up easy.

NUTRITION FACTS

per serving

CALORIES
165

TOTAL FAT
7.2g

TOTAL CARBS
0g

PROTEIN
25g

CHILI LIME SALMON POUCHES

| Makes | 4 servings | Serving size | 4oz (110g) | Prep time | 10 minutes | Cook time | 15 minutes |

INGREDIENTS

1 medium wild salmon filet, approximately 1lb (450g)

2 large limes, sliced into ¼-inch (.5cm) slices (reserve ⅓ of each lime)

2 tsp chili powder

½ tsp salt

1 tsp ground cilantro

DIRECTIONS

1 Preheat the oven to 400°F (204°C). Cut a piece of parchment paper large enough to create a pouch for the salmon. Place the parchment on a large baking sheet.

2 Arrange enough lime slices on the parchment paper to create a bed for the salmon filet. Place the filet, scales-side-down, on top of the lime slices.

3 Squeeze the reserved lime over the filet, discard. Season the filet with the chili powder, salt, and cilantro. Place the remaining lime slices on top of the filet.

4 Fold the parchment paper over the salmon and crimp the edges to form a pouch. Bake for 15 minutes. Serve hot.

PREP TIPS

If you don't have parchment paper, you can use aluminum foil, instead. (The salmon will steam and have a slightly softer texture.)

Store in an airtight container in the refrigerator for up to 2 days.

CHANGE IT UP

Lemons or bitter orange can be used in place of the limes.

For a lighter flavor, substitute 2 tsp dried rosemary for the chili powder and cilantro.

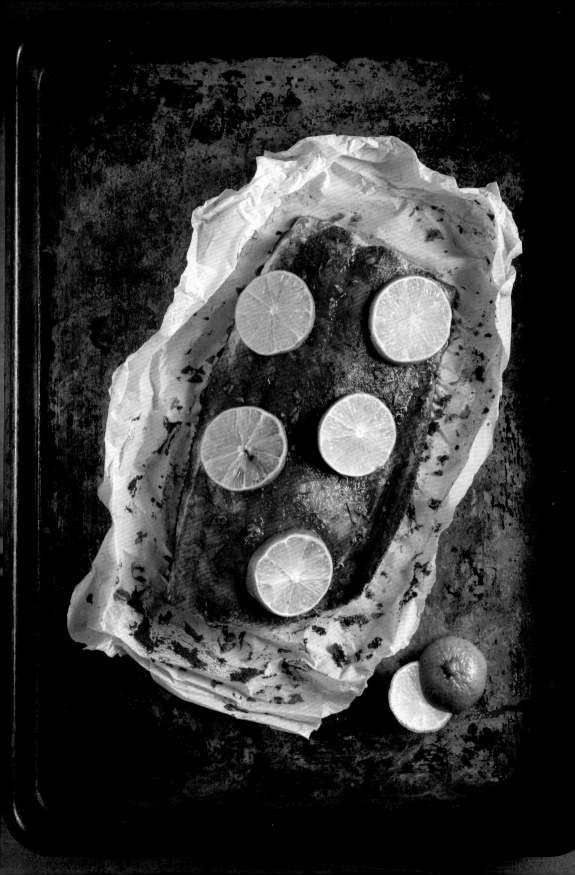

Brining the chicken brings out the flavor and locks in the moisture in this protein-packed classic. Searing the breasts produces a beautiful crust, while finishing them in the oven helps keep this lean protein juicy. You can pair this flavorful chicken with just about any side dish.

PAN-SEARED CHICKEN BREASTS

Makes 8 servings	**Serving size** 4oz (110g)	**Prep time** 10 min + 4 hours	**Cook time** 20 minutes

INGREDIENTS

2 cups water

1 tbsp apple cider vinegar

2 tbsp sriracha hot chili sauce

1 tbsp course ground mustard

½ tsp ground black pepper

2 tbsp salt

1 tsp garlic powder

2lbs (900g) boneless, skinless chicken breasts

DIRECTIONS

1 Preheat the oven to 400°F (204°C). Make the brine by combining the water, vinegar, sriracha sauce, mustard, black pepper, salt, and garlic powder in a large glass bowl. Mix well to combine.

2 Add the chicken breasts to the bowl, ensuring the brine covers the chicken completely. (Add more water to cover the chicken, if needed.) Tightly cover the bowl with plastic wrap and place in the refrigerator to brine for a minimum of 4 hours (or up to 12 hours).

3 Spray a large cast iron grill pan with coconut oil cooking spray and preheat over medium-high heat. Remove the chicken from the brine and rinse under cool water to remove any excess salt.

4 Place the chicken on the pre-heated grill pan. Sear for 3 to 4 minutes per side, then place in the oven to bake for an additional 8 to 10 minutes. The chicken is done when the juices run clear and the internal temperature reaches 165°F (74°C).

NUTRITION FACTS

per serving

CALORIES

140

TOTAL FAT

3g

TOTAL CARBS

0g

PROTEIN

27g

PREP TIPS

You can double this recipe for easy meal prep.

Store in an airtight container in the refrigerator for up to 5 days.

CHANGE IT UP

For a spicier flavor, season the chicken with ½ tsp cayenne pepper powder, ½ tsp paprika, and ½ tsp dried thyme.

APPLE-ROASTED WHOLE CHICKEN

Makes **8 servings** | Serving size **4oz (110g)** | Prep time **10 minutes** | Cook time **1 hour**

INGREDIENTS

1 tsp salt

1 tsp garlic powder

1 tsp ground black pepper

1 small chicken, approximately 2½ to 3lbs (1.2 to 1.4kg), giblets removed

1 medium Granny Smith apple

Coconut oil cooking spray

DIRECTIONS

1 Preheat the oven to 350°F (177°C). Make the rub by combining the salt, garlic powder, and black pepper in a small bowl.

2 Place the chicken in a large roasting pan. Insert the apple into the cavity, and season the outside of the chicken with half of the rub. Place the chicken in the oven and roast for 45 minutes.

3 After 45 minutes, increase the oven temperature to 400°F (204°C). Remove the chicken from the oven, lightly spray with coconut oil spray, and season with the remaining rub.

4 Bake for an additional 15 minutes, or until the internal temperature reaches 165°F (74°C) and the juices run clear when the chicken is pierced with a sharp knife. Slice and serve hot.

CHANGE IT UP

For a bolder flavor, coat the chicken with 3 tbsp mustard before baking, and omit the cooking spray. Or, season with ½ tsp of chipotle powder.

PREP TIPS // *Whole chickens tend to be less expensive than chicken breasts. If you're watching your budget, this recipe goes a long way.*

Store in an airtight container in the refrigerator for up to 6 days.

Turning up the heat during the last 15 minutes of baking helps seal in the juices and crisp the skin to produce this photo-worthy bird. Most meal plans will call for a 50/50 serving of breast and thighs, with the skin removed. Keto plan followers can have the crispy skin and dark meat.

NUTRITION FACTS

per serving

CALORIES

151

TOTAL FAT

4.2g

TOTAL CARBS

0g

PROTEIN

26.4g

Spicy, salty, pungent, and a bit sweet, these skewers hit all the right flavor notes. And, with a cook time of less than 6 minutes, you can prep these ahead and throw a protein-rich meal together in a snap. Shrimp is high in selenium and B12, which can help fight free radicals.

GINGER SOY SHRIMP SKEWERS

| **Makes** 4 servings | **Serving size** 4oz (110g) | **Prep time** 10 min + 1 hour | **Cook time** 6 minutes |

NUTRITION FACTS

per serving

CALORIES
119

TOTAL FAT
1.3g

TOTAL CARBS
2g

PROTEIN
23.9g

INGREDIENTS

1 tsp minced garlic

½ tsp red chili flakes

¼ tsp powdered stevia

3 tbsp soy sauce

½ tsp ground ginger

½ tsp salt

½ tsp ground black pepper

1 pound medium shrimp, peeled, deveined, and tails removed

1 medium lime, sliced into quarters (for serving)

DIRECTIONS

1 In a large, sealable freezer bag, combine the garlic, chili flakes, stevia, soy sauce, ginger, salt, and black pepper. Add the shrimp to the bag, seal, and rotate the bag ensuring all of the shrimp are coated with the marinade. Place in the refrigerator to marinate for up to 1 hour.

2 Set the broiler to low. Thread the shrimp onto skewers, ensuring they line up evenly and lay flat. (If you're using wood skewers, soak them in water for 20 minutes prior to using.)

3 Line a 9 x 13in (23 x 33cm) sheet pan with aluminum foil, and arrange the skewers on the pan. Broil for 2 to 3 minutes, or until the shrimp just begin to turn opaque.

4 Flip the skewers and broil for an additional 2 to 3 minutes, or until the shrimp are opaque. Transfer the skewers to a serving plate and garnish with the lime wedges. Serve warm.

PREP TIPS | *Fresh-frozen shrimp are much less expensive than fresh shrimp, and can be kept frozen for several months.*

Store in an airtight container in the refrigerator for 1 day. (Cooked shrimp is best consumed immediately.)

CHANGE IT UP
Make these keto by adding ¼ cup olive oil to the marinade. The macros will be 239 calories, 14.8g fat, 2g carbs, and 23.9g protein per serving.

SRIRACHA CURRY COCONUT CHICKEN

Makes	8 servings	Serving size	4oz (110g)	Prep time	10 minutes	Cook time	15 minutes

This bold dish is full of flavor and is made with simple, everyday ingredients. Steaming the chicken locks in the flavor and keeps it sumptuously juicy. Sriracha and coconut milk balance the smooth and spicy flavors, and aromatic curry adds warmth and contains beneficial antioxidant compounds.

INGREDIENTS

1 cup light coconut milk

½ cup sriracha hot chili sauce

1 tbsp lime juice

1 tbsp curry powder (Vindaloo is preferred)

½ tsp salt

½ tsp ground black pepper

2lbs (900g) boneless, skinless chicken breasts

DIRECTIONS

1 In a large bowl, combine the coconut milk, sriracha sauce, lime juice, curry powder, salt, and black pepper. Mix well. Add the chicken breasts to the bowl, and toss thoroughly to coat the chicken with the sauce.

2 Spray a medium skillet with non-stick cooking spray and place over medium heat. Add the chicken breasts and cook for 1 to 2 minutes per side, or until the chicken begins to brown.

3 Add the sauce to the skillet, cover, and cook for an additional 10 minutes, flipping the chicken breasts halfway through the cooking time.

4 Adjust the heat to medium-high, uncover, and cook the breasts for an additional 2 to 3 minutes per side, or until the sauce begins to caramelize. The chicken is done when the internal temperature reaches 160°F (71°C) and the juices run clear. Serve hot.

PREP TIPS Store the cooled chicken and sauce in an airtight container in the refrigerator for up to 7 days.

NUTRITION FACTS

per serving

CALORIES
159

TOTAL FAT
4.8g

TOTAL CARBS
2.6g

PROTEIN
25.4g

CHANGE IT UP

Make it keto by replacing the chicken breasts with 2lbs (1kg) bone-in chicken thighs, and replacing the light coconut milk with 1 cup full-fat coconut milk. The macros will be 244 calories, 14.5g fat, 1.6g carbs, and 25.6g protein per serving.

ENTRÉES

This quick and easy entrée features lightly seasoned cod and a tart and citrusy charred tomatillo salsa. Serrano chiles deliver a punch of heat and nice burst of flavor. Earthy cilantro, onions, and lime all add bright flavors to complement this mild and meaty fish.

BROILED COD
WITH CHARRED TOMATILLO SALSA

Makes 2 servings | **Serving size** 4oz (110g) fish, 3 tbsp salsa | **Prep time** 10 minutes | **Cook time** 15 minutes

INGREDIENTS

5 large tomatillos, stems and husks removed

2 serrano chiles, stems and seeds removed, chopped

2 tbsp diced white onion

¼ cup roughly chopped fresh cilantro

½ tsp lime juice

½ tsp salt

½lb (225g) cod fillets (fresh or frozen)

½ tsp garlic powder

½ tsp salt

½ tsp ground black pepper

DIRECTIONS

1 Preheat the broiler to low. Line a small baking pan with aluminum foil and place the tomatillos and serrano chiles in the pan. Place the pan on the top oven rack and roast for 6 to 8 minutes, flipping the tomatillos and chiles halfway through the cooking process. Roast until nicely charred.

2 Add the tomatillos, chiles, onion, cilantro, lime juice, and salt to a blender. Pulse in 10 second intervals until a smooth consistency is achieved. Set aside.

3 Spray a small baking pan with non-stick cooking spray. Place the cod in the pan and season with the garlic powder, salt, and black pepper. Broil for 3 to 4 minutes per side, until the fish is lightly browned and can be flaked with a fork.

4 Transfer the baked cod to a serving platter and spoon the tomatillo salsa over top. Serve hot.

NUTRITION FACTS

per serving

CALORIES

137

TOTAL FAT

1.3g

TOTAL CARBS

3.6g

PROTEIN

25.9g

PREP TIPS // *Save money by purchasing frozen cod fillets instead of fresh. Thaw in the refrigerator 1 day before cooking.*

Store in an airtight container in the refrigerator for up to 2 days.

CHANGE IT UP
You can substitute tilapia, haddock, or roughy for the cod. The macros will be very similar.

CHICKEN HOBO DINNER

Makes **4** *servings* | **Serving size** *1 pouch* | **Prep time** *15 minutes* | **Cook time** *25 minutes*

Cut down on prep time with this easy dinner that's ready in less than 45 minutes. Sweet bell peppers and onions provide an antioxidant boost and season the chicken as it cooks. The cooking process steams the veggies and seals in the flavors in this lighter version of a campfire favorite.

INGREDIENTS

1lb (450g) boneless, skinless chicken breasts, cut into 1-inch (2.5cm) strips

2 large bell peppers, ribs and seeds removed, sliced into ½-inch (1.25cm) strips

1 red onion, sliced crosswise and into ½-inch (1.25cm) slices

1 tsp chili powder

1 tsp ground cumin

1 tsp garlic powder

1 tsp salt

DIRECTIONS

1 Preheat the oven to 400°F (204°C). Lightly spray four 12 x 12in (30 x 30cm) squares of aluminum foil with non-stick cooking spray. In a large bowl, combine the chicken strips, peppers, and onions. Set aside.

2 Make the seasoning mix by combining the chili powder, cumin, garlic powder, and salt in a small bowl. Mix well.

3 Add the seasoning mix to the chicken, peppers, and onions. Toss thoroughly to coat the chicken and peppers with the seasoning.

4 Place equal amounts of the chicken, peppers, and onions onto each foil square. Grasp the corners of the squares, gather the edges at the middle, and crimp tightly together to form pouches.

5 Place the pouches on a large baking sheet and bake for 23 to 25 minutes, or until the juices from the chicken run clear and the internal temperature reaches 165°F (74°C).

6 Remove the pouches from the oven and allow to cool for 10 minutes before serving. (Use caution when opening the pouches, as the steam will be very hot.)

PREP TIPS / *Remove the chicken from the pouches and store in an airtight container in the refrigerator for up to 5 days.*

NUTRITION FACTS

per serving

CALORIES
173

TOTAL FAT
3g

TOTAL CARBS
8.3g
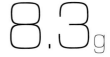

PROTEIN
26.9g
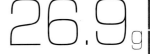

ENTRÉES

Sweet bell peppers and a savory, and slightly spicy beef and onion filling are the stars in this hearty entrée that's ready in less than 30 minutes. Salsa provides an extra kick of flavor without adding lots of excess calories. A quick dip in boiling water ensures that the bell peppers stay tender and flavorful.

SPICY STUFFED PEPPERS

Makes	4 servings	Serving size	1 pepper	Prep time	5 minutes	Cook time	20 minutes

INGREDIENTS

4 medium bell peppers, tops, pith, and seeds removed

1lb (450g) lean ground beef (preferably 92/8 lean-to-fat ratio)

1 cup finely chopped onion

1 tsp celery salt

½ tsp garlic powder

⅛ tsp cayenne pepper

6 tbsp salsa

DIRECTIONS

1 Preheat the oven to 350°F (177°C). Fill a medium stockpot with water to three-quarters full, and bring to a rolling boil.

2 Place the peppers in the pot, bottom-sides up. Boil for 5 minutes, then transfer the peppers to a paper towel to drain, bottom-sides down, for 5 minutes. Set aside.

3 In a medium non-stick skillet, combine the ground beef, onion, celery salt, garlic powder, and cayenne pepper. Cook over medium-high heat for 4 to 6 minutes, stirring frequently, until the ground beef is browned throughout and the onions are soft and translucent. Add 2 tbsp salsa and stir. Remove the pan from the heat and drain off any excess fat.

4 Spray a large baking sheet with non-stick cooking spray. Place the peppers, top-sides up, on the baking sheet. Divide the filling into 4 equal-sized portions and spoon the portions into the peppers. Top each pepper with 1 tbsp salsa.

5 Bake the peppers for 15 minutes, then transfer to a serving platter. Serve hot.

NUTRITION FACTS

per serving

CALORIES
239

TOTAL FAT
9.6g

TOTAL CARBS
18.2g

PROTEIN
23.9g

PREP TIPS // Store the cooled peppers in an airtight container in the refrigerator for up to 5 days.

CHANGE IT UP
Try substituting different varieties of salsa, such as salsa verde or pico de gallo, or for an even bigger punch of heat try a hot habanero salsa.

ENTRÉES

70

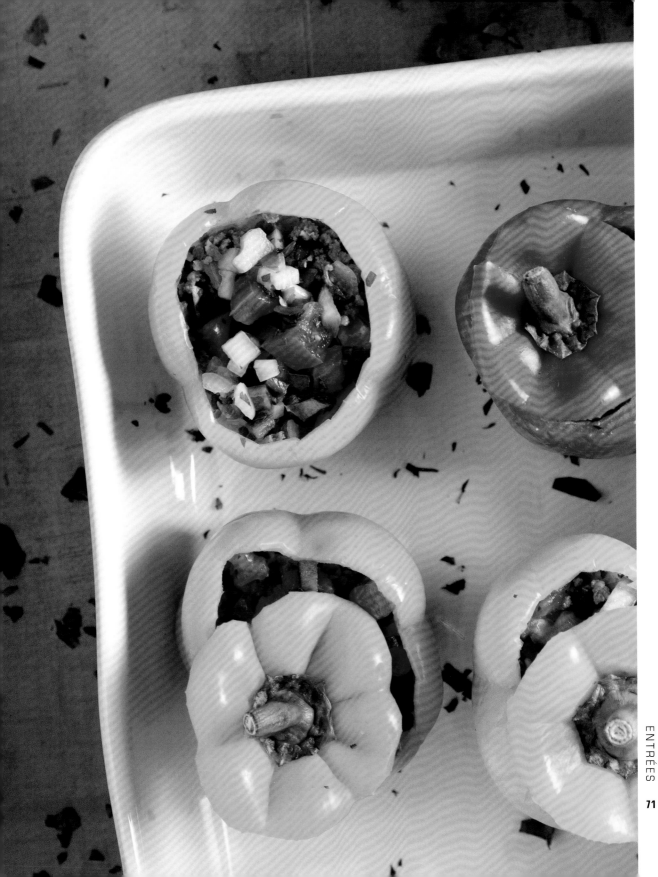

Bold Mediterranean flavors come together in this tangy and spicy chicken dish that's low in fat and high in muscle-building protein. Broiling the chicken seals in the flavor and browns it to perfection, and the bite-sized cubes store well and are perfect as leftovers for quick weekday meals.

NUTRITION FACTS

per serving

CALORIES
145

TOTAL FAT
3.1 g

TOTAL CARBS
1.7 g

PROTEIN
25.9 g

BROILED GREEK CHICKEN KABOBS

Makes	4 servings	Serving size	4oz (110g) or 1 kabob	Prep time	15 min + 30 min	Cook time	15 minutes

INGREDIENTS

1 tbsp minced garlic

2 tbsp dried oregano

1 tsp crushed red pepper flakes

1 tsp ground black pepper

½ tsp salt

½ cup low-sodium chicken broth

¼ cup lemon juice

1lb (450g) boneless, skinless chicken breasts

DIRECTIONS

1 Preheat the broiler to low. Spray a 9 x 13in (23 x 33cm) baking pan with non-stick cooking spray.

2 Make the marinade by combining the garlic, oregano, red pepper flakes, black pepper, salt, chicken broth, and lemon juice in a large glass bowl. Mix well to combine.

3 Using a fork, pierce the chicken breasts on all sides, then cut the breasts into ½-inch (1.25cm) cubes. Add the cubes to the bowl with the marinade, tightly cover with plastic wrap, and place in the refrigerator to marinate for 30 minutes.

4 Carefully thread the chicken cubes onto metal skewers, and place the skewers in the baking pan.

5 Broil for 12 to 16 minutes, flipping the skewers halfway through the cooking process. The chicken is done when the juices run clear and the internal temperature reaches 165°F (74°C). Serve hot.

CHANGE IT UP
For a brighter flavor, substitute 1 tbsp dried parsley for the oregano.

PREP TIPS *Remove the chicken from the skewers and store in an airtight container in the refrigerator for up to 5 days.*

ALMOND-CRUSTED MUSTARD CHICKEN

Makes 4 servings | **Serving size** 5oz (140g) or 3 strips | **Prep time** 15 minutes | **Cook time** 25 minutes

INGREDIENTS

¼ cup liquid egg whites

3 tbsp Dijon mustard

1 cup almond flour

½ tsp paprika

½ tsp dried tarragon

½ tsp ground black pepper

½ tsp salt

1lb (450g) boneless, skinless chicken breasts, cut into 2-inch (5cm) strips

DIRECTIONS

1 Preheat the oven to 400°F (204°C). Line a large baking sheet with aluminum foil.

2 In a small bowl, whisk together the egg whites and mustard. In a separate shallow baking dish, combine the almond flour, paprika, tarragon, black pepper, and salt.

3 Dip the chicken strips in the egg white mixture, then dredge in the almond flour mixture, making sure to evenly coat the strips with the breading. Place the strips on the baking sheet.

4 Bake for 20 to 22 minutes, or until the juices run clear and the internal temperature reaches 165°F (74°C). Allow the chicken strips to rest for 5 minutes. Serve hot.

PREP TIPS

For crunchier strips, bake the chicken on an oven-safe cooling rack, instead of a baking sheet.

Store in an airtight container in the refrigerator for up to 5 days. Reheat on a baking sheet in a 250°F (121°C) oven for 15 minutes.

CHANGE IT UP

For a little extra heat, add ½ tsp chili powder to the almond flour mixture.

Add some brightness by sprinkling the juice of one lemon over the strips just before serving.

Almond flour and egg whites are the secret ingredients for making this chicken crunchy and keeping it juicy. Almonds are rich in vitamins, fiber, and protein, and can help burn fat and control hunger. Dijon mustard adds a tangy kick, and also helps tenderize the chicken.

NUTRITION FACTS

per serving

CALORIES

278

TOTAL FAT

13.8g

TOTAL CARBS

5.1g

PROTEIN

34g

This quick and easy entrée is ready in less than 30 minutes, and features flaky snapper gently poached in a light and simple lemon broth. Snapper is a delicate fish and an excellent source of lean protein. Broccoli is loaded with essential nutrients and powerful antioxidants.

NUTRITION FACTS

per serving

CALORIES
194

TOTAL FAT
2.5g

TOTAL CARBS
9.3g

PROTEIN
34.4g

BROTH-POACHED SNAPPER WITH BROCCOLI

Makes	4 servings	Serving size	4oz (110g) fish + 4oz (110) broccoli	Prep time	15 minutes	Cook time	10 minutes

INGREDIENTS

1 cup low-sodium chicken broth

½ white onion, sliced crosswise

1 lemon, sliced crosswise

1lb (450g) fresh snapper fillets, skin on

1 12oz (340g) package frozen broccoli florets, thawed

Pinch of salt

DIRECTIONS

1 In a large stock pot, combine the chicken broth, onion slices, and lemon slices. Carefully place the snapper fillets in the pot, skin-side down, making sure the fillets are partially submerged in the broth.

2 Cover, and bring to a simmer over medium-low heat. Cook for 5 to 6 minutes, or until the fish is firm and flaky and the flesh is opaque. Using a spatula, carefully transfer the cooked fillets to a plate.

3 Keeping the pot at a simmer, add the broccoli florets, cover, and cook for 5 minutes, or until the florets develop a bright green color and become slightly soft.

4 Use a slotted spoon to remove the broccoli, onion slices, and lemon slices from the pot. Discard the lemon slices, and spoon the broccoli and onions over the fillets. Season with a pinch of salt. Serve hot.

PREP TIPS // *Frozen fillets are less expensive and can be used for this recipe. Thaw frozen fish in the refrigerator one day before cooking.*

This recipe is best when prepared and consumed immediately, but can be stored in an airtight container in the refrigerator for 1 day.

CHANGE IT UP

Other firm white fish, such as flounder, grouper, cod, or tilapia, can be substituted for the snapper. The macros will be about the same.

SLOW COOKER BBQ PULLED CHICKEN

Makes	4 servings	Serving size	4oz (110g)	Prep time	15 minutes	Cook time	4.5–8.5 hours

All of the flavors of the smokehouse come together in this recipe—but without all the extra fat and sugar. The chicken is slow cooked to perfection, and the sauce is a bit bold yet incredibly simple to make. The macros are clean enough that you can use this recipe for meals throughout the week.

INGREDIENTS

2 cups bone broth or low-sodium chicken broth

2 tbsp dried onion flakes

1 tbsp garlic powder

2lbs (900g) boneless, skinless chicken breasts

⅔ cup no-sugar-added ketchup

½ cup apple cider vinegar

2 tbsp Worcestershire sauce

1 tsp paprika

1 tsp kosher salt

1 tsp ground black pepper

¼ tsp chipotle powder (optional)

DIRECTIONS

1 In a large slow cooker, combine the broth, onion flakes, and garlic powder. Add the chicken breasts to the broth, ensuring they are completely covered in the liquid. Cover, and cook on low for 8 hours, or on high for 4 hours.

2 After the cook time has passed, use two forks to gently shred the chicken. Adjust the heat to high and allow the chicken to cook in the broth for an additional 30 minutes.

3 Make the sauce by combining the ketchup, vinegar, Worcestershire sauce, paprika, kosher salt, black pepper, and chipotle powder (if using) in a large bowl. Mix well to combine.

4 Use a slotted spoon to transfer the chicken from the slow cooker to the bowl containing the sauce. Toss the chicken in the sauce to coat thoroughly. Serve warm.

CHANGE IT UP

Make a Carolina-style sauce combining ½ cup plain nonfat Greek yogurt, ¼ cup spicy Dijon mustard, ½ tsp salt, and ½ tsp dried thyme in a large bowl. The impact on the macros will be minimal.

PREP TIPS *Store the cooled chicken and sauce in an airtight container in the refrigerator for up to 7 days.*

NUTRITION FACTS

per serving

CALORIES
152

TOTAL FAT
3g

TOTAL CARBS
2.2g

PROTEIN
26.8g

ENTRÉES

This easy entrée features wild-caught salmon, which is high in omega-3 fats, can help reduce inflammation, and increases mood-elevating serotonin levels. It can be assembled in less than 45 minutes for a tasty weekday dinner option that's budget-friendly and loaded with protein.

NUTRITION FACTS

per serving

CALORIES
179

TOTAL FAT
4.5g

TOTAL CARBS
5.2g

PROTEIN
29.7g

SPICY SALMON BURGERS

Makes	2 servings		Serving size	2 burgers		Prep time	25 minutes		Cook time	10 minutes

INGREDIENTS

2 5oz (140g) cans wild-caught salmon, rinsed and drained

1 tbsp lemon juice

1 large egg

1 tbsp cornmeal

1 tbsp dried onion flakes

½ tsp ground black pepper

4 tsp hot sauce (optional)

DIRECTIONS

1 In a medium bowl, combine the salmon, lemon juice, egg, cornmeal, onion flakes, and black pepper. Mix well, and allow to rest for 15 minutes to help the ingredients bind.

2 Using clean hands, form the mixture into 4 equal-sized patties.

3 Generously spray a medium non-stick frying pan with non-stick cooking spray. Cook the patties over medium-high heat for 4 to 5 minutes per side, or until the patties are lightly browned on each side.

4 Drizzle 1 tsp hot sauce (if using) over each patty. Serve hot.

PREP TIPS // This recipe can be doubled for easy meal prep.

Store in an airtight container in the refrigerator for up to 4 days.

CHANGE IT UP

For a spicier burger, add ½ tsp red pepper flakes to the burger mixture.

For a more herbal flavor, omit the black pepper and hot sauce, and add 1 tbsp finely chopped fresh dill and 2 tbsp Dijon mustard.

REVERSE-SEARED SIRLOIN STEAK

This simple, yet flavorful steak is protein-packed and contains zero carbs! The steak is cooked in the oven at low temperature to ensure even cooking, and a quick sear on the stovetop seals in the juices. The end result is a beautifully crusted steak that is moist, tender, and delicious.

Makes	4 servings	Serving size	4oz (120g)	Prep time	30 minutes	Cook time	45–60 minutes

INGREDIENTS

1lb (450g) sirloin steak

1 tsp salt

1 tsp ground black pepper

DIRECTIONS

1 Preheat the oven to 275°F (135°C). Place an oven-safe cooling rack atop a large, foil-lined baking sheet.

2 Season both sides of the steak with salt and pepper, and allow to rest at room temperature for 30 minutes.

3 Place the steak on the cooling rack and place in the oven. Bake for 30 minutes if the steak is 1 to 2 inches thick (2.5 to 5cm), or 45 minutes if the steak is 3 to 4 inches thick (7.5 to 10cm).

4 Remove the steak from the oven and allow to rest for 15 minutes.

5 Spray a large cast iron skillet with coconut oil cooking spray and preheat over high heat. Place the steak in the skillet and sear for approximately 1 minute per side. The steak is done when it's pink in the middle and the internal temperature reaches 145°F (63°C). Serve hot.

PREP TIPS Store in an airtight container in the refrigerator for up to 5 days.

CHANGE IT UP

For a Southwestern twist, season the steak with ½ tsp garlic powder, ½ tsp cumin, and ½ tsp paprika.

NUTRITION FACTS

per serving

CALORIES
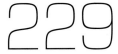
229

TOTAL FAT

9.1 g

TOTAL CARBS
0 g

PROTEIN

34.4 g

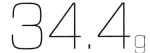

ENTRÉES

77

Pork tenderloin is packed with protein and provides the perfect canvas for sweet and spicy flavors. Cooking the tenderloin on a cast iron skillet imparts a golden crust and seals in the juices. Tenderloin typically costs less per pound than chicken breasts, so it's a budget-friendly option.

NUTRITION FACTS

per serving

CALORIES
233

TOTAL FAT
9.3g

TOTAL CARBS
1.1g

PROTEIN
33.7g

VIETNAMESE-STYLE PORK TENDERLOIN

Makes 8 servings	**Serving size** 4oz (110g)	**Prep time** 10 min + 4–8 hrs	**Cook time** 6 minutes

INGREDIENTS

1 tbsp powdered stevia

¼ cup green onions, finely sliced (green ends only)

3 tsp minced garlic

1 tbsp lime juice

1 tbsp fish sauce (Vietnamese or Thai)

½ tsp salt

1lb (450g) pork tenderloin, trimmed, silver skin removed, and sliced crosswise into ½-inch-thick (1.25cm) medallions

DIRECTIONS

1 Make the marinade by combining the stevia, half the green onions, garlic, lime juice, fish sauce, and salt in a large glass bowl. Mix well. Add the tenderloin medallions to the marinade, cover tightly, and place in the refrigerator to marinate for 4 to 8 hours.

2 Preheat a cast iron skillet over medium heat. Place the tenderloin medallions in the skillet and cook for 2 to 3 minutes per side. The meat is done when the internal temperature reaches 160°F (71°C) degrees and the juices run clear.

3 Transfer the cooked medallions to a serving plate and garnish with the remaining green onions. Serve warm.

PREP TIPS // *You can marinate a whole tenderloin for up to 24 hours and slice after cooking. To do so, cook in the skillet over medium heat for 20 minutes, turning frequently. Allow the whole tenderloin to rest for 5 minutes before slicing.*

Avoid buying pre-marinated pork tenderloin, which can be loaded with preservatives and sodium.

Store in an airtight container in the refrigerator for up to 5 days. (Reserve the scallions and add to the reheated tenderloin just before serving.)

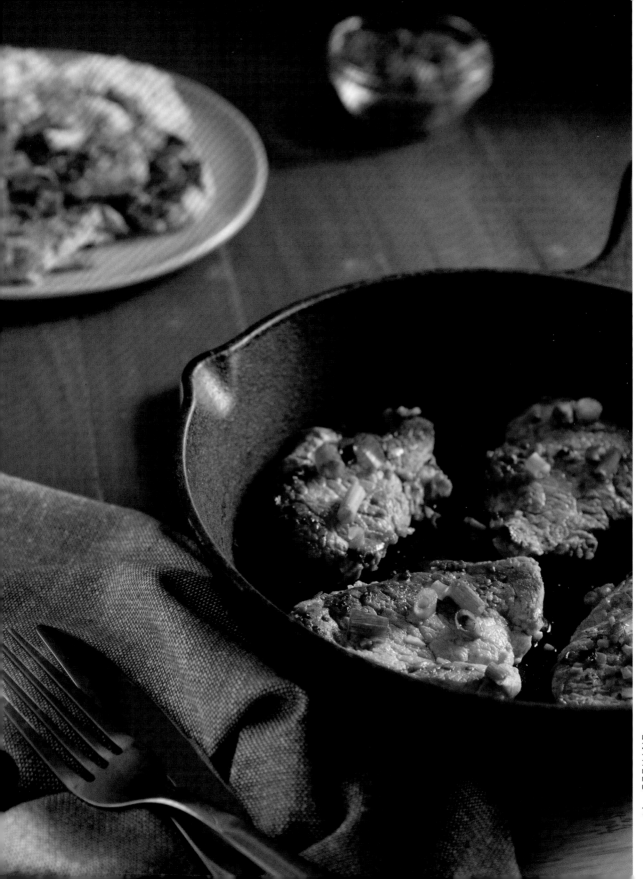

These fajitas are protein-packed and feature tender skirt steak, meaty mushrooms, and sweet onions. Lime adds brightness and helps tenderize the steak, and the fajita seasoning adds just the right amount of spice. Ready in less than 30 minutes, these are perfect for a weeknight meal!

NUTRITION FACTS

per serving

CALORIES
299

TOTAL FAT
8.6g

TOTAL CARBS
26.5g

PROTEIN
27.9g

TEX-MEX FAJITAS

Makes 4 servings | **Serving size** 2 fajitas | **Prep time** 15 minutes | **Cook time** 20 minutes

INGREDIENTS

2 tsp chili powder

1½ tsp ground cumin

1 tsp ground paprika

½ tsp ground coriander

1 tsp salt

½ tsp ground black pepper

1lb (450g) skirt steak, cut against the grain into ¼-inch (.5cm) slices

1 cup sliced Portobello mushrooms, sliced into ½-inch (1.25cm) strips

1 medium red onion, sliced into 1-inch (2.5cm) wedges

¼ cup lime juice

8 6-inch (15.25cm) corn tortillas

¼ cup chopped fresh cilantro

½ cup salsa

DIRECTIONS

1 Preheat the oven to 400°F (204°C). Line a large baking sheet with aluminum foil.

2 Make the seasoning mix by combining the chili powder, cumin, paprika, coriander, salt, and black pepper in a small bowl. Mix well.

3 In a large bowl, combine the steak strips, mushrooms, onions, lime juice, and seasoning mix. Toss the ingredients, ensuring that the steak, mushrooms, and onions are thoroughly coated with the seasonings. Place the contents on the baking sheet, and bake for 20 minutes. Transfer to a serving bowl.

4 Wrap the tortillas in aluminum foil and place them in the oven during the final 5 minutes of the baking time.

5 Transfer the warmed tortillas to a plate. Top each tortilla with 4oz (110g) steak, 2oz (55g) vegetables, and 2 tbsp salsa. Garnish each with a pinch of cilantro. Serve warm.

PREP TIPS / Store the cooled filling in an airtight container in the refrigerator for up to 5 days.

CHANGE IT UP

Make it a bowl by omitting the corn tortillas, and adding the fillings to a bowl along with 1 cup fresh baby spinach and ½ cup cooked white rice. The macros will be about the same.

SLOW COOKER PORK ROAST

Makes **8** servings / Serving size **4oz (110g)** / Prep time **5 minutes** / Cook time **3–8 hours**

Cooking this roast low and slow makes it fall-apart tender, and just a touch of honey, soy sauce, and ketchup create an addicting and tangy glaze. Pork is budget-friendly, high in protein, and keeps well in the fridge. Prep and assemble in the morning for a ready-made dinner in the evening.

INGREDIENTS

1 cup low fat chicken broth

¼ cup balsamic vinegar

¼ cup light soy sauce

1 tbsp no-sugar-added ketchup

2 tbsp honey

2 tsp minced garlic

2lbs (900g) boneless pork loin, trimmed of excess fat

DIRECTIONS

1 In a medium bowl, combine the chicken broth, vinegar, soy sauce, ketchup, honey, and garlic. Mix well. Pour approximately ¼ cup of the glaze into a large slow cooker.

2 Add the pork loin to the slow cooker. Pour the remaining glaze over top of the pork, cover, and cook for 6 to 8 hours on low, or 3 to 4 hours on high.

3 Transfer the cooked roast to a cutting board and slice crosswise into ½-inch (1.25cm) slices. Serve warm.

CHANGE IT UP

For a more savory glaze, add 2 tbsp dried oregano.

PREP TIPS // For easier meal prep, divide the roast into single serving portions, and seal in small zipper lock storage bags.

Store in an airtight container in the refrigerator for up to 5 days.

NUTRITION FACTS

per serving

CALORIES

192

TOTAL FAT

6.5g

TOTAL CARBS

3.9g

PROTEIN

27.7g

ENTRÉES

High quality steaks are prized for their fat marbling, but that fat can also add lots of unnecessary calories. The flavorful coffee rub in this recipe uses expresso powder, spices, and salt to tenderize and season the meat, while the broiling process seals in the juices. You won't miss the fat!

NUTRITION FACTS

per serving

CALORIES

150

TOTAL FAT

4.4g

TOTAL CARBS

0g

PROTEIN

25.8g

COFFEE-RUBBED STEAK

Makes	4 servings		Serving size	4oz (110g)		Prep time	10 min + 30 min		Cook time	15 minutes

INGREDIENTS

1lb (450g) sirloin or eye of round steak, trimmed of excess fat

1 tbsp instant espresso powder

1 tsp garlic powder

½ tsp salt

¼ tsp ground cumin

¼ tsp dried oregano

¼ tsp chili powder

¼ tsp ground black pepper

DIRECTIONS

1 Preheat the broiler to high. Line an 8 x 8in (20 x 20cm) baking pan with aluminum foil. Allow the steak to rest at room temperature for 30 minutes before patting dry with a paper towel.

2 In a medium bowl, combine the espresso powder, garlic powder, salt, cumin, oregano, chili powder, and black pepper. Mix well.

3 Generously season the steak with the rub, using your fingertips to gently press the rub into both sides of the steak.

4 Place the steak in the oven and broil for 2 to 3 minutes per side for medium rare, 3 to 4 minutes per side for medium, and 4 to 5 minutes per side for medium well.

5 Allow the steak to rest for 5 minutes before slicing against the grain, and into four equal-sized servings. Serve warm.

PREP TIPS
Store any unsliced steak in an airtight container in the refrigerator for up to 3 days. (Unsliced steak will retain more moisture.)

Store any leftover rub in an airtight jar at room temperature for up to 2 months.

CHANGE IT UP

This recipe also works great on the grill. Set the grill to high heat, and cook for 3 to 5 minutes per side, depending on preferred level of doneness.

RIDICULOUSLY EASY PORK ROLL-UPS

Makes 4 servings | **Serving size** 4oz (110g) | **Prep time** 20 minutes | **Cook time** 20 minutes

Pork provides the perfect canvas for a zesty spinach and tomato filling that is full of nutrients. The fillings also help keep you full, and keep the pork juicy and tender. These simple roll-ups are a snap to prepare, and will provide a delicious protein punch with virtually zero carbs.

INGREDIENTS

1lb (450g) pork tenderloin, trimmed, silver skin removed, and cut into 4 equal-sized pieces

2 large handfuls fresh baby spinach

⅓ cup no-sugar-added tomato sauce

2 tbsp minced garlic

¼ cup grated parmesan cheese

Salt and pepper to taste

DIRECTIONS

1 Preheat the oven to 400°F (204°C). Spray a large baking sheet with non-stick cooking spray.

2 Using a meat tenderizer or rolling pin, pound each tenderloin flat to about ¼-inch (.5cm) thickness. Place the tenderloins on the baking sheet and set aside.

3 In a medium non-stick frying pan, combine the spinach, tomato sauce, and garlic. Cook over medium heat for 6 to 8 minutes, or until the spinach is tender. Drain.

4 Divide the spinach mixture into even portions and spoon over top of each tenderloin. Grasp the edge of each tenderloin and roll it up, being careful to keep the ingredients inside. Secure each roll-up with a toothpick or baking twine, and season with 1 tbsp parmesan cheese.

5 Bake for 20 minutes. The pork is done when the internal temperature reaches 145°F (63°C). Serve warm.

PREP TIPS *Although fresh spinach is better for this recipe, you can also use 1 cup frozen spinach that's been thawed and drained.*

These roll-ups can be made ahead of time, stored in the refrigerator, and cooked when you're ready. Uncooked, they'll keep in the refrigerator for up to 2 days.

NUTRITION FACTS

per serving

CALORIES
261

TOTAL FAT
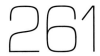
10.9g

TOTAL CARBS
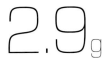
2.9g

PROTEIN

36g

ENTRÉES

Spice up plain old chicken with this tangy and spicy, Caribbean-inspired recipe that features classic jerk seasonings. Fresh thyme and aromatic spices form a highly aromatic spice paste, and the soy sauce and lime juice tenderize the chicken to ensure the meat stays juicy and tender.

GRILLED JERK CHICKEN BREASTS

Makes	4 servings		Serving size	4oz (110g)		Prep time	15 min + 4–6 hours		Cook time	12 minutes

NUTRITION FACTS

per serving

CALORIES
145

TOTAL FAT
3.1g

TOTAL CARBS
0.8g

PROTEIN
26.8g

INGREDIENTS

1 small jalapeño pepper, stem and seeds removed

½ medium red onion, roughly chopped

2 tsp minced garlic

2 tbsp fresh thyme

1 tsp ground allspice

1 tsp ground ginger

⅛ tsp ground cloves

2 tbsp light soy sauce

2 tbsp lime juice

1 lb (450g) boneless, skinless chicken breasts

DIRECTIONS

1 Combine the jalapeño, onion, garlic, thyme, allspice, ginger, cloves, soy sauce, and lime juice in a blender. Pulse until the mixture resembles a uniform paste.

2 Spoon the mixture into a large zipper lock bag. Add the chicken breasts, and squeeze the bag to massage the seasonings into the chicken. Place in the refrigerator to marinate for 4 to 6 hours.

3 Preheat a grill to medium. Grill the chicken for 4 to 6 minutes per side. The chicken is done when the juices run clear and the internal temperature reaches 165°F (74°C). Allow the cooked chicken to rest for 5 minutes before serving.

PREP TIPS // *The spice paste can be made in advance and stored in the refrigerator for up to 4 days.*

Store in an airtight container in the refrigerator for up to 6 days, or in the freezer for up to 2 months. To reheat, place on a baking sheet in a 250°F (121°C) oven for 15 minutes. (Thaw in the refrigerator 1 day before reheating.)

CHANGE IT UP

For a sweeter heat, add 1 tsp stevia to the dry ingredients.

For more heat, only remove the stem from the jalapeño and keep the seeds intact.

GRILLED SOUTHWESTERN PORK MEDALLIONS

Bursting with Southwestern flavors, these medallions can be prepared and cooked in 30 minutes, and a single serving packs in over 30 grams of protein! Pork tenderloin has a mild flavor and leanness that lends itself nicely to the zesty spices in this recipe.

Makes	4 servings	Serving size	4oz (110g)	Prep time	15 minutes	Cook time	15 minutes

INGREDIENTS

1lb (450g) pork tenderloin, trimmed, silver skin removed, and sliced into 2-inch-thick (5cm) medallions

1 tsp chili powder

1 tsp paprika

1 tsp garlic powder

1 tsp cumin

1/2 tsp dried oregano

1/2 tsp salt

DIRECTIONS

1 Prior to starting the grill, spray the grill grate with non-stick cooking spray. Preheat grill to medium.

2 In a small bowl, combine the chili powder, paprika, garlic powder, cumin, oregano, and salt. Mix well.

3 Sprinkle the seasoning over the medallions. Use your fingertips to gently press the seasonings into both sides of the medallions.

4 Grill for 4 to 5 minutes per side. The medallions are done when the internal temperature reaches 145°F (63°C). Serve warm.

NUTRITION FACTS

per serving

CALORIES
186

TOTAL FAT
5.5 g

TOTAL CARBS
0 g

PROTEIN
31.9 g

CHANGE IT UP

Kick up the heat by adding 1/2 tsp chipotle powder to the seasoning mix.

For a bolder garlic flavor, increase the garlic powder to 2 tsp.

PREP TIPS
Store in an airtight container in the refrigerator for up to 5 days.

Juicy chicken breast pairs with the traditional Southwestern flavors of onion, cumin, and paprika to create a quick, tasty entrée that is ready in less than 30 minutes. Corn tortillas have fewer carbs than traditional flour tortillas, and chicken breast is an excellent source of protein.

SOUTHWESTERN CHICKEN STREET TACOS

Makes **4** servings | Serving size **2** tacos | Prep time **10** minutes | Cook time **15** minutes

NUTRITION FACTS

per serving

CALORIES
260

TOTAL FAT
4.6g

TOTAL CARBS
24.7g

PROTEIN
28.1g

INGREDIENTS

1lb (450g) boneless, skinless chicken breasts

½ tbsp minced garlic

1 tsp ground cumin

1 tsp paprika

1 tsp salt

½ tsp ground black pepper

1 medium red onion, sliced into ¼-inch (.5cm) wedges

½ cup pico de gallo

8 small corn tortillas

1 lime, sliced into quarters

DIRECTIONS

1 Spray a medium cast iron skillet with non-stick cooking spray and place over medium-high heat. Season the chicken breasts with the garlic, cumin, paprika, salt, and black pepper.

2 Add the chicken breasts and onion wedges to the skillet. Cook the breasts for 4 to 5 minutes per side, or until the juices run clear and the internal temperature reaches 165°F (74°C). Remove the skillet from the heat and allow the breasts to rest in the skillet for an additional 5 minutes.

3 Transfer the onions to a bowl, then transfer the chicken breasts to a cutting board and slice into ½-inch (1.25cm) strips.

4 Briefly place the tortillas in the hot skillet to warm. Assemble the tacos by spooning 1 tbsp salsa into each tortilla, followed by 2oz (55g) chicken, the onion wedges, and a squeeze of lime juice over top. Serve warm.

PREP TIPS // Store the sliced chicken and onions in an airtight container in the refrigerator for up to 5 days. Assemble the tacos just before serving.

CHANGE IT UP

Make these keto by substituting lettuce wraps for the tortillas, and replacing the onion wedges with avocado slices. The macros will be 309 calories, 16.6g fat, 13.5g carbs, and 28.6g protein per serving.

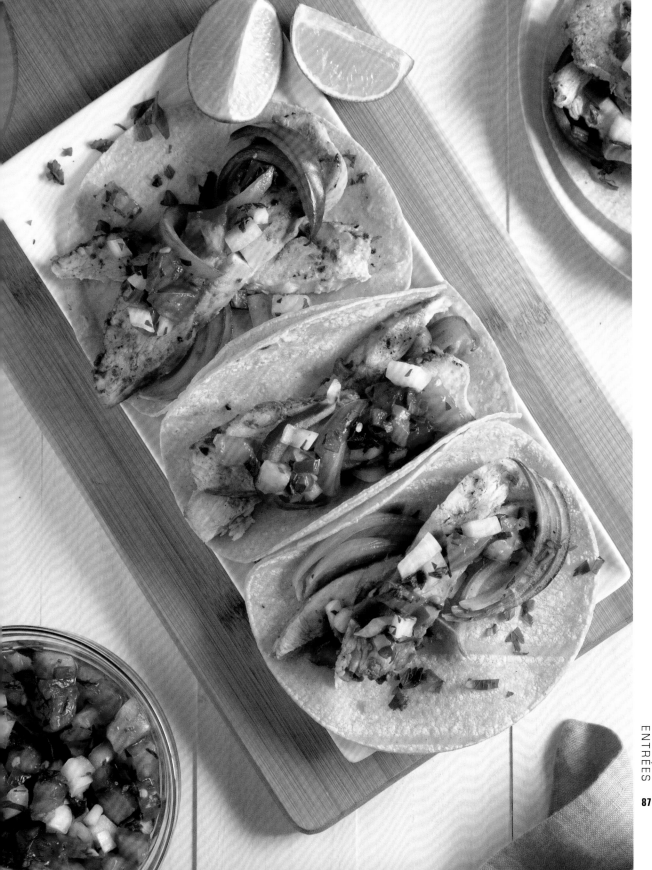

The slow cooker is an absolute necessity in any bodybuilder's kitchen, and is also the secret weapon for creating this fork-tender roast. Fragrant rosemary blends beautifully with the beef and onion, and the coconut oil is the ideal choice for searing the meat at a high temperature.

SLOW COOKER ROSEMARY POT ROAST

Makes 8 servings | **Serving size** 4oz (110g) roast + ¼ cup onions | **Prep time** 15 minutes | **Cook time** 4–8 hours

NUTRITION FACTS

per serving

CALORIES
222

TOTAL FAT
12 g

TOTAL CARBS
1.4 g

PROTEIN
25 g

INGREDIENTS

1 tbsp coconut oil

2lbs (1kg) top round steak or sirloin roast

1 tsp sea salt

3 tbsp chopped fresh rosemary

2 cups bone broth

1 medium onion, sliced into 1-inch (2.5cm) wedges

DIRECTIONS

1 Add the coconut oil to a large cast iron skillet and preheat over high heat. Season the roast with the sea salt and rosemary.

2 Place the roast in the hot skillet and brown for 1 to 2 minutes per side, depending on the thickness of the roast.

3 Pour the bone broth into the slow cooker. Add the roast. Add the onion wedges, ensuring they are completely covered in the liquid.

4 Cover. Cook on high for 4 hours, or on low for 8 hours, until the roast is tender and can easily be pulled apart with a fork. Transfer to a serving platter and slice into ½–inch (1.25cm) portions. Serve hot.

PREP TIPS // *Leaner cuts of beef, such as strip loin, sirloin, top round, or eye of round are usually less expensive, and all will stand up well to the longer cooking times of this recipe.*

Store in an airtight container in the refrigerator for up to 5 days.

CHANGE IT UP

Substitute 1 tbsp Fines herbs or 1 tbsp Mediterranean herbs for the fresh rosemary.

For a subtle sweetness, add ½ tsp dried basil when seasoning the roast.

You can substitute beef broth or chicken broth for the bone broth.

ENTRÉES

88

CHICKEN CACCIATORE

Makes	8 servings	Serving size	4oz (120g)	Prep time	10 minutes	Cook time	40 minutes

Clean eating and comfort food come together in this simpler version of an old classic. Fresh veggies, a robust tomato sauce, and tender chicken are all stars in this dish, and while this recipe features a number of pantry staples, fresh basil is used to finish the dish with a pop of flavor.

INGREDIENTS

1 16oz (450g) jar no-sugar-added tomato sauce

½ cup bone broth

1 cup cherry tomatoes, sliced into halves

½ white onion, diced

1 8oz (225g) can sliced mushrooms

4 tbsp minced garlic

1 tsp salt

½ tsp dried oregano

½ tsp ground black pepper

2lbs (900g) boneless, skinless chicken breasts

2 tbsp chopped fresh basil

DIRECTIONS

1 Preheat the oven to 400°F (204°C). Spray a 9 x 13in (23 x 33cm) baking dish with non-stick cooking spray.

2 In a large bowl, combine the tomato sauce, bone broth, cherry tomatoes, onion, mushrooms, garlic, basil, salt, oregano, and black pepper. Mix well. Pour approximately one third of the sauce into the baking dish.

3 Add the chicken to the baking dish in a single layer. Pour the remaining sauce over the chicken, cover tightly with aluminum foil, and bake for 20 minutes.

4 Remove the foil and bake for an additional 15 to 20 minutes. Sprinkle the basil over top. Serve hot.

PREP TIPS *Store in an airtight container in the refrigerator for up to one week.*

NUTRITION FACTS

per serving

CALORIES

161

TOTAL FAT

4.2g

TOTAL CARBS

4.2g

PROTEIN

26g

ENTRÉES

Add the ingredients to a slow cooker in the morning and this comforting chili will be ready when you walk in the door at night. The lean chicken breast becomes pull-apart tender, green chiles and a cayenne pepper add a bit of heat, and a dollop of Greek yogurt brings a cool balance.

WHITE CHICKEN CHILI

Makes	4 servings	Serving size	4oz (110g) chicken + ½ cup beans	Prep time	10 minutes	Cook time	3–8 hours

INGREDIENTS

1½ cups low fat chicken broth

1 medium white onion, roughly chopped

1 4oz (110g) can diced green chiles

1 15oz (420g) can cannellini beans, drained and rinsed

1 tsp garlic powder

1 tsp cumin

½ tsp dried oregano

½ tsp dried cilantro

⅛ tsp cayenne pepper powder

1lb (450g) boneless, skinless chicken breasts

4 tbsp plain, nonfat Greek yogurt

DIRECTIONS

1 In a large slow cooker, combine the chicken broth, onion, green chiles, cannellini beans, garlic powder, cumin, oregano, cilantro, and cayenne pepper. Stir well.

2 Add the chicken breasts, ensuring they're completely covered in the liquid. Cook on low for 6 to 8 hours, or on high for 3 to 4 hours.

3 To serve, transfer one 4oz (110g) chicken breast and ½ cup of the beans to a serving bowl. Use a fork to shred the chicken, and top each serving with 1 tbsp Greek yogurt. Serve warm.

NUTRITION FACTS

per serving

CALORIES
221

TOTAL FAT
3.6g

TOTAL CARBS
12.4g

PROTEIN
33.1g

PREP TIPS Store in an airtight container in the refrigerator for up to 5 days.

CHANGE IT UP

Make this keto by omitting the canned beans, and adding 2 tbsp coconut oil to the slow cooker before adding the other ingredients. One hour before serving, pour ½ cup heavy cream into the slow cooker and stir. Serving size will be 3oz (85g) chicken, and ½ cup onions and cream. The macros will be 270 calories, 18.3g fat, 2g carbs, and 19.9g protein per serving.

MUSCLE-BUILDING MEATLOAF

Makes **4** servings | Serving **size** **1** loaf | Prep **time** 10 minutes | Cook **time** 35 minutes

These satisfying, personal-sized meatloaves are packed with protein and veggies. The secret ingredient is the almond flour, which holds the loaves together and helps keep them juicy. Sun-dried tomato, sweet onion, and fresh parsley all lend a wonderful depth of flavor.

INGREDIENTS

1lb (450g) lean ground beef (preferably 92/8 lean-to-fat ratio)

1 medium egg

½ cup chopped fresh mushrooms

⅓ cup finely chopped onion

¼ cup finely chopped sun-dried tomatoes

¼ cup chopped fresh parsley

½ tsp salt

½ tsp ground black pepper

⅓ cup almond flour

DIRECTIONS

1 Preheat the oven to 375°F (191°C). Line a 9 x 13in (23 x 33cm) baking sheet with parchment paper.

2 In a large bowl, combine the ground beef, egg, mushrooms, onion, sun-dried tomatoes, parsley, salt, and black pepper. Mash the ingredients together with a fork until just incorporated. Sprinkle the almond flour over top, and continue to mash until all ingredients are well incorporated.

3 Form the mixture into 4 equal-sized, oval-shaped loaves. Place the loaves on the baking sheet, allowing at least ½-inch (1.25cm) between each loaf.

4 Bake for 30 to 35 minutes, or until the internal temperature reaches 165°F (74°C). Serve hot.

CHANGE IT UP
You can substitute ground chicken breast for the ground beef. The macros will be 209 calories, 7g fat, 5g carbs, and 29g protein per serving.

PREP TIPS *Double this recipe and freeze the cooked loaves for up to 2 months. Reheat in a 250°F (121°C) oven for 15 minutes. (Thaw the loaves in the refrigerator 1 day before reheating.)*

Store in an airtight container in the refrigerator for up to 5 days.

NUTRITION FACTS
per serving

CALORIES
232

TOTAL FAT
13.7g

TOTAL CARBS
5.2g

PROTEIN
24.6g

This dish will have you feasting on delicious spaghetti squash and savory turkey meatballs for under 200 calories per serving. Squash is high in vitamins and loaded with fiber, so this recipe will leave you feeling full for longer. Ground turkey breast packs in the protein, with almost no added fat.

NUTRITION FACTS

per serving

CALORIES

180

TOTAL FAT

1.7 g

TOTAL CARBS

12.8 g

PROTEIN

30.6 g

SPAGHETTI SQUASH AND MEATBALL BOATS

| Makes | 4 servings | Serving size | 1 boat | Prep time | 15 minutes | Cook time | 1 hour |

INGREDIENTS

2 medium spaghetti squash, halved lengthwise, seeds removed

1 tsp salt

1 tsp ground black pepper

1 cup low-sodium chicken broth

1lb (450g) lean ground turkey breast

1 tbsp liquid egg whites

1 tsp garlic powder

½ cup diced fresh tomato

¼ cup diced white onion

¼ cup diced green pepper

DIRECTIONS

1 Preheat the oven to 350°F (177°C). Spray a medium baking dish with non-stick cooking spray. In a small bowl, combine the tomato, onion, and green pepper. Set aside.

2 Season the squash with ½ tsp salt and ½ tsp black pepper. Place the squash in the baking dish, flesh-side down, and fill the dish with ½ cup chicken broth. Bake for 40 to 50 minutes. Set aside to cool.

3 While the squash is cooling, combine the turkey breast, egg whites, garlic powder, and the remaining salt and black pepper in a large bowl. Mix well. Use clean hands to form the mixture into 8 equal-sized meatballs.

4 Place a large non-stick frying pan over medium-high heat. Add the meatballs and brown for 3 minutes, turning the meatballs halfway through the cooking process. Pour the remaining chicken broth into the pan, cover, and reduce the heat to low. Steam for an additional 8 to 10 minutes.

5 Using a fork, create the "spaghetti" by scraping the flesh from the sides of the squash, being careful not to break through the outer skin of the squash.

6 Add 2 meatballs to each squash boat and top with a spoonful of the diced vegetables. Serve hot.

PREP TIPS // *These are great for using up any leftover lean protein. Store in an airtight container in the refrigerator for up to 5 days.*

GINGER BEEF AND BOK CHOY STIR FRY

Makes	4 servings		Serving size	4oz (110g) beef + 2oz (55g) bok choy		Prep time	15 minutes		Cook time	15 minutes

This budget-friendly dish features crunchy bok choy, bright fresh ginger, and lean sirloin steak. A touch of coriander intensifies the ginger, while red pepper adds a subtle hint of heat. Slicing the sirloin against the grain keeps it tender, and soy sauce acts as an umami-flavored tenderizer.

INGREDIENTS

1 tbsp fresh ginger, minced

1 tsp garlic, minced

½ cup white onion, diced

1lb (450g) beef sirloin, sliced against the grain into ¼-inch (.5cm) strips

½ tsp red pepper flakes

½ tsp ground cumin

½ tsp ground coriander

1 tbsp low sodium soy sauce (or liquid aminos)

1 large bok choy stalk, washed and sliced into ½-inch (1.25cm) strips

DIRECTIONS

1 Generously spray a medium skillet with non-stick cooking spray and place over medium heat. Add the ginger, garlic, and onion to the skillet, and cook until the onions are soft and translucent, stirring frequently.

2 Increase the heat to medium-high and add the sirloin strips, red pepper flakes, cumin, and coriander. Cook for 2 to 3 minutes, or until the meat is browned. Add the soy sauce, and continue to cook for an additional 1 to 2 minutes, stirring frequently.

3 Reduce the heat to low. Add the bok choy, cover, and steam for 5 minutes. Remove the lid, and continue to cook on low for an additional 2 to 3 minutes, or until the liquid is reduced. Serve hot.

PREP TIPS Store in an airtight container in the refrigerator for up to 5 days.

CHANGE IT UP

For a different taste with similar macros, substitute 2 cups shredded cabbage for the bok choy.

For a bit more crunch, top each serving with a small pinch of sesame seeds. This will not add any appreciable calories.

NUTRITION FACTS

per serving

CALORIES

242

TOTAL FAT

9.1g

TOTAL CARBS

2.8g

PROTEIN

35.7g

ENTRÉES

Crush cravings with this low carb, protein-packed twist on pizza. Ground turkey provides the perfect crust, as it binds together well and holds up to a mountain of fresh veggie toppings. Tomato sauce, just a hint of parmesan cheese, and fresh chopped basil all add wonderful pops of flavor.

MEATZA

Makes	4 servings	Serving size	1 slice	Prep time	10 minutes	Cook time	45 minutes

INGREDIENTS

1 lb (450g) lean ground turkey breast

¼ cup liquid egg whites

1 tsp dried oregano

1 tsp salt

1 tsp ground black pepper

1 tsp garlic powder

½ cup no-sugar-added tomato sauce

½ cup sliced fresh mushrooms

½ cup sliced zucchini

½ cup sliced yellow squash

2 tbsp roughly chopped fresh basil

2 tbsp finely grated parmesan cheese

DIRECTIONS

1 Preheat the oven to 350°F (177°C). In a large bowl, combine the ground turkey, egg whites, oregano, salt, pepper, and garlic powder. Using clean hands, mix the ingredients until well incorporated, then shape the mixture into a tight ball.

2 Spray a medium oven-safe frying pan with non-stick cooking spray. Using wet hands, add the mixture to the pan and form the crust by using the palm of your hand to press the mixture into the bottom of the pan, and into the shape of a pizza crust that is about ½-inch (1.25cm) thick.

3 Bake the crust for 25 minutes. Remove from the oven and allow to cool for 10 minutes.

4 Spread the tomato sauce across the top of the crust, then evenly distribute the mushrooms, zucchini, and squash over top of the sauce. Bake for 13 to 15 minutes, or until the toppings begin to brown.

5 Remove from the oven and evenly sprinkle the basil and parmesan cheese over top. Cut into four equal-sized slices. Serve hot.

NUTRITION FACTS

per serving

CALORIES
167

TOTAL FAT
2.8g

TOTAL CARBS
4.8g

PROTEIN
29.8g

CHANGE IT UP
For a Southwest-style meatza, omit the oregano and top the crust with ½ cup salsa.

PREP TIPS *Store in an airtight container in the refrigerator for up to 6 days.*

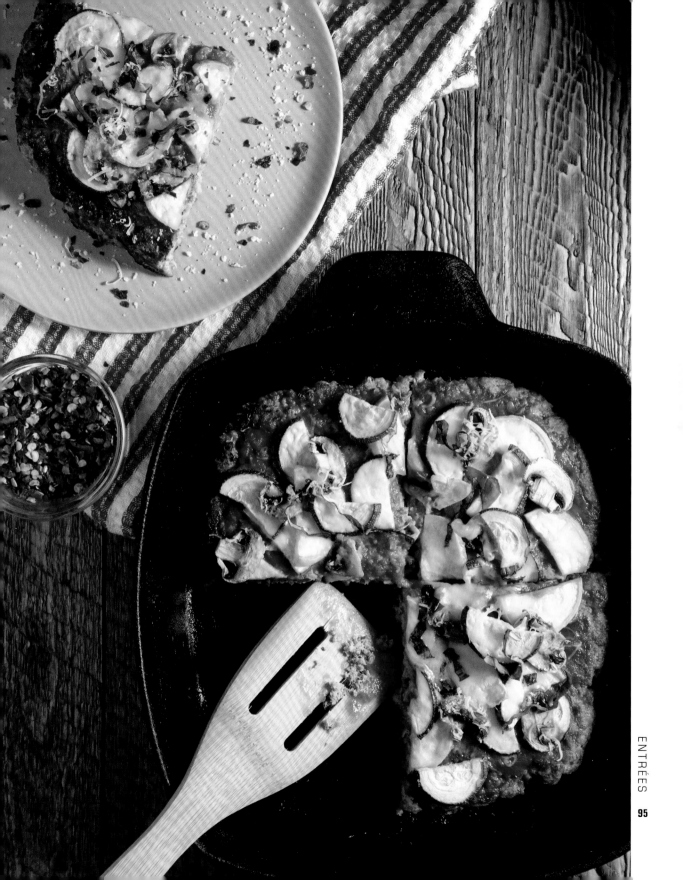

This Indian-inspired one pot wonder is ready in 15 minutes. The shrimp are complemented by smooth coconut and warm curry flavors, and lime awakens the palate and adds touches of acidity and brightness. This ultra low carb option is also low in fat and packed with protein.

COCONUT CURRY SHRIMP

Makes	4 servings	Serving size	4oz (110g)	Prep time	10 minutes	Cook time	5 minutes

INGREDIENTS

1 14oz (400g) can light coconut milk

1 tbsp fresh-squeezed lime juice

1 tbsp curry powder

2 tsp freshly grated ginger

1 tsp salt

1 tsp ground black pepper

1lb (450g) shrimp, peeled and deveined

DIRECTIONS

1 In a medium saucepan, combine the coconut milk, lime juice, curry powder, ginger, salt, and black pepper. Simmer over low heat for 8 to 10 minutes, allowing the mixture to thicken slightly.

2 Add the shrimp to the pan and cook for an additional 3 to 5 minutes, or until the shrimp just turn opaque. (Do not overcook the shrimp, as they can become rubbery.) Serve hot.

NUTRITION FACTS

per serving

CALORIES
124

TOTAL FAT
2.3 g

TOTAL CARBS
0.5 g

PROTEIN
23.7 g

PREP TIPS // Cook fresh shrimp within 1 day of purchasing.

Store in an airtight container in the refrigerator for up to 2 days.

CHANGE IT UP

For a little extra heat, add ½ tsp cayenne powder.

For a tangier dish with a milder shrimp flavor, marinate the shrimp in 2 tbsp lime juice for 30 minutes prior to cooking.

You can substitute an equal amount of cooked chicken breast for the shrimp.

BLACKENED BAKED TILAPIA

Makes **5** servings | Serving **size** 6oz (170g) | Prep **time** 25 minutes | Cook **time** 15 minutes

New Orleans flavors come alive with this low fat, high protein version of traditional blackened tilapia. The spices are kicked up a notch to compensate for the extra fat that would be present in a more traditional version. Tilapia is a mild fish and provides a perfect canvas for the spices.

INGREDIENTS

1 tbsp paprika

2 tsp dried thyme

1 tsp cumin

1 tsp dried oregano

1 tsp garlic powder

1 tsp onion powder

1 tsp salt

½ tsp ground black pepper

½ tsp red pepper flakes

2lbs (1kg) tilapia fillets (fresh or frozen)

DIRECTIONS

1 Preheat the oven to 400°F (204°C). Make the rub by combining the paprika, thyme, cumin, oregano, garlic powder, onion powder, salt, black pepper, and red pepper flakes in a small bowl. Mix well.

2 Rinse the tilapia fillets and pat dry with a paper towel. Season both sides of the fillets with the rub, using your fingers to gently press the seasonings into both sides of the fillets. Allow the fillets to sit at room temperature for 15 minutes to allow the flavors to develop.

3 Spray a 9 x 13in (22 x 33cm) baking pan with non-stick cooking spray. Place the fillets in the pan and lightly spray the tops with the non-stick cooking spray.

4 Bake for 10 to 12 minutes, or until the fish is firm and flaky, and the flesh is opaque. Serve hot.

NUTRITION FACTS

per serving

CALORIES
146

TOTAL FAT
2.7g

TOTAL CARBS
0g

PROTEIN
32g

CHANGE IT UP

Brighten the flavor by adding a squeeze of fresh lemon juice to the fillets just after cooking.

If you prefer a little more heat, increase the red pepper flakes to 1 tsp.

PREP TIPS Tilapia is inexpensive and a muscle-building favorite, but you can also substitute any lean white fish, or equal amounts of cooked chicken breast, for the tilapia.

Store in an airtight container in the refrigerator for up to 5 days.

SALADS & SIDES

No meal is complete without nutritious sides! Sides provide key nutrients, antioxidants, vitamins, and fiber, and also give volume to the plate, which is important since we eat with our eyes first. Sides also provide fuel for your workouts and your recovery, and help provide the energy you need throughout the day. This chapter features a wide variety of recipes, many of which can be made in advance to help make your meal prep easier.

The roasting process brings out the sweetness in these potatoes and creates a delectable finger food that can be eaten as a side or a snack. Sweet potato is anti-inflammatory, low glycemic, and rich in vitamins—making it a great choice for replenishing energy stores and aiding recovery.

ROASTED SWEET POTATO MEDALLIONS

Makes	4 servings		Serving size	6oz (170g)		Prep time	10 minutes		Cook time	50 minutes

INGREDIENTS

2 large white or purple sweet potatoes, washed and peeled

Coconut oil cooking spray

1 tsp salt

Pinch of cinnamon

½ tsp ground chipotle powder

½ tsp paprika

DIRECTIONS

1 Preheat the oven to 400°F (204°C). Generously spray a 9 x 13in (23 x 33cm) baking pan with coconut oil cooking spray.

2 Slice the potatoes crosswise into ½-inch (1.25cm) medallions. Place the medallions in a large bowl and lightly spray with coconut oil cooking spray.

3 Season the potatoes with the salt, cinnamon, chipotle powder, and paprika. Toss to evenly distribute the spices over the potatoes. Arrange the medallions in a single layer in the baking pan.

4 Roast for 40 to 50 minutes, flipping the potatoes halfway through the cooking time. The potatoes are done when they begin to brown and become soft in the center. Serve hot.

NUTRITION FACTS

per serving

CALORIES

150

TOTAL FAT

0g

TOTAL CARBS

33g

PROTEIN

5g

PREP TIPS // *If you can't find white or purple sweet potatoes, you can use the yellow variety (cook up to one hour longer). Round potatoes tend to roast better than oblong.*

Store in an airtight container in the refrigerator for up to 6 days.

CHANGE IT UP

For a more savory flavor, omit the cinnamon, chipotle, and paprika, and add 1 tsp dried rosemary.

To enhance the sweetness of the potatoes, top the cooked medallions with 2 to 3 tsp powdered stevia.

COCONUT CAYENNE SMASHED SWEET POTATOES

This powerhouse tuber fuels workouts and aids in recovery, so it's a staple in most meal plans, but it's often prepared bland and boring. However, the addition of a few simple ingredients can transform the simple sweet potato into a deliciously rich side that packs just a hint of heat.

Makes 6 servings **/** **Serving size** 6oz (170g) **/** **Prep time** 30 minutes **/** **Cook time** 1 hour

INGREDIENTS
2lbs (1kg) sweet potatoes, washed and ends trimmed

½ cup light coconut milk

2 tsp ground cinnamon

½ tsp ground cayenne pepper

DIRECTIONS
1 Preheat the oven to 400°F (204°C). Pierce the sweet potatoes with a fork and individually wrap in aluminum foil. Place directly on the oven rack and bake for 1 hour, turning the potatoes halfway through the baking time.

2 Remove the potatoes from the oven and allow to cool for 20 minutes. Once cooled, remove the foil and peel the skin from the potatoes.

3 In a large bowl, combine the peeled sweet potatoes, coconut milk, cinnamon, and cayenne pepper.

4 Using a fork or immersion blender, thoroughly smash the ingredients together until a smooth consistency is achieved, and no lumps remain. Serve warm.

PREP TIPS // Save time on meal prep by baking an extra pound of sweet potatoes when you make this recipe. They will keep well in the refrigerator and can be used in other recipes.

Store in an airtight container in the refrigerator for up to 6 days.

CHANGE IT UP
For a tangier flavor, omit the cayenne and add ½ cup Greek yogurt and 1 tsp ground ginger.

NUTRITION FACTS
per serving

CALORIES
139

TOTAL FAT
0.7 g

TOTAL CARBS
31.7 g

PROTEIN
2.1 g

SALADS & SIDES

The texture of these potatoes is totally addicting—crisp and gently browned on the edges, while the centers melt in your mouth—and the spicy crema provides a satisfying twist. The kicker is that these delicious potatoes are virtually fat free, so they're perfect as a snack or as a meal.

NUTRITION FACTS

per serving

CALORIES
151

TOTAL FAT
0.4g

TOTAL CARBS
34g

PROTEIN
3.3g

HASSELBACK SWEET POTATOES
WITH SPICY CREMA

Makes	5 servings	Serving size	6oz (170g)	Prep time	15 minutes	Cook time	1 hour

INGREDIENTS

2lbs (1kg) sweet potatoes (look for round shapes, rather than oblong)

Coconut oil cooking spray

1/2 tsp salt

For the crema

1/3 cup nonfat Greek yogurt

3 tbsp jarred red enchilada sauce

1/2 tsp fresh-squeezed lime juice

1/4 tsp powdered stevia

DIRECTIONS

1 Preheat the oven to 400°F (204°C). Spray a medium baking dish with coconut oil cooking spray.

2 Slice the sweet potatoes crosswise, about three fourths of the way through. The slices should be approximately 1/4-inch (.5cm) thick. Place the sliced sweet potatoes in the baking dish and lightly spray with the coconut oil cooking spray, and season with the salt.

3 Tightly cover the dish with aluminum foil and bake for 45 minutes. Uncover and bake for an additional 15 minutes. Remove from the oven and allow to cool for 10 minutes.

4 While the sweet potatoes cool, prepare the crema by combining the Greek yogurt, enchilada sauce, lime juice, and stevia in a medium bowl. Mix well to combine.

5 Drizzle the crema over top of the potatoes. Serve warm.

PREP TIPS *Store the sweet potatoes in an airtight container in the refrigerator for up to one week. Store the crema in an airtight container in the refrigerator for up to 4 days. (Reserve the crema until you're ready to serve.)*

CHANGE IT UP
For a sweet and smoky snack with a little more heat, omit the enchilada sauce and sprinkle 1/2 tsp chipotle powder over the baked potatoes.

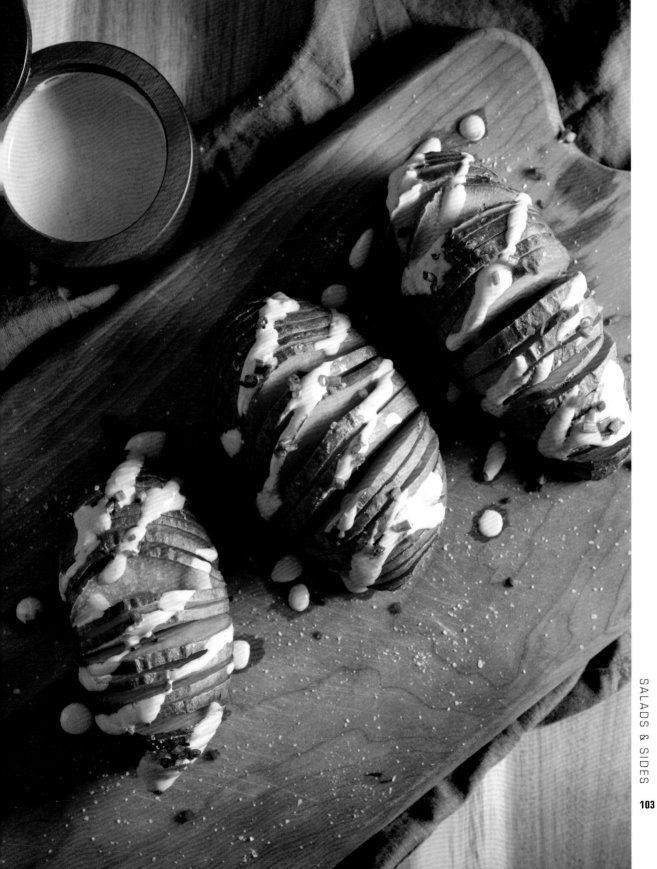

Vibrant colors and bold flavors come together in this exciting side. Quinoa provides a blank canvas for the spices, and savory chicken broth adds depth and balances nicely with sweet pops of corn. Black beans add complex carbs and fiber, and the jalapeño adds just a hint of heat.

NUTRITION FACTS

per serving

CALORIES

154

TOTAL FAT

2.4g

TOTAL CARBS

28.5g

PROTEIN

5.6g

SPICY BLACK BEANS AND QUINOA

Makes	8 servings	Serving size	1 cup	Prep time	5 minutes	Cook time	20 minutes

INGREDIENTS

1 jalapeño pepper, seeds and stem removed, finely diced

2 tsp minced garlic

2 cups low fat chicken broth

1½ cups uncooked white quinoa, rinsed 3 to 4 times

1 15oz (420g) can diced fire-roasted tomatoes, not drained

½ tsp chipotle powder

1 tsp ground cumin

1 tsp onion powder

1 tsp paprika

1 15oz (420g) can black beans, drained and rinsed

1 cup frozen corn kernels

DIRECTIONS

1 Spray a large skillet with non-stick cooking spray and place over medium heat. Add the jalapeño and garlic to the pan and cook for 1 minute, or until the garlic starts to soften and becomes fragrant. Stir frequently.

2 Add the chicken broth, quinoa, tomatoes, chipotle powder, cumin, onion powder, and paprika to the pan. Increase the heat to high and bring to a boil, stirring constantly. As soon as the mixture reaches a boil, reduce the heat to low, cover, and cook for 15 minutes.

3 Add the black beans and corn. Stir, cover, and continue to cook for an additional 4 to 5 minutes, or until the quinoa is tender. Serve hot.

PREP TIPS *Make sure to rinse the quinoa in cold water before cooking. Rinsing removes the saponins, which can impart a bitter flavor.*

Store in an airtight container in the refrigerator for up to one week.

CHANGE IT UP

For a firmer texture and nuttier flavor, substitute 1½ cups red quinoa for the white quinoa.

CARB CUTTER TWICE-BAKED POTATOES

Makes **4** servings | Serving size **½** potato | Prep time **10** minutes | Cook time **1 hour 30 min**

INGREDIENTS

2 medium russet potatoes

1 cup broccoli florets, chopped

2 cups cauliflower florets

½ cup unflavored coconut milk

½ tbsp white vinegar

1 tbsp dried chives

1 tsp salt

½ tsp ground black pepper

8 tbsp low fat shredded cheddar cheese

DIRECTIONS

1 Preheat the oven to 400°F (204°C). Pierce the potatoes with a fork, individually wrap in aluminum foil, and place on the middle oven rack. Bake for 1 hour.

2 While the potatoes bake, fill a large pot with 1 inch (2.5cm) water, and place a steamer tray in the bottom of the pot. Place the broccoli and cauliflower in the pot, cover, and steam for 10 minutes. Use a slotted spoon to remove only the broccoli to a small bowl. Steam the cauliflower for an additional 10 minutes.

3 Remove the potatoes from the oven and allow to cool for 15 minutes. Once cooled, unwrap the potatoes and remove the foil, slice lengthwise, and use a small spoon to scoop the flesh out into a large bowl. Reserve the skins and set the bowl aside.

4 Add the cooked cauliflower to the potato, and use a fork or immersion blender to thoroughly mash the ingredients together. Add the coconut milk, vinegar, chives, salt, and black pepper, and continue to mash until all ingredients are well incorporated and smooth texture is achieved.

5 Scoop the cauliflower and potato mixture into the reserved skins. Top each with the broccoli and 2 tbsp cheddar cheese. Place back in the oven and bake for an additional 15 minutes. Serve hot.

PREP TIPS / *Store in an airtight container in the refrigerator for up to 5 days.*

Creative seasonings add a tangy kick to this low fat side. This recipe cuts the carbs by combining steamed cauliflower with the potato, which adds volume without adding a lot of additional calories. The result is a larger serving size with fewer overall carbs and calories.

NUTRITION FACTS

per serving

CALORIES
118

TOTAL FAT
1.2 g

TOTAL CARBS
24.5 g

PROTEIN
4.4 g

SALADS & SIDES

These craveable, addictive fries are full of flavor and have only 75 calories per serving! Spiced parmesan cheese forms a satisfying and flavorful crust, and zucchini is a perfect low carb substitute for potato. This simple side is perfect for weekday meals, and is ready in 30 minutes.

BAKED ZUCCHINI FRIES

Makes 2 servings | **Serving size** 4 fries | **Prep time** 10 minutes | **Cook time** 20 minutes

NUTRITION FACTS

per serving

CALORIES
74

TOTAL FAT
3.3 g

TOTAL CARBS
5.1 g

PROTEIN
7.7 g

INGREDIENTS

2 large zucchini, ends trimmed and sliced lengthwise into 8 wedges

¼ cup liquid egg whites

½ cup grated parmesan cheese

½ tsp garlic powder

½ tsp ground black pepper

DIRECTIONS

1 Preheat the oven to 425°F (218°C). Line a 9 x 13-inch (23 x 33cm) baking sheet with aluminum foil. Place an oven-safe cooling rack on top of the foil, and spray with non-stick cooking spray.

2 Pour the egg whites into a small bowl. In a separate small bowl, combine the parmesan cheese, garlic powder, and black pepper. Mix well to combine.

3 Dip the zucchini wedges in the egg whites, then dredge them in the parmesan mixture. Place the fries on the cooling rack.

4 Bake for 18 to 20 minutes, or until the fries turn golden brown. Serve hot.

PREP TIPS // *These are best eaten fresh from the oven, but can be stored in an airtight container in the refrigerator for up to 3 days.*

To bring back the crunch, place on a baking sheet and reheat in a 250°F (121°C) oven for 10 minutes.

CHANGE IT UP

If you crave a little more heat, add ¼ tsp cayenne pepper powder to the parmesan mixture.

For a more herbal flavor, add ½ tsp oregano to the parmesan mixture.

SALADS & SIDES

106

CURRIED RICE PILAF

Makes	4 servings		Serving size	½ cup		Prep time	10 minutes		Cook time	40 minutes

Simple brown rice is transformed from boring to bold in this quick and easy recipe. Onions and curry enhance the nutty notes of the rice, and turmeric complements the rich curry while adding anti-inflammatory benefits. Cooked and cooled rice is high in resistant starch, which may help burn fat.

INGREDIENTS

1 medium white onion, diced

1 cup low-sodium chicken broth

1¼ cups water

1 cup uncooked brown rice

1 tsp curry powder

¼ tsp ground black pepper

¼ tsp ground turmeric

DIRECTIONS

1 Spray a large pot with non-stick cooking spray. Add the onion to the pot and cook over medium heat, stirring frequently, until the onion becomes soft and translucent.

2 Add the broth and water, and use a wooden spoon to gently scrape the bottom of the pot to release any bits. Add the rice, curry powder, black pepper, and turmeric. Stir well.

3 Bring the mixture to a rolling boil, stirring frequently, then reduce the heat to low, cover, and simmer until the rice is cooked, approximately 35 to 40 minutes. Fluff the rice with a fork and serve hot.

PREP TIPS This recipe can be doubled for easy meal prep. Store in an airtight container in the refrigerator for up to 5 days.

CHANGE IT UP

For a bolder flavor, add 1 tsp garlic powder and ¼ tsp ground cinnamon to the rice, and top with 1 tbsp chopped fresh cilantro.

NUTRITION FACTS

per serving

CALORIES

179

TOTAL FAT

1.6 g

TOTAL CARBS

35.7 g

PROTEIN

4 g

SALADS & SIDES

This delicious low-carb veggie side uses riced cauliflower in place of white rice, which is high in calories and carbs. Traditional fried rice ingredients give this dish an authentic taste and feel, but with almost zero fat and a fraction of the carbs and calories of traditional fried rice.

NUTRITION FACTS

per serving

CALORIES
71

TOTAL FAT
0.4 g

TOTAL CARBS
13.1 g

PROTEIN
5.9 g

CAULIFLOWER "FRIED RICE"

Makes	4 servings	Serving size	1 ½ cups	Prep time	10 minutes	Cook time	15 minutes

INGREDIENTS

1 medium cauliflower head, rinsed and cut into small florets

½ white onion, finely diced

4 large green onions, sliced and separated into green and white pieces

½ tsp garlic powder

½ tsp ground ginger

½ tsp ground black pepper

1 cup frozen peas and carrots

2 tbsp light soy sauce

¼ cup liquid egg whites

DIRECTIONS

1 In small batches, add the cauliflower florets to a food processor or blender and pulse until it resembles the size and consistency of rice, stirring often. Place the riced cauliflower in a medium bowl and set aside.

2 Spray a large skillet with non-stick cooking spray and place over medium heat. Add the onion, green onion (white ends), garlic powder, ginger, and black pepper, and cook until the onions are soft and translucent.

3 Add the peas and carrots, and cook for an additional 3 to 5 minutes, stirring frequently. Move the mixture to one side of the skillet and add the egg whites. Scramble the egg whites, then gently incorporate into the vegetables.

4 Add the riced cauliflower and soy sauce, and continue to cook for an additional 3 to 5 minutes, or until the cauliflower just begins to soften. (Be careful not to overcook the cauliflower, as it can become soggy.)

5 Transfer the rice to a serving platter and garnish with the remaining green onions. Serve hot.

PREP TIPS *You can save prep time by buying frozen, pre-riced cauliflower.*

Store in an airtight container in the refrigerator for up to one week.

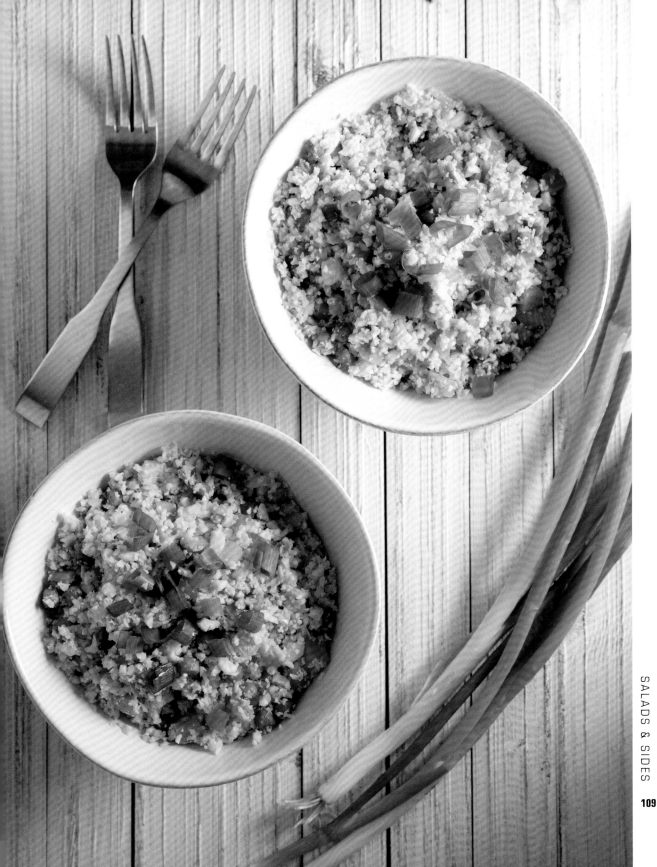

Rice is a staple of any bodybuilding kitchen, yet too often it's overcooked, gummy, or clumpy. This recipe will help you cook fluffy rice perfectly every time. Hearty Basmati rice holds up well to cooking and boasts a slightly nutty flavor, and avocado oil adds a delicate touch of flavor.

FLUFFY BASMATI RICE

Makes	8 servings		Serving size	¾ cup		Prep time	10 minutes		Cook time	30 minutes

INGREDIENTS

2 cups Basmati rice, rinsed and drained

4 cups water

1 tsp avocado oil

1 tsp salt

DIRECTIONS

1 In a large pot, combine the rice, water, avocado oil, and salt. Bring to a boil over high heat, stirring once, then cover, reduce the heat to low, and cook for 15 minutes.

2 Remove the pot from the heat and allow the rice to rest for 15 minutes. Fluff the cooked rice with a fork. Serve hot.

NUTRITION FACTS

per serving

CALORIES

170

TOTAL FAT

2 g

TOTAL CARBS

33.4 g

PROTEIN

3.2 g

PREP TIPS // *Store the cooled rice in an airtight container in the refrigerator for up to 6 days. To reheat, place the rice in a microwave-safe bowl, cover with a damp paper towel, and heat on high for 1 minute.*

CHANGE IT UP
For a richer flavor, omit the salt and substitute 2 cups chicken broth for the water.

SALADS & SIDES

ROASTED CABBAGE STEAKS

| Makes | 4–6 servings | Serving size | 1 steak | Prep time | 5 minutes | Cook time | 45 minutes |

INGREDIENTS

1 medium green cabbage

2 tbsp garlic, minced

½ tsp salt

½ tsp ground black pepper

DIRECTIONS

1 Preheat the oven to 350°F (177°C). Line a 9 x 13in (23 x 33cm) baking sheet with aluminum foil and lightly spray with non-stick cooking spray.

2 Slice the cabbage crosswise into ½-inch-thick (1.25cm) steaks. Place the steaks on the baking sheet and lightly spray with non-stick cooking spray. Evenly spread the garlic over the steaks, and season with the salt and black pepper.

3 Bake for 35 to 45 minutes, or until the steaks become soft and translucent and begin to brown around the edges. Serve hot.

PREP TIPS // *Store in an airtight container in the refrigerator for up to 3 days. These can be reheated, or eaten cold. (When eaten cold, they have a taste and texture similar to sauerkraut.)*

CHANGE IT UP

For a more umami flavor, omit the salt and spray liquid aminos evenly over the cabbage steaks. (Approximately 6 sprays has 0 calories, and adds a soy sauce-like flavor.)

Amp up the heat by adding ½ tsp red pepper flakes.

Add volume to your plate with this easy-to-make, nutrient-packed side that's super low in calories, fat, and carbs. Roasting the cabbage mellows the flavor, while garlic adds a kick. Cabbage is high in vitamins C and K, contains anti-aging compounds, and is high in fiber to help keep you full.

NUTRITION FACTS

per serving

CALORIES

38

TOTAL FAT

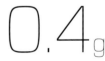
0.4 g

TOTAL CARBS

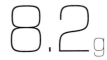
8.2 g

PROTEIN

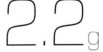
2.2 g

When the carb cravings strike, strike back with this light and airy bread alternative that will satisfy those nagging cravings! The key is to whip the egg whites to a light peak, then gently fold in the egg yolks for a chewiness and crust that could easily be mistaken for the real thing!

CLOUD BREAD

| Makes | 3 servings | Serving size | 4 pieces | Prep time | 15 minutes | Cook time | 25 minutes |

INGREDIENTS

4 large eggs, warmed to room temperature

½ tsp cream of tartar

Pinch of salt

4 tbsp light cream cheese, softened and warmed to room temperature

DIRECTIONS

1 Preheat the oven to 350°F (177°C). Line two 9 x 13in (23 x 33cm) baking sheets with parchment paper.

2 Separate the egg yolks from the egg whites, placing the yolks in a medium bowl and the whites in a large glass or metal mixing bowl. (Do not use a plastic bowl for the egg whites.)

3 Add the cream of tartar to the egg whites. Using a hand mixer, beat the egg whites on high speed until they form stiff peaks that don't collapse when the mixer blade is lifted from the bowl.

4 Add the salt and cream cheese to the egg yolks, and whisk until all ingredients are well incorporated. Use a rubber spatula to gently fold the egg yolk mixture into the egg whites.

5 Use a ½ cup measuring cup to measure the batter into individual mounds on the baking sheet, maintaining at least 1 inch (2.5cm) between each mound.

6 Bake for 20 to 25 minutes, rotating the baking sheets halfway through the baking process to ensure the bread bakes evenly. Allow the bread to cool on the baking sheets.

NUTRITION FACTS

per serving

CALORIES

119

TOTAL FAT

8.1 g

TOTAL CARBS

1.5 g

PROTEIN

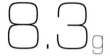

8.3 g

PREP TIPS // *Insert sheets of parchment paper between each piece and store in an airtight container in the refrigerator for up to 7 days,*

CHANGE IT UP

For a richer flavor, season the unbaked batter mounds with ½ tsp dried rosemary, ½ tsp garlic powder, and 1 tsp parmesan cheese. This will add only a few calories per serving.

SALADS & SIDES

112

HERB-ROASTED VEGETABLES

Makes	4 servings	Serving size	2 cups	Prep time	10 minutes	Cook time	30 minutes

This dish is ideal for weekly meal prep. It's simple to make, and the leftovers taste even better the next day! The roasting process brings out the natural sweetness of the squash and carrots, while mellowing and caramelizing the onion. Zucchini and squash are both high in fiber and vitamins.

INGREDIENTS

2 large zucchini squash, sliced crosswise into ½-inch (1.25cm) slices

2 large yellow squash, sliced crosswise into ½-inch (1.25cm) slices

1 cup baby carrots

1 medium red onion, sliced into 1-inch (2.5cm) wedges

Non-stick cooking spray

1 tsp garlic powder

1 tsp dried thyme

1 tsp dried parsley

1 tsp dried rosemary

1 tsp salt

DIRECTIONS

1 Preheat the oven to 400°F (204°C). Line a large baking sheet with parchment paper.

2 In a large bowl, combine the zucchini, squash, carrots, and onion wedges. Lightly spray the vegetables with non-stick cooking spray.

3 Make the seasoning by combining the garlic powder, thyme, parsley, rosemary, and salt in a small bowl. Mix well. Sprinkle the seasoning mix over the vegetables and toss thoroughly to coat.

4 Spread the vegetables in an even layer on the baking sheet. Roast for 15 minutes.

5 Using tongs, flip the vegetables and roast for an additional 15 minutes, or until the vegetables are soft and slightly caramelized. Serve hot.

PREP TIPS // The vegetables can be prepped in advance and refrigerated for up to 2 days prior to roasting.

Store in an airtight container in the refrigerator for up to 6 days.

CHANGE IT UP

For a heartier texture, substitute 1 cup diced eggplant for either the zucchini or the squash. The macros will be very similar.

You can substitute 1 cup halved Brussels sprouts for the carrots. This will not impact the macros.

NUTRITION FACTS

per serving

CALORIES

45

TOTAL FAT

0.2 g

TOTAL CARBS

9.4 g

PROTEIN

1.8 g

These noodles have the look and texture of traditional pasta, but contain only a fraction of the carbs and calories! The veggie volume will fill you up without throwing off your meal plan, and an inexpensive spiralizer is all you'll need to make these delectable, low carb noodles.

ZESTY ZOODLES

Makes	4 servings		Serving size	1 cup		Prep time	5 minutes		Cook time	none

INGREDIENTS

1 tbsp olive oil mayonnaise

1 tsp lemon juice

2 tbsp large grain mustard

½ tsp salt

½ tsp ground black pepper

4 medium zucchini, washed and ends trimmed

DIRECTIONS

1 In a large bowl, make the dressing by combining the mayonnaise, lemon juice, mustard, salt, and black pepper. Mix well.

2 Create the zoodles by running each zucchini through a spiralizer, making sure to discard the seeds. (Alternatively, you can use a julienne peeler or potato peeler to make ribbons.)

3 Add the zoodles to the dressing, and toss thoroughly to ensure the zoodles are fully coated in the dressing. Serve chilled, or at room temperature.

NUTRITION FACTS

per serving

CALORIES
44

TOTAL FAT
1.1g

TOTAL CARBS
7.6g

PROTEIN
1.2g

PREP TIPS // *Store in an airtight container in the refrigerator for up to 4 days.*

CHANGE IT UP

For a Mediterranean flavor, omit the mustard and add 1 tsp ground oregano and 1 tsp garlic powder to the dressing.

If you prefer the zoodles more al dente, steam for 5 minutes before tossing with the dressing.

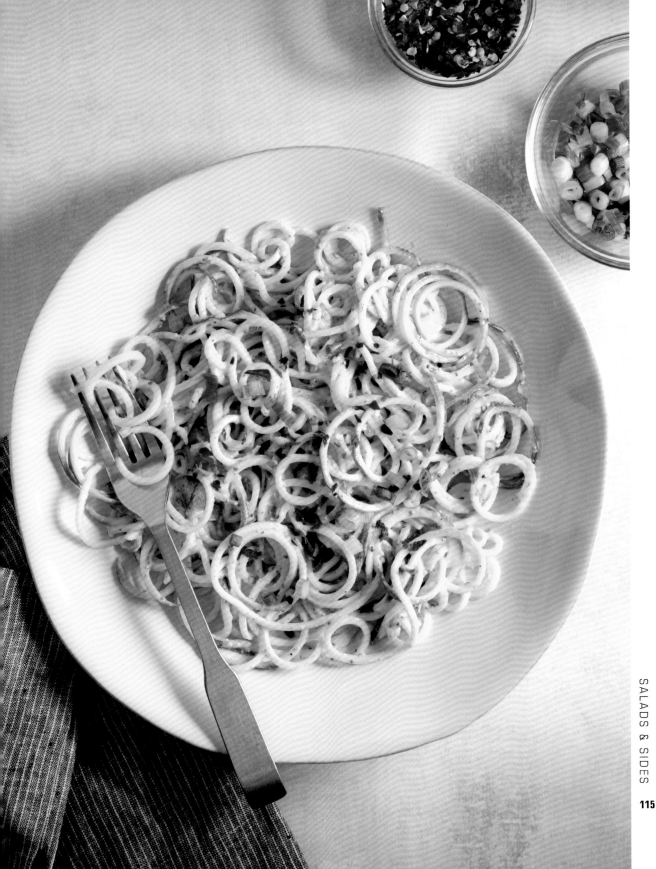

Fragrant rosemary livens up this simple dish, and contrasts beautifully with hearty beefsteak tomatoes. Allowing the tomatoes to soak up the seasonings will make them tender and enhance their sweetness. This simple side is a snap to prepare, and is ready to serve in under 30 minutes.

ROSEMARY BEEFSTEAK TOMATOES

Makes	4 servings		Serving size	4oz (110g)		Prep time	25 minutes		Cook time	none

INGREDIENTS

4 medium beefsteak tomatoes, sliced into quarters, skin and seeds left intact

1 tsp chopped fresh rosemary

¼ tsp garlic powder

¼ tsp paprika

¼ tsp salt

¼ tsp ground black pepper

DIRECTIONS

1 In a small bowl, combine the rosemary, garlic powder, paprika, and salt. Mix well.

2 In a large bowl, combine the tomatoes and seasonings. Gently toss to thoroughly coat the tomatoes with the seasonings.

3 Allow the tomatoes to rest for 15 to 20 minutes to absorb the seasonings before serving. Serve at room temperature.

NUTRITION FACTS

per serving

CALORIES

26

TOTAL FAT

0.1g

TOTAL CARBS

5.7g

PROTEIN

1g

PREP TIPS // *This dish is best made and served immediately, as the tomatoes can become mealy when stored in the refrigerator.*

CHANGE IT UP
For a different herbal twist, substitute 1 tsp chopped fresh basil for the rosemary.

SALADS & SIDES

116

CITRUS KALE SALAD

Makes	4 servings	Serving size	6oz (170g)	Prep time	15 minutes	Cook time	none

Vibrant pops of color invite you to dig into this nutrient-dense salad. Oranges add just a touch of sweetness, perfectly complementing the slightly bitter kale, which is packed with antioxidants, vitamins, and fiber. Poppy seeds add a nutty element, which pairs well with the onion.

INGREDIENTS

2 cups kale, washed, ribs removed, and chopped into ½-inch (1.25cm) strips

½ naval orange, peeled, separated into wedges, and cut into thirds

¼ medium onion, thinly sliced

1 tsp canola oil

2 to 3 drops liquid stevia

1 tsp lime juice

1 tsp apple cider vinegar

⅛ tsp salt

1 tsp poppy seeds

DIRECTIONS

1 In a large bowl, combine the kale strips, orange segments, and onion slices. Set aside.

2 In a medium bowl, combine the canola oil, stevia, lime juice, vinegar, salt, and poppy seeds. Whisk to combine.

3 Pour the dressing over the salad and gently toss to coat. Serve immediately.

PREP TIPS // *You can buy pre-sliced onions and bagged kale for easier meal prep.*

This recipe is best prepared and served fresh. The dressing can be made ahead of time and stored in an airtight container in the refrigerator for up to one week.

CHANGE IT UP

Other leafy greens, such as spinach, arugula, or butter lettuce, can be substituted for the kale.

For a tangier kick, add 1 tsp dijon mustard to the dressing.

NUTRITION FACTS

per serving

CALORIES

43

TOTAL FAT

1.4 g

TOTAL CARBS

5.3 g

PROTEIN

1.6 g

This simple, nutrient-dense salad features deep, vibrant greens, pops of plump red cherry tomatoes, and a light and refreshing dressing. Spinach is packed with potassium, fiber, and contains anti-inflammatory properties to help your body recover from tough workouts.

NUTRITION FACTS

per serving

CALORIES

23

TOTAL FAT

0.3g

TOTAL CARBS

2.5g

PROTEIN

2.5g

WILTED SPINACH AND CHERRY TOMATO SALAD

Makes	4 servings	Serving size	4oz (110g)	Prep time	5 minutes	Cook time	3 minutes

INGREDIENTS

1 tsp minced garlic

12 ounces fresh baby spinach

1 cup cherry tomatoes

½ tsp lemon juice

½ tsp salt

½ tsp ground black pepper

DIRECTIONS

1 Spray a large skillet with non-stick cooking spray and place over medium heat. Add the garlic and cook for 2 to 3 minutes, or until it begins to soften and becomes fragrant.

2 Add the spinach to the skillet in small handfuls, tossing repeatedly for 2 to 3 minutes to ensure that the leaves are evenly cooked. Transfer the cooked spinach to a serving bowl.

3 Add the tomatoes, lemon juice, salt, and black pepper to the spinach. Gently toss to thoroughly coat the spinach in the dressing. Serve warm.

PREP TIPS *This salad is best when prepared and served fresh, as it can become mushy in the refrigerator.*

CHANGE IT UP

You can substitute ½ cup of diced onions for the garlic. Sauté the onions in the skillet for 5 to 6 minutes, or until they become soft and translucent.

FRESH VEGGIE STIR FRY

Makes 4 servings | *Serving size* 2 cups | *Prep time* 5 minutes | *Cook time* 12 minutes

Eastern flavors and loads of fresh vegetables transform this simple stir fry into a satisfying, low calorie side. The broccoli becomes sweet and fork tender, while bok choy adds balance, and the cabbage adds fiber to keep you full. Fresh ginger brightens the flavors and aids with digestion.

INGREDIENTS

2 tsp grated fresh ginger root

2 tsp minced garlic

2 cups roughly chopped bok choy

1 cup broccoli florets, fresh or frozen

3 cups shredded green cabbage

2 tbsp light soy sauce

½ cup sliced fresh button mushrooms

¼ cup low-sodium chicken broth

DIRECTIONS

1 Spray a large frying pan with non-stick cooking spray and place over medium-high heat. Add the ginger and garlic to the pan and cook for 1 to 2 minutes, or until the garlic softens and becomes fragrant.

2 Add the bok choy, broccoli, cabbage, and soy sauce. Cook for 2 to 3 minutes, stirring frequently.

3 Add the sliced mushrooms and cook for an additional 2 minutes, stirring frequently.

4 Add the chicken broth, cover, and reduce the heat to low. Steam for 4 to 5 minutes, or until the broccoli is tender and can be pierced with a knife. Serve hot.

NUTRITION FACTS

per serving

CALORIES

34

TOTAL FAT

0.2 g

TOTAL CARBS

6 g

PROTEIN

3 g

CHANGE IT UP

Make this keto by adding 4 tbsp toasted sesame oil to the pan before cooking the vegetables. This will add 120 calories and 12g fat per serving.

For an even more filling side, omit the bok choy and use 3 cups broccoli florets. The macros will be about the same.

PREP TIPS // *If using frozen broccoli florets, make sure to thaw them in the refrigerator 1 day before using.*

Store in an airtight container in the refrigerator for up to 6 days.

SALADS & SIDES

This twist on deviled eggs offers heart-healthy fats, and palate-awakening flavors. Lime juice adds a surprising kick, while paprika brings color and a hint of heat. Healthy fats aid in satiety, while the egg whites provide protein and a vessel for the yolky-guacamole goodness.

GUACAMOLE DEVILED EGGS

Makes	3 servings		Serving size	4 eggs		Prep time	10 minutes		Cook time	10 minutes

NUTRITION FACTS

per serving

CALORIES

192

TOTAL FAT

14g

TOTAL CARBS

3.3g

PROTEIN

13.2g

INGREDIENTS

6 hard-boiled eggs, halved lengthwise

1 medium avocado

2 tsp lime juice

2 tbsp chopped fresh cilantro

1 tsp dried onion flakes

⅛ tsp garlic powder

½ tsp salt

½ tsp ground black pepper

½ tsp paprika

DIRECTIONS

1 Separate the egg yolks from the egg white halves. Place the yolks in a large bowl, and place the whites in a separate, medium bowl.

2 Slice the avocado in half, remove the seed, and scoop the flesh into the bowl containing the yolks. Add the lime juice, cilantro, onion flakes, garlic powder, salt, and black pepper.

3 Use a fork or potato masher to thoroughly mash the ingredients together until a smooth consistency is achieved and no lumps remain.

4 Arrange the egg white halves on a serving platter, sliced sides up, and spoon equal amounts of the filling into each egg white half. Sprinkle the paprika over top of the eggs. Serve chilled.

PREP TIPS

For perfectly boiled eggs, place the eggs in a large pot of water and bring to a rolling boil. Once boiling, turn off the burner and allow the eggs to sit in the water for 10 minutes, then use a slotted spoon to transfer them to a bowl of ice water.

Store in an airtight container in the refrigerator for up to 3 days.

CHANGE IT UP

For a punchier flavor, swap lemon juice for the lime juice, and top with ½ tsp chipotle powder instead of paprika.

SALADS & SIDES

120

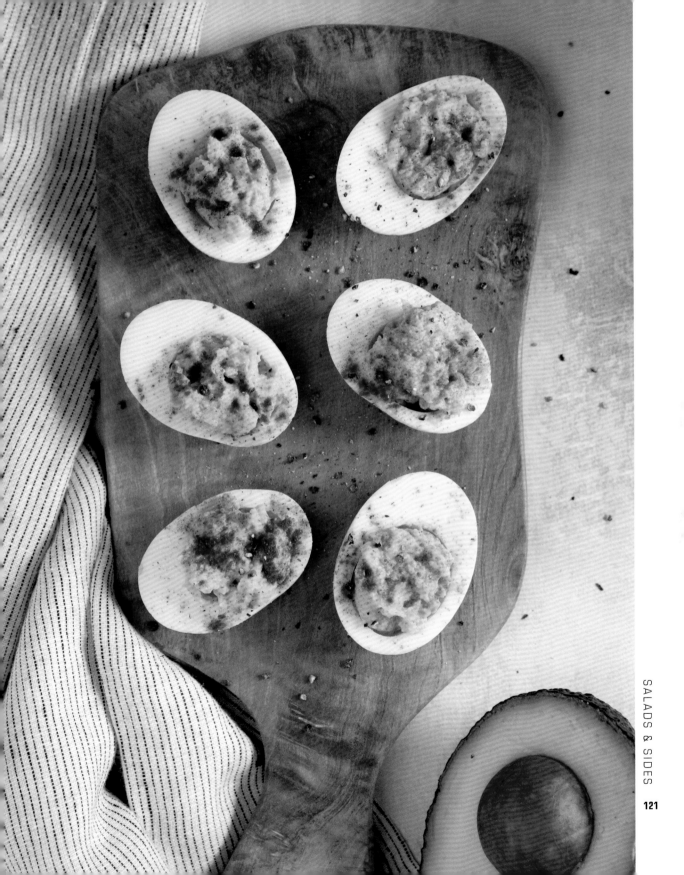

Brussels sprouts and fennel aren't at the top of everyone's list of favorite sides, but this dish will change that! Both are low in fat, and packed with beneficial nutrients and antioxidants. Roasting caramelizes the exteriors, while keeping the insides delicate and sweet.

NUTRITION FACTS

per serving

CALORIES
46

TOTAL FAT
0.3g

TOTAL CARBS
9.7g

PROTEIN
3.3g

ROASTED BRUSSELS SPROUTS AND FENNEL

Makes	4 servings	Serving size	6oz (170g)	Prep time	10 minutes	Cook time	30 minutes

INGREDIENTS

16oz (450g) Brussels sprouts, ends trimmed and halved lengthwise

2 fennel bulbs, cores removed and thinly sliced

Non-stick cooking spray

1 tbsp minced garlic

1 tsp salt

1 tsp ground black pepper

DIRECTIONS

1 Preheat the oven to 400°F (204°C). Line a large baking sheet with aluminum foil.

2 In a large bowl, combine the Brussels sprouts and fennel slices, and lightly spray with non-stick cooking spray.

3 Add the garlic, salt, and black pepper, and gently toss to coat the vegetables with the seasonings.

4 Spread the vegetables in a single layer on the baking sheet. Roast for 25 to 30 minutes, tossing every 10 minutes to ensure the vegetables are evenly cooked. Serve hot.

PREP TIPS Store in an airtight container in the refrigerator for up to 5 days.

CHANGE IT UP

For even more caramelization and crunch, instead of roasting the vegetables, toss them into a preheated cast iron skillet and cook over medium heat for 10 to 15 minutes, stirring frequently.

LEMONY GRILLED ASPARAGUS

Makes	2 servings	Serving size	10 spears	Prep time	5 min + 30 mins	Cook time	10 minutes

INGREDIENTS

1 bunch young asparagus (approximately 20 spears),
woody ends trimmed

Juice of 2 lemons

1 tsp lemon zest

1 tsp onion powder

1 tsp garlic powder

½ tsp salt

½ tsp ground black pepper

DIRECTIONS

1 In a large bowl, combine the asparagus spears and lemon juice. Toss to coat, and allow to rest at room temperature for 30 minutes.

2 Preheat a grill to medium. Transfer the asparagus to a plate and pat dry with a paper towel. Spray the spears with non-stick cooking spray and season with the onion powder, garlic powder, salt, and black pepper.

3 Grill the spears for 2 to 3 minutes per side, or until they form a nice char and have good caramelization. Transfer to a serving platter and garnish with the lemon zest. Serve hot.

CHANGE IT UP
You can also make this recipe in the oven. Move the rack to the middle, and set the oven to low broil. Place the asparagus on an aluminum foil-lined 9 x 13in (22 x 33cm) baking sheet. Broil for 6 to 8 minutes, shaking the pan every few minutes to flip the asparagus.

PREP TIPS
You can double or triple this recipe for easy meal prep.

Store in an airtight container in the refrigerator for up to 5 days.

Mild, earthy asparagus is jazzed up with fresh lemon, while onion and garlic add savory sharpness, and fresh lemon zest adds vibrant contrast to this dish. Asparagus is high in fiber, nutrients, and detoxifying compounds. This is a simple side that keeps well and can be made ahead for meal prep.

NUTRITION FACTS
per serving

CALORIES
42

TOTAL FAT
0.3g

TOTAL CARBS
9.3g

PROTEIN
3.7g

This recipe satisfies the need to snack on something crunchy, without derailing your meal plan. Blanching the beans prevents them from becoming dull and rubbery. Instead, they're crisp and refreshing, and when paired with the seasonings they're a tasty, healthy alternative to chips.

SNAPPY GINGER GREEN BEANS

Makes	4 servings	Serving size	4oz (110g)	Prep time	15 minutes	Cook time	20 minutes

INGREDIENTS

1 cup reduced-sodium chicken broth

2 cups fresh green beans, rinsed and ends trimmed

2 tsp freshly grated ginger root

1 tbsp sesame seeds

½ tsp salt

1 tsp lemon juice

½ tsp minced garlic

DIRECTIONS

1 In a large pot, bring the chicken broth to a low boil over medium heat.

2 Add the green beans to the pot and blanche for 5 to 7 minutes. With a slotted spoon, immediately transfer the beans to a large bowl filled with ice water. Set aside to cool.

3 In a small bowl, make the ginger sauce by combining the ginger root, sesame seeds, salt, lemon juice, and garlic. Mix well.

4 Drain the ice water from the green beans. Pour the ginger sauce over the green beans, and toss gently to coat. Serve immediately.

NUTRITION FACTS

per serving

CALORIES

66

TOTAL FAT

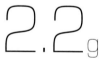

2.2 g

TOTAL CARBS

9 g

PROTEIN

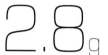

2.8 g

PREP TIPS // Always use fresh green beans for this recipe. Frozen or canned beans won't have the same snap or flavor.

Store in an airtight container in the refrigerator for up to 2 days.

CHANGE IT UP

To reduce the fat content even more, omit the sesame seeds, ginger, and lemon, and replace with 1 tsp apple cider vinegar and ½ tsp ground black pepper.

SALADS & SIDES

124

CRUNCHY AVOCADO SALAD

Makes	4 servings	Serving size	1 cup	Prep time	15 minutes	Cook time	none

Creamy avocado and sweet cherry tomatoes come together in this refreshing, antioxidant-rich salad that features a satisfying crunch and just a hint of heat. The avocado and olive oil provide healthy monounsaturated fats, which can help reduce inflammation and aid recovery.

INGREDIENTS

2 large ripe avocados, halved lengthwise, seed removed, and cut into ½-inch (1.25cm) cubes

1 cup cherry tomatoes, sliced into halves

1 seedless cucumber, cut into ½-inch (1.25cm) cubes

½ medium red onion, finely diced

¼ cup finely chopped fresh cilantro

2 tbsp lemon juice

½ tsp salt

1 tbsp olive oil

DIRECTIONS

1 In a large bowl, combine the avocado, tomatoes, cucumber, onion, and cilantro. Mix well.

2 Sprinkle the lemon juice over top and season with the salt. Add the olive oil, and gently toss with a rubber spatula until all ingredients are well combined. Serve immediately.

PREP TIPS // *Store in an airtight container in the refrigerator for up to 3 days.*

CHANGE IT UP
If you're not a fan of cilantro, you can use 2 tbsp finely chopped parsley, instead.

NUTRITION FACTS
per serving

CALORIES
183

TOTAL FAT
16.9g

TOTAL CARBS
9.3g

PROTEIN
2.0g

SALADS & SIDES

SNACKS & POWER BARS

This chapter is full of recipe ideas to sustain you throughout the day and through your workouts. A variety of homemade power bars will give you a boost of protein, and cost just pennies to make compared to store-bought bars. And the snacks are simple to make, energy sustaining, and most importantly—they're delicious!

The aroma of fresh rosemary will fill your kitchen as these bake! These keto-friendly bars are packed with healthy fats and have just the right amount of protein for a snack, or for recovery after a hard workout. Almonds contain vitamin E, fiber, and can help keep you feeling full for longer.

SAVORY ROSEMARY ALMOND BARS

Makes	8 servings		Serving size	1 bar		Prep time	10 minutes		Cook time	30 minutes

INGREDIENTS

2 cups whole almonds, finely chopped

2 tbsp coconut flour

½ cup almond flour

2 tbsp finely chopped fresh rosemary

1 tsp garlic powder

1 tsp onion flakes

1½ tsp salt

½ cup liquid egg whites

3 tbsp coconut oil

DIRECTIONS

1 Preheat the oven to 300°F (149°C). Line an 8 x 8in (20 x 20cm) baking dish with aluminum foil.

2 In a large bowl, combine the almonds, coconut flour, almond flour, rosemary, garlic powder, onion flakes, and salt. Mix well.

3 Add the egg whites and coconut oil. Using clean hands, mix the ingredients until they form a rough dough. Press the dough into the baking dish, ensuring the thickness is uniform throughout.

4 Bake for 30 minutes, or until the bars are lightly browned around the edges. Slice into 8 equal-sized bars.

NUTRITION FACTS

per serving

CALORIES

269

TOTAL FAT

22.3g

TOTAL CARBS

7.4g

PROTEIN

14g

PREP TIPS Individually wrap the bars in plastic wrap and store in an airtight container at room temperature for up to 10 days.

CHANGE IT UP

For an even more savory flavor, add 1 tsp dried thyme and ½ tsp dried sage to the dough.

PUMPKIN AND OAT BARS

| Makes | 6 servings | Serving size | 1 bar | Prep time | 10 minutes | Cook time | 25 minutes |

INGREDIENTS

1 cup oat flour

1/2 cup vanilla whey protein powder

1 tsp baking powder

1/2 tsp salt

2 tsp ground cinnamon

1/2 tsp allspice

1/2 tsp ground ginger

1/3 cup powdered stevia

1/3 cup liquid egg whites

1 cup canned pumpkin purée (not pumpkin pie mix)

1 tsp vanilla extract

DIRECTIONS

1 Preheat the oven to 350°F (177°C). Spray an 8 x 8in (20 x 20cm) baking pan with non-stick cooking spray.

2 In a large bowl, combine the oat flour, protein powder, baking powder, salt, cinnamon, allspice, ginger, and stevia. Mix well.

3 In a separate large bowl, combine the egg whites, pumpkin purée, and vanilla extract. Mix well.

4 Make the batter by adding the wet ingredients to the dry ingredients. Mix well to combine.

5 Pour the batter into the baking pan. Bake for 20 to 25 minutes, or until a toothpick inserted in the middle comes out clean. Slice into 6 equal-sized bars.

CHANGE IT UP

Try substituting mashed sweet potato or squash for the pumpkin.

PREP TIPS

If you don't have oat flour, you can make your own by milling dry oats in a blender until they reach a flour-like consistency.

Individually wrap the bars in plastic wrap and store in an airtight container in the refrigerator for up to one week.

Pricey store-bought bars often contain loads of sugar and preservatives. These spiced bars are healthier, and are great as a snack or for a post-workout refuel. Pumpkin keeps the bars moist, and oat flour adds whole grain nutrition and fiber. This bar does some heavy lifting!

NUTRITION FACTS

per serving

CALORIES
153

TOTAL FAT
0.5g

TOTAL CARBS
24.7g

PROTEIN
11.9g

SNACKS & POWER BARS

129

Creamy almond butter, hearty oats, and whey protein powder create a balanced bar that's perfect for taking off the edge. These simple-to-make bars also provide you with whole grain carbohydrates for fuel, healthy fats for satiety, and a healthy boost of muscle-building protein.

NUTRITION FACTS

per serving

CALORIES
215

TOTAL FAT
10g

TOTAL CARBS
17.3g

PROTEIN
14.3g

NO-BAKE ALMOND AND OATS BARS

Makes 12 servings / **Serving size** 1 bar / **Prep time** 10 min + 30 min / **Cook time** none

INGREDIENTS

2 cups quick oats

3 scoops whey protein powder

½ cup creamy almond butter

⅔ cup almond milk

1 tsp vanilla extract

2 tbsp powdered stevia

DIRECTIONS

1 In a large bowl, combine the oats, protein powder, almond butter, almond milk, vanilla extract, and stevia. Mix well until the ingredients form a dough.

2 Press the dough into a 9 x 13in (23 x 33cm) baking pan. Place the pan in the refrigerator for 30 minutes to harden the bars.

3 Cut into 8 equal-sized bars, and individually wrap in parchment paper. Seal the wrapped bars in a plastic storage bag.

PREP TIPS // *Store in an airtight container in the refrigerator for up to one week.*

CHANGE IT UP
Punch up the flavor by adding 1 tsp cinnamon and 1 tbsp cocoa powder to the dough. These additions will add just a few calories to each bar.

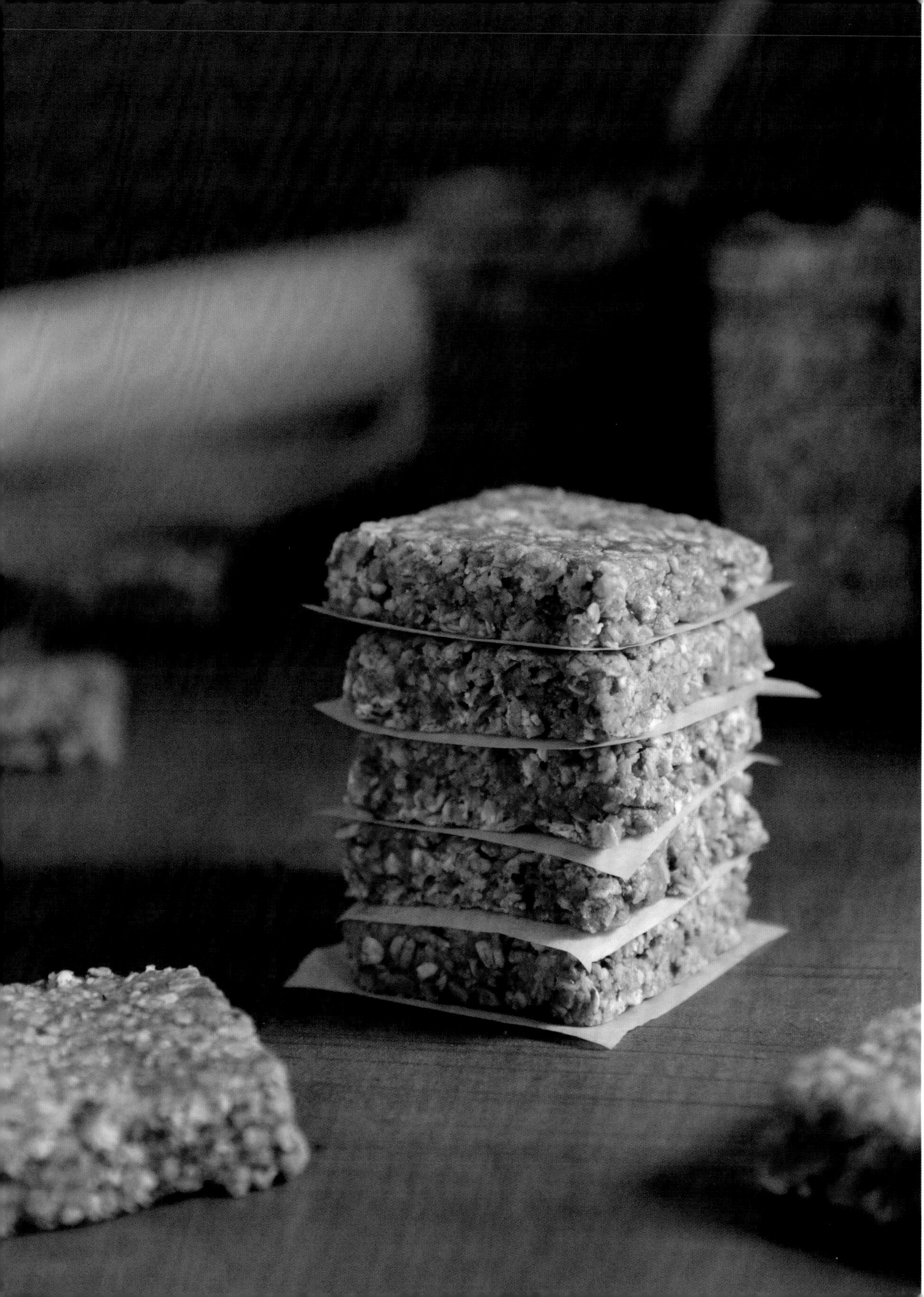

This leaner version of a traditional rice crispy treat is every bit as sticky, crunchy, and chewy as the original, but with less sugar. Almond butter replaces the marshmallows, while protein powder and honey add sweetness, and help bind the bars. These are addicting, so avoid overindulging!

LEAN RICE CRISPY TREATS

| Makes | 12 servings | Serving size | 1 square | Prep time | 25 minutes | Cook time | none |

INGREDIENTS

⅔ cup natural almond butter

½ cup raw honey

½ cup vanilla whey protein powder

1 tbsp ground cinnamon

3 cups toasted brown rice cereal

DIRECTIONS

1 In a large glass bowl, combine the almond butter and honey. Warm in the microwave on medium for 30 to 45 seconds, stir, then add the protein powder and cinnamon. Stir well.

2 Add the brown rice cereal and gently fold it into the mixture. Pour into a 9 x 13in (23 x 33cm) baking dish and use a spoon to flatten the mixture and form a uniform surface.

3 Place in the refrigerator to harden for 15 minutes before cutting into 12 equal-sized squares.

NUTRITION FACTS

per serving

CALORIES

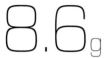

183

TOTAL FAT

8.4g

TOTAL CARBS

20g

PROTEIN

8.6g

PREP TIPS Individually wrap the treats in plastic wrap and store in an airtight container at room temperature for 3 days, or in the refrigerator for up to 1 week. (If stored in the refrigerator, allow the bars to soften at room temperature for 15 minutes before eating.)

CHANGE IT UP

Try substituting different flavors of protein powder, or substituting different nut butters, such as peanut butter or cashew butter.

QUICK AND EASY EGG BITES

Makes	3 servings	Serving size	2 bites	Prep time	10 minutes	Cook time	20 minutes

These bite-sized bundles of protein are a snap to make, and can be modified to fit your tastes and meal plan. You can experiment with a variety of vegetables and spices, they're easier to make and more portable than an omelet, and they store well in the refrigerator.

INGREDIENTS

3 cups liquid egg whites

½ cup diced tomato

½ cup diced white onion

1 tsp salt

1 tsp ground black pepper

DIRECTIONS

1 Preheat the oven to 350°F (177°C). Spray a large muffin tin with non-stick cooking spray.

2 In a large bowl, combine the egg whites, tomato, onion, salt, and black pepper. Mix well.

3 Pour equal amounts of the egg white mixture into six muffin cups. Bake for 18 to 20 minutes, or until the centers are set and firm. Serve warm.

NUTRITION FACTS

per serving

CALORIES
136

TOTAL FAT
0.1g

TOTAL CARBS
3.7g

PROTEIN
28.6g

CHANGE IT UP

Make these keto by replacing the egg whites with 6 large eggs, and adding ½ cup shredded sharp cheddar cheese. The macros will be 223 calories, 15.7g fat, 2.6g carbs, and 16.8g protein per serving.

Make post-workout muffins by omitting the salt, pepper, tomatoes, and onions, and adding 1 tsp cinnamon and 1½ cups quick oats. Allow to sit for 15 minutes, then bake for 18 to 20 minutes. Macros will be 286 calories, 3.1g fat, 30.7g carbs, and 33.6g protein per serving.

PREP TIPS // *Double this recipe and keep the muffins on hand as a quick snack.*

Store in an airtight container in the refrigerator for up to one week.

This simple yet refreshing muscle-building snack creates a delightful flavor and textural contrast when the cottage cheese is paired with the grilled melon. Watermelon is refreshing, hydrating, and also high in lycopene, which is a key antioxidant compound.

NUTRITION FACTS

per serving

CALORIES
260

TOTAL FAT
3.7 g

TOTAL CARBS
28.1 g

PROTEIN
30 g

GRILLED BALSAMIC MELON AND CHEESE

Makes	1 serving	Serving size	4 slices + 1 cup cheese	Prep time	5 minutes	Cook time	4 minutes

INGREDIENTS

4 slices watermelon, rind on, sliced into 1-inch-thick (2.5cm) triangles

1 cup 1% cottage cheese

1 tbsp roughly chopped fresh basil

1 tbsp balsamic vinegar

Coconut oil cooking spray

Pinch of salt

DIRECTIONS

1 Preheat a grill to high. Lightly spray each watermelon slice with coconut oil cooking spray, and evenly drizzle the balsamic vinegar over each watermelon slice.

2 Grill the watermelon slices for 1 to 2 minutes per side, or until they are lightly seared and develop grill marks on each side.

3 Transfer the watermelon slices to a plate. Lightly season the slices with the salt, and top with the basil. Add the cottage cheese to the plate. Serve chilled.

PREP TIPS // *This recipe is best when prepared and served fresh.*

For meal prep, you can grill the watermelon ahead of time and store it tightly sealed in plastic wrap in the refrigerator. Add the cottage cheese and basil just before serving.

CHANGE IT UP

In a pinch, you can substitute 1 tbsp light vinaigrette dressing for the salt and balsamic vinegar. Changes to the macros will be negligible.

Substitute 1% ricotta cheese in place of the cottage cheese. Macros will be 271 calories, 2.3g fat, 30.1g carbs, and 29.0g protein per serving.

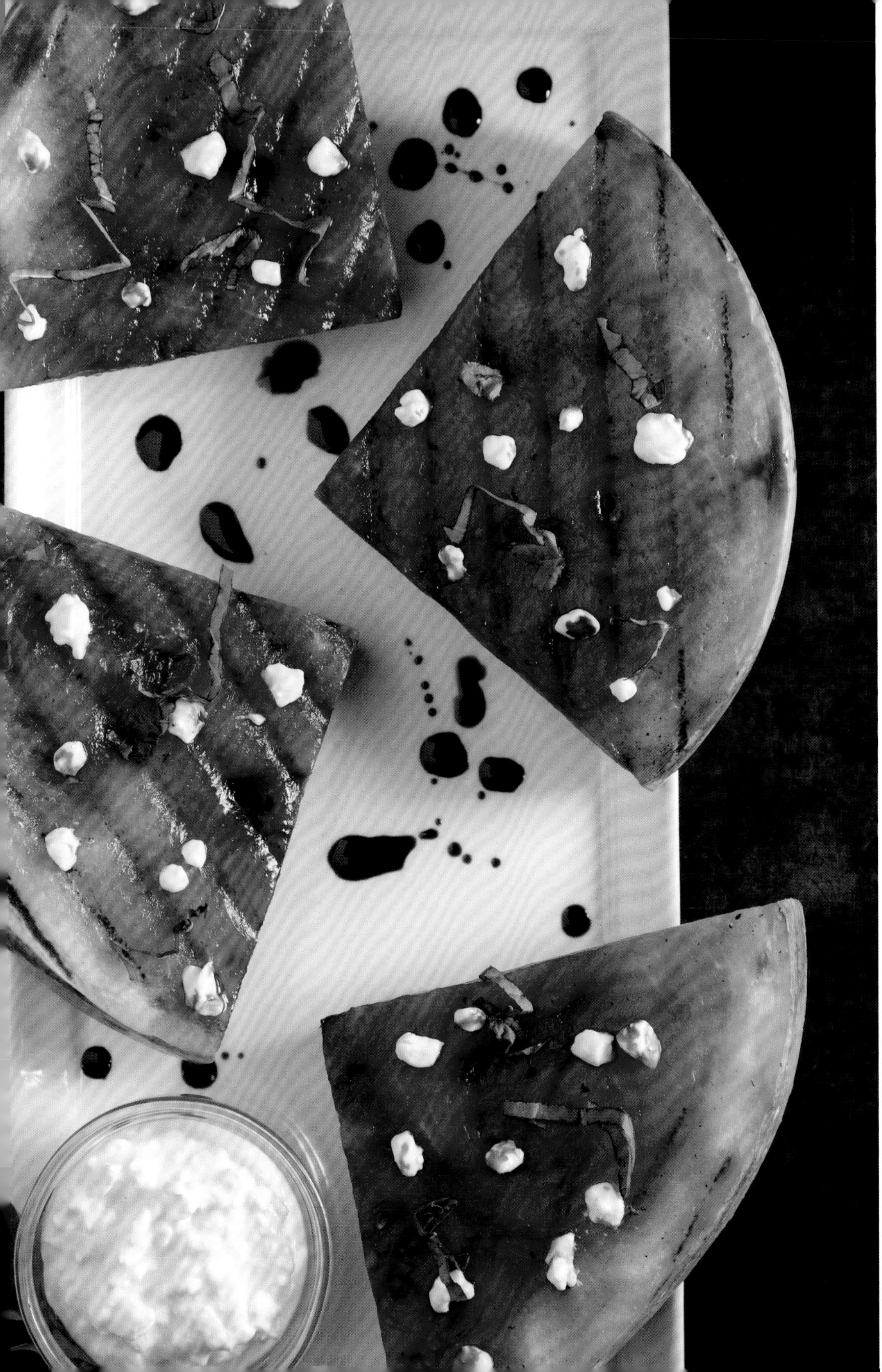

Silky smooth with a punch of lemon, this hummus is a light and balanced snack. Greek yogurt adds tartness, and also increases the serving size without drastically increasing the calories. Chickpeas are high in fiber and vitamins, and also a good source of vegetarian protein.

GREEK YOGURT HUMMUS

| Makes | 4 servings | Serving size | ½ cup | Prep time | 10 minutes | Cook time | none |

INGREDIENTS

2 15oz (420g) cans chickpeas, drained and rinsed

½ cup plain nonfat Greek yogurt

Juice of 1 lemon

½ tsp garlic powder

¼ tsp cumin

½ tsp paprika

¼ tsp salt

For serving

1 small seedless cucumber, thinly sliced

1 small carrot, peeled and sliced lengthwise into sticks

NUTRITION FACTS

per serving

CALORIES
152

TOTAL FAT
2.0g

TOTAL CARBS
26.2g

PROTEIN
8.5g

DIRECTIONS

1 In a blender or food processor, combine the chickpeas, Greek yogurt, lemon juice, garlic powder, cumin, paprika, and salt. Pulse at 15 second intervals until the ingredients are well incorporated and no lumps remain.

2 Scrape the sides of the blender with a rubber spatula and blend on high for an additional 60 seconds, or until a smooth and creamy consistency is achieved. (If the hummus is too thick, add additional water, 1 tbsp at a time, until the desired consistency is reached.)

3 Transfer to a serving bowl. Serve chilled with the carrot sticks and cucumber slices on the side.

PREP TIPS // Store in an airtight container in the refrigerator for up to 4 days.

CHANGE IT UP
For a more aromatic twist, add ½ tsp dried parsley.

NO-BAKE COCOA AND OATS BARS

Makes	3 servings		Serving size	1 bar		Prep time	10 minutes		Cook time	none

INGREDIENTS

½ cup old-fashioned oats

½ cup oat bran

3 tbsp almond flour

3 tbsp unsweetened cocoa powder

1 tbsp powdered stevia

½ cup vanilla protein powder (whey and casein blend)

¼ cup unsweetened vanilla almond milk

1 tsp vanilla extract

DIRECTIONS

1 Spray a small, sealable food storage container (approximately 8 x 8in (20 x 20cm)) with non-stick cooking spray.

2 In a medium bowl, combine the oats, oat bran, almond flour, cocoa powder, stevia, and protein powder. Mix well to combine. In a separate medium bowl, combine the almond milk and vanilla extract. Mix well to combine.

3 Make the batter by adding the dry ingredients to the wet ingredients. Mix the ingredients until a thick, uniform consistency is achieved.

4 Spoon the batter into the prepared container, and use a spoon to smooth and flatten the mixture. Refrigerate for 15 minutes before slicing into 3 bars.

PREP TIPS // A whey and casein protein blend works best for this recipe, as the casein will absorb the almond milk and thicken the batter.

Individually wrap the bars in plastic wrap and store in an airtight container in the refrigerator for up to one week.

CHANGE IT UP

For a more intense chocolate flavor, substitute ½ cup chocolate whey protein powder for the vanilla whey protein powder.

This bar tastes like a dessert, but still fits the macros for most bodybuilding meal plans. The unsweetened cocoa powder offers a potent antioxidant and energy boost, and the oats and oat bran add complex carbs for energy. Pop one of these into your bag for a quick snack between meals!

NUTRITION FACTS

per serving

CALORIES

235

TOTAL FAT

7.1g

TOTAL CARBS

21.3g

PROTEIN

28.1g

SNACKS & POWER BARS

Everyone craves crunchy snacks, but all too often they're off limits on most bodybuilding meal plans. These crackers will fit into most meal plans, and will also satisfy those cravings for some crunch. Flax and sesame seeds provide healthy fats and create a texture that's perfect for dipping!

PALEO PROTEIN CRACKERS

Makes 12 servings	**Serving size** 2 crackers	**Prep time** 15 minutes	**Cook time** 25 minutes

NUTRITION FACTS

per serving

CALORIES
220

TOTAL FAT
17.7 g

TOTAL CARBS
9.2 g

PROTEIN
9.3 g

INGREDIENTS

½ cup liquid egg whites

3 cups almond flour

1 cup flax meal

2 tbsp sesame seeds

1 tbsp dried parsley

1 tbsp dried tarragon

½ tbsp dried chives

½ tbsp ground thyme

1 tsp sea salt

DIRECTIONS

1 Preheat the oven to 350°F (177°C). Line a large baking sheet with parchment paper.

2 In a large bowl, combine the egg whites, almond flour, flax meal, sesame seeds, parsley, tarragon, chives, thyme, and sea salt.

3 Using clean hands, mix the ingredients until a dough is formed, then shape the dough into a ball. (If the dough is too crumbly, add more egg whites, one tablespoon at a time, until the desired consistency is reached.)

4 Place the dough on the baking sheet. Place another sheet of parchment paper over top of the dough, and use a rolling pin to roll the dough out as thin as possible. Score the dough into 24 even-sized squares.

5 Bake for 20 to 25 minutes, or until the crackers turn golden brown. Allow to cool, and break the crackers into even-sized pieces.

PREP TIPS Store in an airtight container at room temperature for up to one week.

CHANGE IT UP

Substitute pumpkin seeds for the sesame seeds. The macros will be about the same.

Substitute hemp hearts for the flax meal. The macros will be very similar.

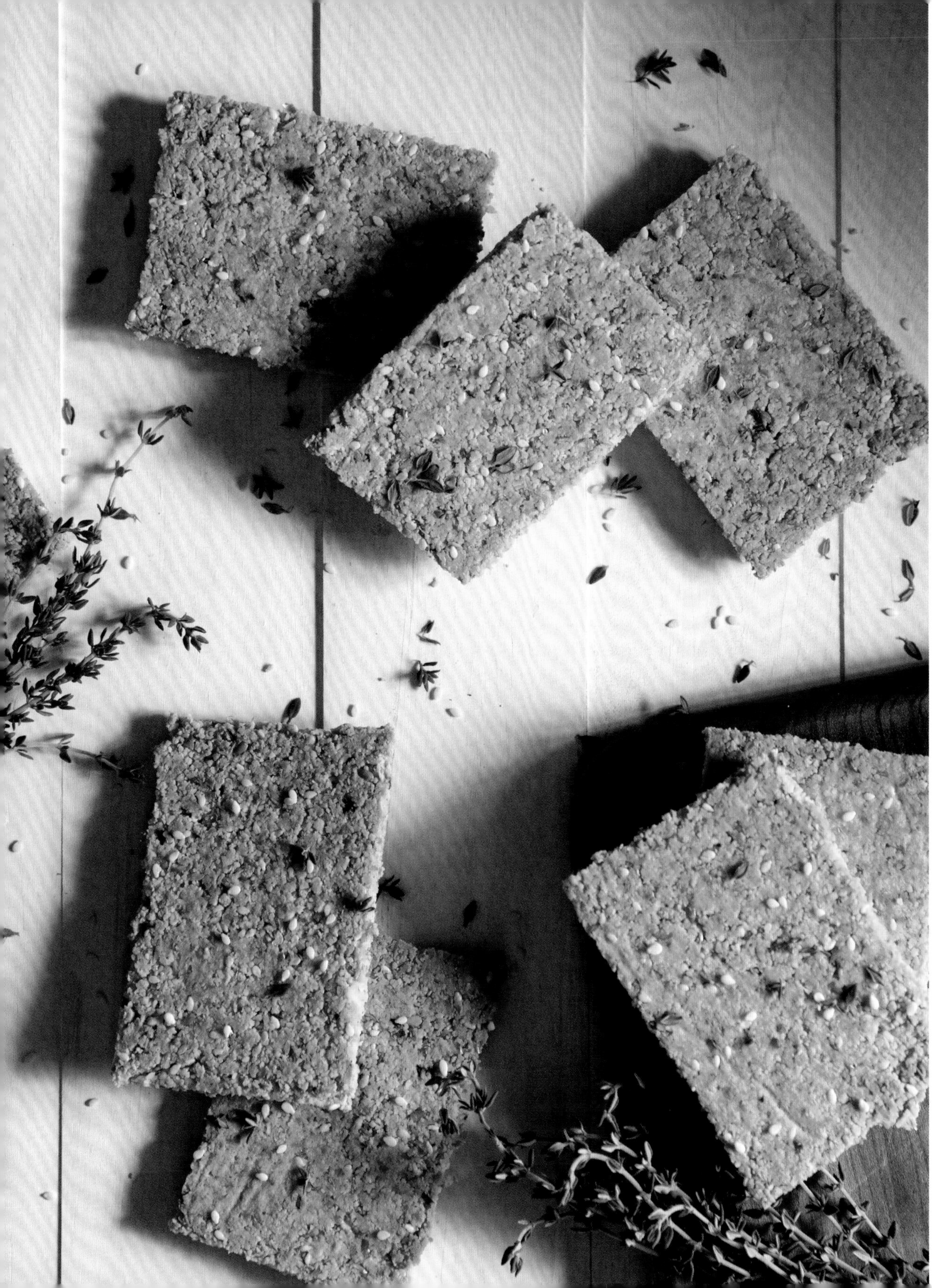

Kick those nagging sweet tooth cravings to the curb and get a shot of protein with this personal-sized mug cake that is full of chocolatey goodness. Cocoa powder satisfies the palate and provide a little kick of caffeine, while protein powder and egg whites feed the muscles.

NUTRITION FACTS

per serving

CALORIES
190

TOTAL FAT
2.1g

TOTAL CARBS
9.2g

PROTEIN
34.3g

CHOCOLATE PROTEIN SNACK MUG

| Makes | 1 serving | Serving size | 1 mug | Prep time | 5 minutes | Cook time | 2 minutes |

INGREDIENTS

1 tbsp unsweetened cocoa powder
1 tbsp coconut flour
¼ cup vanilla whey protein powder

½ tsp baking powder
¼ cup liquid egg whites
¼ cup unsweetened almond milk

DIRECTIONS

1 In a microwave-safe, medium-sized mug, combine the cocoa powder, coconut flour, protein powder, and baking powder. Stir well.

2 Add the egg whites and almond milk. Mix all ingredients well.

3 Microwave on high for 1 to 2 minutes, checking every 15 seconds for doneness. The cake is done when the center is set and no longer appears shiny. (Make sure not to overcook the cake, as it can quickly become rubbery and dry.) Serve warm.

PREP TIPS // *Make the mix ahead of time by combining the cocoa powder, coconut flour, protein powder, and baking powder, and storing the mix in individual portions in zipper lock bags. When you're ready for a snack, just pour the ingredients in a mug, and add the egg whites and almond milk.*

CHANGE IT UP

Make a post-workout mug by using a slightly larger mug, and adding ⅓ cup quick oats to the dry ingredients, and adding an additional ¼ cup liquid egg whites. The macros will be 287 calories, 4.5g fat, 25.6g carbs, and 37.6g protein.

ZESTY TUNA SNACK BOWL

Makes | 1 serving | / | Serving size | 1 bowl | / | Prep time | 10 minutes | / | Cook time | none

INGREDIENTS

1 5oz (140g) can light tuna packed in water, rinsed and drained

⅓ cup diced celery

¼ cup diced carrot

1 tsp minced garlic dill pickle

1 tsp lemon juice

1 tsp creamy Dijon mustard

¼ cup nonfat plain Greek yogurt

DIRECTIONS

1 In a small glass bowl, combine the tuna, celery, carrot, pickle, lemon juice, mustard, and Greek yogurt.

2 Stir well to incorporate all ingredients. Serve chilled.

CHANGE IT UP

For a non-dairy option, omit the Greek yogurt. This will eliminate 27 calories, 2.1g carbs, and 4.5g protein.

Make it keto by adding half a medium avocado to the bowl. Total macros per serving wil be 324 calories, 13.8g fat, 12.1g carbs, and 38g protein.

PREP TIPS / *Store in an airtight container in the refrigerator for up to 5 days.*

Canned tuna is an inexpensive source of protein and a great way to maximize your training budget. This low fat take on traditional tuna salad features naturally sweet vegetables, garlicky pickles, and tangy condiments that will all help keep the macros on track. You won't miss the mayo!

NUTRITION FACTS

per serving

CALORIES

194

TOTAL FAT

1.8g

TOTAL CARBS

7.1g

PROTEIN

37.3g

Stave off cravings with this salty and crunchy snack that's low in fat, and ready in less than 10 minutes. Lean turkey keeps you full and delivers muscle-building protein, while juicy tomato, crunchy spinach, and crisp cucumber all come together to create a light and delicate roll.

TURKEY AND VEGGIE ROLL-UP

| Makes | 1 serving | | Serving size | 1 roll-up | | Prep time | 10 minutes | | Cook time | none |

INGREDIENTS

4oz (110g) sliced all natural deli turkey

1 large cucumber

½ cup chopped tomato

½ cup fresh baby spinach

1 tbsp creamy Dijon mustard

DIRECTIONS

1 Using a vegetable peeler, slice the cucumber lengthwise into long, thin strips. Arrange the cucumber strips in a row on a sheet of plastic wrap, overlapping them slightly to form a square. Place the turkey slices on top of the cucumber strips.

2 Spread the mustard in a thin layer over the turkey. Add the spinach in a thin layer, then spoon the chopped tomato in a narrow column near one edge of the wrap.

3 Create the roll-up by grasping the plastic wrap at the end with the tomatoes, and rolling the ingredients into a tight roll. (Make sure not to roll the plastic wrap into the roll-up.)

4 Discard the plastic wrap. Secure the ingredients by inserting a toothpick at each end, and carefully transferring the roll-up to a plate. Serve immediately.

NUTRITION FACTS

per serving

CALORIES
160

TOTAL FAT
1.4g

TOTAL CARBS
11.4g

PROTEIN
26.3g

PREP TIPS This recipe is best prepared and served immediately, as the cucumber can become soggy quickly.

CHANGE IT UP

For a little more crunch, substitute ¼ cup thinly sliced bell peppers for the tomatoes. The macros will be the same.

For a milder flavor, substitute ½ cup butter lettuce for the spinach. Make sure to tear the butter lettuce into small pieces before placing it on the wrap.

BAKED CHEESEBURGER BITES

Makes **4** servings | Serving **size** **2** bites | Prep **time** **10** minutes | Cook **time** **25** minutes

These yummy cheeseburger bites are juicy and filled with gooey cheese. Coconut flour adds fiber and helps keep them moist, while tangy ketchup and mustard add sweet and spicy notes. These low carb bites are a snap to make and store well, so this recipe can easily be doubled for meal prep.

INGREDIENTS

1lb (450g) lean ground sirloin

2 tbsp coconut flour

2 large eggs

2 tbsp no-sugar-added ketchup

2 tsp spicy brown mustard

½ cup low-fat shredded mozzarella cheese

¼ cup diced white onion

DIRECTIONS

1 Preheat oven to 350°F (177°C). Spray an 8-cup muffin tin with non-stick cooking spray.

2 In a large bowl, combine the ground sirloin, coconut flour, eggs, ketchup, mustard, mozzarella cheese, and onion. Mix the ingredients until just incorporated. (Do not over mix, as the burgers can become tough.)

3 Spoon equal amounts of the mixture into the muffin cups. Bake for 20 minutes, or until the internal temperature reaches 160°F (71°C). Serve hot.

PREP TIPS // *Store in an airtight container in the refrigerator for up to 5 days, or in the freezer for up to 2 months. To reheat, place the thawed bites on a baking sheet and heat in a 250°F (121°C) oven for 10 minutes.*

NUTRITION FACTS

per serving

CALORIES

242

TOTAL FAT

13 g

TOTAL CARBS

3.1 g

PROTEIN

28.3 g

SNACKS & POWER BARS

SHAKES & DESSERTS

The quickest and easiest way to ensure effective post-workout nutrition and recovery is through protein shakes. But the recipes in this chapter go well beyond just adding protein powder to water, and instead will have you looking forward to breaking out the blender! And no meal is complete without dessert! The dessert recipes in this chapter will help crush cravings, but still keep you on track toward meeting your training goals.

Greek yogurt and banana make up the creamy base of this shake. Cardamom's citrus scent intensifies the carrot flavor, while ginger adds a sweet heat.

CARROT CAKE SHAKE

Makes	1 serving	Serving size	16oz (450g)	Prep time	10 minutes	Cook time	none

NUTRITION FACTS

per serving

CALORIES	PROTEIN
290	33.4g

FAT	CARBS
1.7g	37.2g

INGREDIENTS

1 cup shredded carrots

½ cup unsweetened vanilla almond milk

½ cup plain nonfat Greek yogurt

3 tbsp vanilla whey protein powder

½ medium frozen banana

⅛ tsp ground cardamom

¼ tsp ground ginger

¼ tsp ground cinnamon

1 tsp powdered stevia

DIRECTIONS

1 Place the carrots in a microwave-safe dish, cover with a damp paper towel, and microwave on high for 1 minute. Allow to cool for 5 minutes.

2 Combine all ingredients in a blender. Blend on high for one minute. Scrape the sides of the blender with a rubber spatula, and blend on high for 1 additional minute. Transfer to a glass and serve immediately.

Channel "The King" with this recipe, except here Elvis has a six pack and trains six days a week. Powdered peanut butter and banana will rock your taste buds, without racking up the calories.

ELVIS SHAKE

Makes	1 serving	Serving size	12oz (340g)	Prep time	10 minutes	Cook time	none

NUTRITION FACTS

per serving

CALORIES	PROTEIN
260	34.1g

FAT	CARBS
4.9g	23g

INGREDIENTS

½ medium banana

¼ cup powdered peanut butter

1 cup unsweetened almond milk

¼ cup vanilla whey protein powder

½ tsp vanilla extract

½ tsp powdered stevia

1 cup crushed ice

DIRECTIONS

1 Combine the banana, powdered peanut butter, almond milk, protein powder, vanilla, stevia, and ice in a blender. Blend on low for 30 seconds.

2 Scrape the sides of the blender with a rubber spatula. Blend on high for an additional 30 seconds to 1 minute, or until the ice is crushed and the shake is smooth and creamy. Transfer to a glass and serve immediately.

PREP TIPS *For a thicker shake, omit the ice and use a frozen banana (make sure to peel and slice the banana before freezing).*

SHAKES & DESSERTS

146

GOLDEN MILK SHAKE

Golden milk is touted for its anti-inflammatory, digestive, and recovery benefits. MCTs (medium-chain triglycerides) from the coconut oil provide energy.

Makes	1 serving	Serving size	10oz (285g)	Prep time	10 minutes	Cook time	none

INGREDIENTS

1 cup unsweetened vanilla coconut milk

¼ cup vanilla whey protein powder

½ cup 2% low sodium cottage cheese

½ tbsp coconut oil

1 tsp ground ginger

½ tsp ground turmeric

½ tsp ground cinnamon

¼ tsp ground black pepper

2 tsp powdered stevia

½ cup crushed ice

DIRECTIONS

1 Combine the coconut milk, protein powder, cottage cheese, coconut oil, ginger, turmeric, cinnamon, black pepper, stevia, and ice in a blender. Blend on low for 30 seconds, or until the ingredients are well incorporated.

2 Scrape the sides of the blender with a rubber spatula. Blend on high for one additional minute, or until the shake is smooth and creamy. Transfer to a glass and serve immediately.

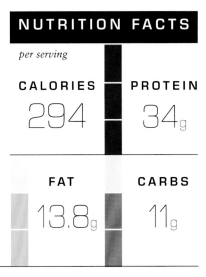

NUTRITION FACTS

per serving

CALORIES 294

PROTEIN 34g

FAT 13.8g

CARBS 11g

KEY LIME SHAKE

Tart lime, coconut, and vanilla flavors give this shake a delectable tropical flavor. You'll reap the nutritional benefits of a full serving of spinach, but you won't taste it at all!

Makes	1 serving	Serving size	14oz (400g)	Prep time	5 minutes	Cook time	none

INGREDIENTS

½ cup nonfat plain Greek yogurt

3 tbsp vanilla whey protein powder

2 tbsp lime juice

1 cup unsweetened vanilla coconut milk

2 tsp powdered stevia

1 cup fresh baby spinach

½ cup crushed ice

DIRECTIONS

1 Combine the Greek yogurt, protein powder, lime juice, coconut milk, stevia, spinach, and ice in a blender. Blend on low for 1 minute.

2 Scrape the sides of the blender with a rubber spatula. Blend on high for an additional 30 seconds to 1 minute, or until the shake is smooth and creamy. Transfer to a glass and serve immediately.

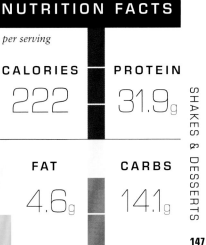

NUTRITION FACTS

per serving

CALORIES 222

PROTEIN 31.9g

FAT 4.6g

CARBS 14.1g

SHAKES & DESSERTS

Juicy blueberries combine with tart Greek yogurt to create a shake that tastes like a decadent dessert. The Greek yogurt, protein powder, and almond milk all power the protein up to over 30g per serving. This shake is delicious when made with virtually any type of sweet berry.

BLUEBERRY CHEESECAKE SHAKE

| Makes | 1 serving | | Serving size | 12oz (340g) | | Prep time | 10 minutes | | Cook time | none |

INGREDIENTS

1 cup blueberries (fresh or frozen)

¼ cup vanilla whey protein powder

½ cup fat free plain Greek yogurt

½ tsp vanilla extract

½ cup unsweetened almond milk

1 cup crushed ice

DIRECTIONS

1 Combine the blueberries, protein powder, Greek yogurt, vanilla extract, almond milk, and ice in a blender. Pulse for 15 second intervals until the ingredients are well incorporated.

2 Scrape the sides of the blender with a rubber spatula. Blend on high for 1 additional minute, or until the ice is crushed and the shake is smooth and creamy. Transfer to a glass and serve immediately.

NUTRITION FACTS

per serving

CALORIES

266

TOTAL FAT

1.3g

TOTAL CARBS

32g

PROTEIN

32.5g

PREP TIPS / *Buy frozen fruit in bulk and store it in your freezer. Frozen fruit is often just as delicious as fresh, and is usually less expensive. Most fresh fruit also freezes well.*

CHANGE IT UP

Make a strawberry cheesecake shake by substituting 1 cup strawberries for the blueberries, and adding ½ tsp lemon juice.

For a post-workout shake, add ½ banana. The macros will be 319 calories, 3.49g fat, 45.48g carbs, and 33.1g protein per serving.

SHAKES & DESSERTS

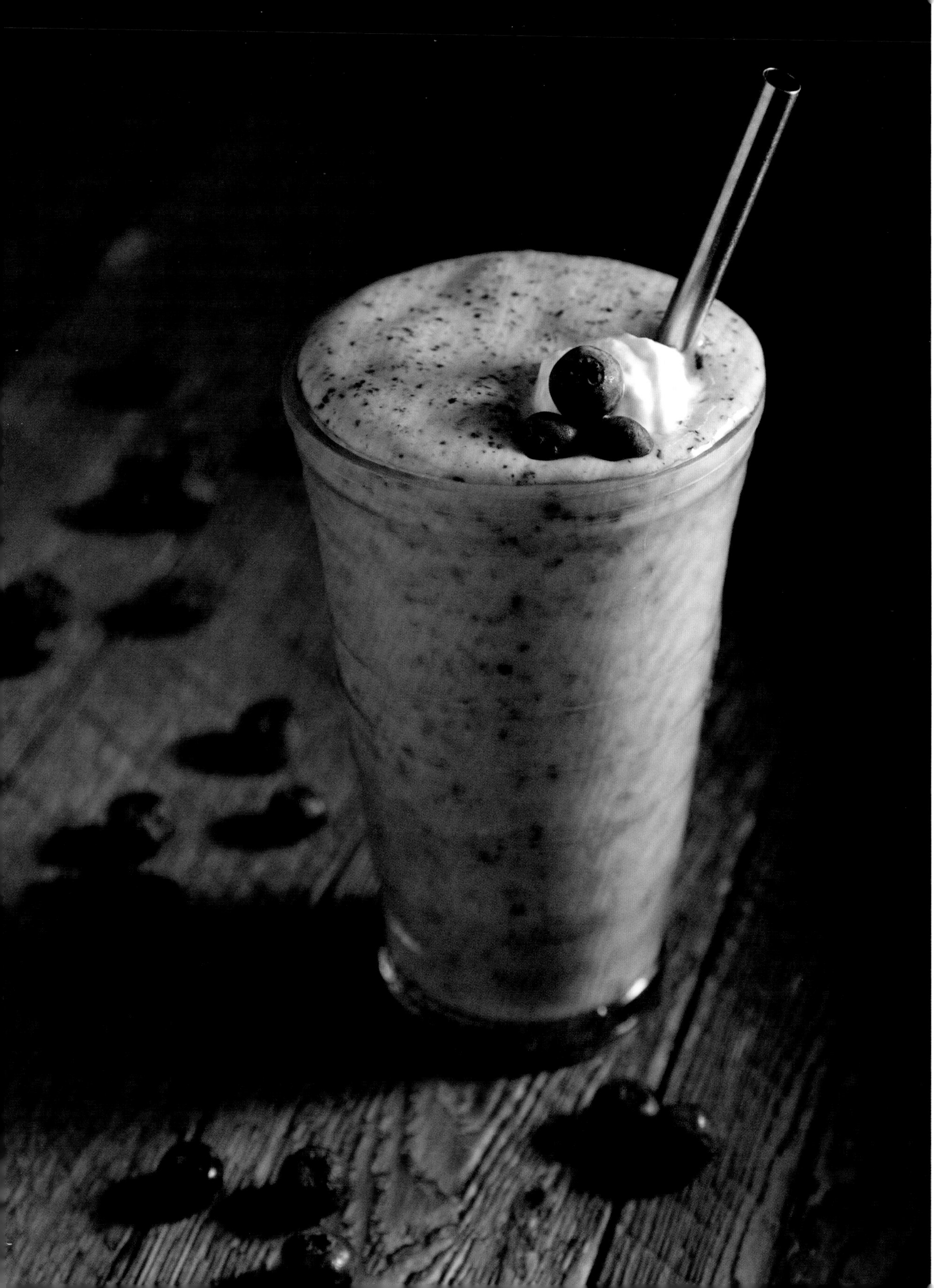

This tart and sweet shake is elevated by juicy orange and a touch of orange zest, while Greek yogurt adds protein and creates an ice cream-like consistency.

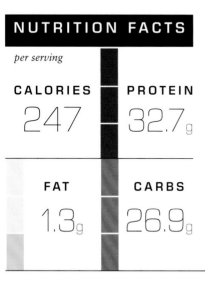

NUTRITION FACTS

per serving

CALORIES	PROTEIN
247	32.7g

FAT	CARBS
1.3g	26.9g

ORANGE CREAMSICLE SHAKE

Makes	1 serving		Serving size	14oz (400g)		Prep time	10 minutes		Cook time	none

INGREDIENTS

1 tsp orange zest

1 orange, peeled and cut into segments, seeds and pith removed

¼ cup vanilla whey protein powder

½ cup nonfat plain Greek yogurt

½ cup unsweetened vanilla almond milk

½ tsp vanilla extract

2 tsp powdered stevia

½ cup crushed ice

DIRECTIONS

1 Combine the orange zest, orange segments, protein powder, Greek yogurt, almond milk, vanilla extract, stevia, and ice in a blender. Blend on low for 30 seconds.

2 Scrape the sides of the blender with a rubber spatula. Blend on high for an additional 1 to 2 minutes, or until the shake is smooth and creamy. Transfer to a glass and serve immediately.

This shake is more satisfying than a candy bar! Healthy fats from the almond butter and coconut keep the carbs low, and antioxidant-rich cocoa powder provides an extra boost of energy.

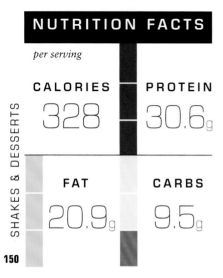

NUTRITION FACTS

per serving

CALORIES	PROTEIN
328	30.6g

FAT	CARBS
20.9g	9.5g

COCO-CHOCO ALMOND SHAKE

Makes	1 serving		Serving size	14oz (400g)		Prep time	10 minutes		Cook time	none

INGREDIENTS

1 cup unsweetened vanilla almond milk

¼ cup chocolate whey protein powder

1 tbsp almond butter

1 tbsp unsweetened cocoa powder

2 tbsp unsweetened shredded coconut

3 tsp powdered stevia

1 tbsp slivered almonds

DIRECTIONS

1 Combine the almond milk, protein powder, almond butter, cocoa powder, coconut, and stevia in a blender. Blend on high for 30 seconds.

2 Scrape the sides of the blender with a rubber spatula, and blend on high for 1 additional minute.

3 Transfer to a glass and top with the slivered almonds. Serve immediately.

SHAKES & DESSERTS

HULK SHAKE

Smash cravings with this green powerhouse! Fiber from the spinach will keep you feeling full, and a touch of tart lemon juice adds balance to the sweet banana.

| Makes | 1 serving | Serving size | 12oz (340g) | Prep time | 5 minutes | Cook time | none |

INGREDIENTS

1 cup unsweetened vanilla almond milk

2 cups fresh baby spinach

1 tsp lemon juice

1 medium banana, frozen

¼ cup vanilla whey protein powder

1 tsp powdered stevia

½ tsp ground cinnamon

DIRECTIONS

1 Add the almond milk, spinach, lemon juice, and banana to a blender. Blend on high for 1 minute.

2 Scrape the sides of the blender with a rubber spatula. Add the protein powder, stevia, and cinnamon. Blend for 1 minute, or until the shake is smooth and creamy. Transfer to a glass and serve immediately.

PREP TIPS This shake can be made ahead and refrigerated for up to 2 days.

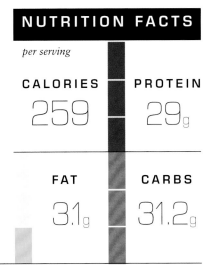

NUTRITION FACTS

per serving

CALORIES 259

PROTEIN 29g

FAT 3.1g

CARBS 31.2g

OATMEAL RAISIN COOKIE PROTEIN SHAKE

A cookie in shake form? Yes! Replenish glycogen stores and calm your sweet tooth with this shake. Fast-digesting and complex carbs will provide you with instant fuel and sustained energy.

| Makes | 1 serving | Serving size | 16oz (450g) | Prep time | 10 minutes | Cook time | none |

INGREDIENTS

½ banana

1 cup unsweetened almond milk

¼ cup old-fashioned oats

¼ cup vanilla or chocolate protein powder

1 tbsp raisins

½ tsp ground cinnamon

1 cup crushed ice (optional)

DIRECTIONS

1 Place the banana, almond milk, oats, protein powder, raisins, cinnamon, and ice into a blender. (If you are using a frozen banana, you can omit the ice.) Blend on low for 30 seconds to 1 minute.

2 Scrape the sides of the blender with a rubber spatula. Blend on high for one additional minute, or until the shake looks uniform in texture and color. Transfer to a glass and serve immediately.

PREP TIPS For a thicker shake, use ½ frozen banana. (Make sure to peel and slice the banana before freezing.)

NUTRITION FACTS

per serving

CALORIES 277

PROTEIN 29.1g

FAT 2.9g

CARBS 34.8g

Cocoa powder and avocado pair up to create a velvety, decadent mousse. Avocado provides healthy fats and anti-inflammatory benefits, while cocoa powder gives the mousse a boost of antioxidants. The richness of the cocoa powder is the star—while the avocado provides creaminess.

CHOCO-CADO MOUSSE

Makes 4 servings | Serving size 3oz (85g) | Prep time 10 minutes | Cook time none

NUTRITION FACTS

per serving

CALORIES

142

TOTAL FAT

12 g

TOTAL CARBS

7 g

PROTEIN

3 g

INGREDIENTS

2 medium avocados, halved lengthwise, seeds removed

⅓ cup unsweetened cocoa powder

1 tsp vanilla extract

Pinch of salt

¼ cup powdered stevia

½ cup unsweetened coconut milk

DIRECTIONS

1 Using a spoon, scoop the avocado flesh into a blender. Add the cocoa powder, vanilla extract, salt, and stevia.

2 With the lid off, begin blending the ingredients on low while simultaneously adding the coconut milk in a steady stream. Continue blending until all ingredients are well incorporated.

3 Scrape the sides of the blender with a rubber spatula. Cover, and blend on high for an additional 30 seconds to 1 minute, or until a smooth and creamy texture is achieved. Serve chilled.

PREP TIPS // *This is best when prepared and served immediately, but will keep in an airtight container in the refrigerator for up to 2 days.*

CHANGE IT UP

For a spicier twist, add ½ tsp ground chipotle powder.

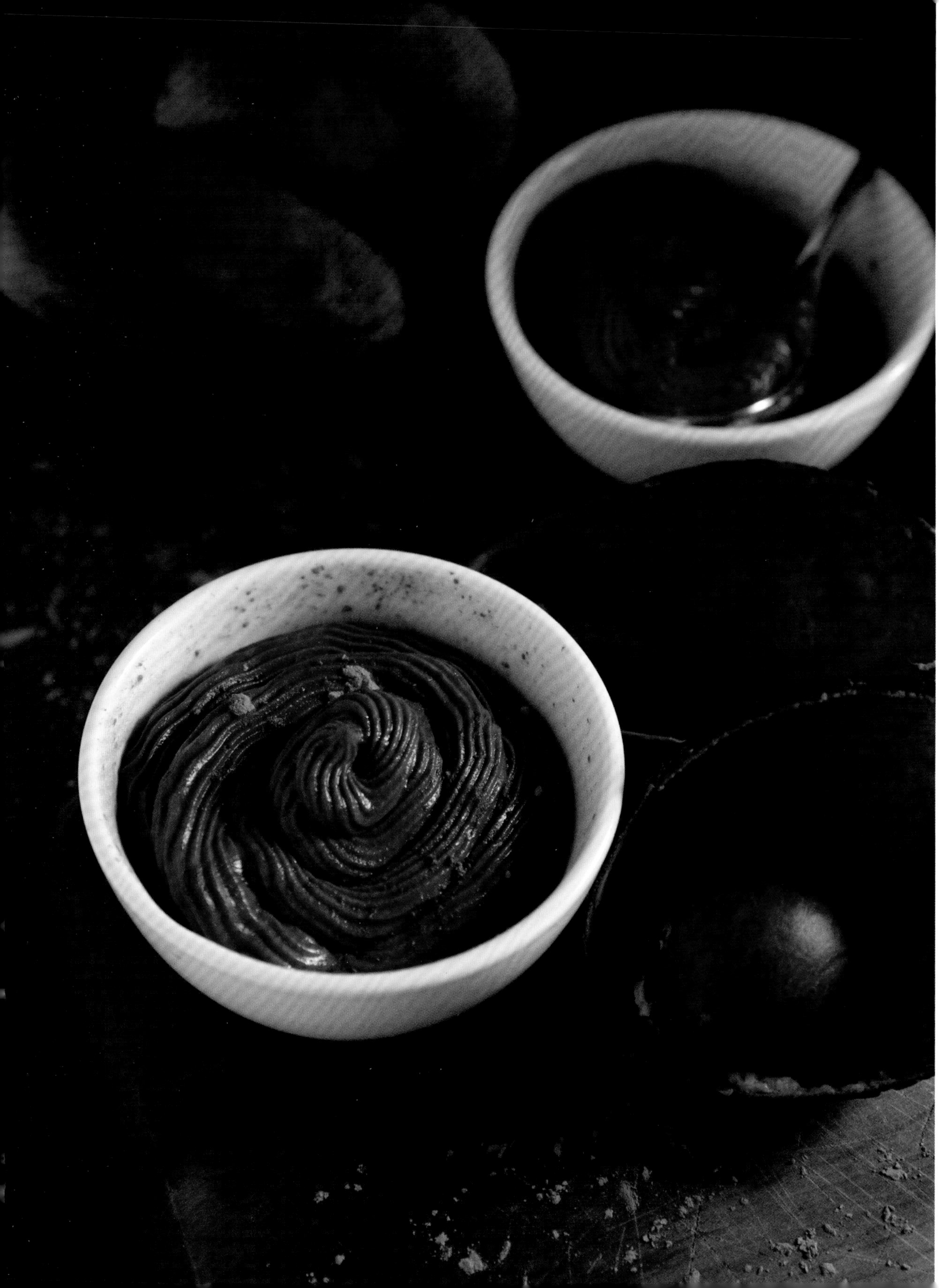

This satisfyingly creamy dessert is reminiscent of flan, but with a fraction of the calories and sugar. The egg whites still add a custard-like texture, but without the yolks. This low-fat treat can be whipped up in less than an hour, so it's a great option for when sweet cravings strike.

EGG WHITE CUSTARDS

Makes 2 servings | **Serving size** 2 ramekins | **Prep time** 10 minutes | **Cook time** 40 minutes

NUTRITION FACTS

per serving

CALORIES

135

TOTAL FAT

3.8 g

TOTAL CARBS

6 g

PROTEIN

18.5 g

SHAKES & DESSERTS

154

INGREDIENTS

1 cup liquid egg whites

¾ cup nonfat dry milk powder

3 tsp powdered stevia

½ tsp vanilla extract

2 cups unsweetened vanilla almond milk

½ tsp ground cinnamon

⅛ tsp ground nutmeg

DIRECTIONS

1 Preheat the oven to 350°F (177°C). Fill a large glass casserole dish with 1 inch (2.5cm) of water. Spray 4 large ramekins with non-stick cooking spray.

2 In a large bowl, combine the egg whites, milk powder, stevia, vanilla extract, and almond milk. Mix until well incorporated.

3 Pour equal amounts of the mixture into each ramekin. Sprinkle equal amounts of the cinnamon and nutmeg over top of each ramekin.

4 Place the ramekins in the casserole dish and carefully place the casserole dish in the oven. Bake for 35 to 40 minutes, or until the middles of the custards are set. (Use caution when removing the casserole dish from the oven.) Serve warm.

PREP TIPS // Cover the cooled ramekins with plastic wrap and store in the refrigerator for up to 6 days.

CHANGE IT UP

For a chocolatey twist, add 1 tbsp unsweetened cocoa powder and 1 tsp powdered stevia to the custard mix. This will add only 3 calories to each serving.

For an added indulgence, top the cooked custards with 1 tbsp finely chopped almonds. This will add 56 calories, 5g fat, 2g carbs, and 2g protein per serving.

GAINS GLAZED DONUTS

Makes 4 servings | **Serving size** 4 donuts | **Prep time** 10 minutes | **Cook time** 12 minutes

You'll make sweet gains with these low-carb, protein-glazed donuts! Coconut flour gives them a cake-like texture, and the proteins will all be digested at different speeds, so you can enjoy these as a snack or even after a workout. These are perfect for a sweet protein boost.

INGREDIENTS

1 cup vanilla protein powder (whey and casein blend)

⅓ cup coconut flour

2 tsp baking powder

½ tsp ground cinnamon

1 tbsp powdered stevia

pinch of salt

2 tbsp coconut oil, melted

3 tbsp liquid egg whites

1 tsp vanilla extract

⅓ cup unsweetened almond milk

For the glaze

¼ cup almond milk

⅓ cup vanilla whey protein powder

DIRECTIONS

1 Preheat the oven to 350°F (177°C). Spray a donut pan with non-stick cooking spray.

2 In a large bowl, combine the protein powder, coconut flour, baking powder, cinnamon, stevia, and salt. Mix well. In a separate medium bowl, combine the coconut oil, egg whites, vanilla extract, and almond milk. Mix well.

3 Make the batter by adding the wet ingredients to the dry ingredients. Mix until all ingredients form a smooth, pourable batter. (If the batter is too thick, add more almond milk, 1 tbsp at a time, until the desired consistency is achieved.)

4 Pour the batter into four donut cups. Bake for 9 to 12 minutes. The donuts are done when a toothpick inserted in the middle comes out clean. Remove the donuts from the pan and place on a cooling rack. Repeat the steps with the remaining batter.

5 Make the glaze by combining the almond milk and protein powder in a small bowl. Mix thoroughly, and allow to thicken for 5 minutes.

6 Drizzle the glaze over the cooled donuts. Serve warm.

PREP TIPS // *Store in an airtight container at room temperature for up to 6 days.*

NUTRITION FACTS

per serving

CALORIES

237

TOTAL FAT

5.8g

TOTAL CARBS

14.3g

PROTEIN

31.3g

SHAKES & DESSERTS

INDEX

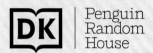

Publisher Mike Sanders
Associate Publisher Billy Fields
Senior Editor Brook Farling
Book Designer Rebecca Batchelor
Photographer Kelley Jordan
Food Stylist Savannah Norris
Prepress Technician Brian Massey
Proofreader Laura Caddell
Indexer Heather McNeill

First American Edition, 2018
Published in the United States by DK Publishing
6081 E. 82nd Street, Indianapolis, Indiana 46250

Copyright © 2018 Dorling Kindersley Limited
A Penguin Random House Company
21 22 23   10 9 8
008–308493–March/2018

Published in the United States by Dorling Kindersley Limited.

ISBN: 978-1-4654-6997-7
Library of Congress Catalog Number: 2017952281

Note: This publication contains the opinions and ideas of its author(s).
It is intended to provide helpful and informative material on the subject
matter covered. It is sold with the understanding that the author(s) and
publisher are not engaged in rendering professional services in the
book. If the reader requires personal assistance or advice, a competent
professional should be consulted. The author(s) and publisher
specifically disclaim any responsibility for any liability, loss, or risk,
personal or otherwise, which is incurred as a consequence, directly or
indirectly, of the use and application of any of the contents of this book.

Trademarks: All terms mentioned in this book that are known to be or
are suspected of being trademarks or service marks have been
appropriately capitalized. Alpha Books, DK, and Penguin Random House
LLC cannot attest to the accuracy of this information. Use of a term in
this book should not be regarded as affecting the validity of any
trademark or service mark.

DK books are available at special discounts when purchased in bulk for
sales promotions, premiums, fund-raising, or educational use. For
details, contact: DK Publishing Special Markets, 345 Hudson Street,
New York, New York 10014 or SpecialSales@dk.com.

Printed and bound in China

All images © Dorling Kindersley Limited
For further information see: www.dkimages.com

A WORLD OF IDEAS:
SEE ALL THERE IS TO KNOW
www.dk.com

ABOUT THE AUTHOR
Erin Stern is a professional bodybuilder and two-time
Ms. Figure Olympia who has won 14 IFBB
(International Federation of Bodybuilding and Fitness)
titles, including the 2012 Arnold Classic Europe.
She has been featured on over 20 fitness and
bodybuilding magazine covers, and has created
training programs that have helped thousands of
people reach their fitness and bodybuilding goals.
Her mission is to empower, educate, and enrich the
lives of people through fitness and healthy living.
Find Erin online at www.erinstern.com.

AUTHOR'S ACKNOWLEDGMENTS
I would like to thank Alpha Books and DK Publishing
for choosing to work with me. I have long dreamed
of sharing healthy, delicious recipes, and with their
help, I can.

Editing a book by a woman who picks heavy things
up and puts them back down again was no easy feat.
Brook Farling did a fantastic job of streamlining
recipes, perfecting the flow of the chapters, and
catching every last detail.

Becky Batchelor created the most stunning
and easy-to-read layouts for each page. Without
her artistic touch, the book would just be words
on paper.

Lastly, I want to thank my parents for being my
taste testers and for giving me honest feedback.